9/20/02

AMPHETAMINE SYNTHESES

REVISED INDUSTRIAL EDITION

by Otto Snow

Hi Eileen, Wish you happiness + great health,

Otto Snow

THOTH PRESS
P.O. Box 6081
Spring Hill, Fl 34611

Created and Printed in the United States of America

ISBN: 0-9663128-3-X
LCCN: 2002093827

Cover design graphics by Ted Stockowski
Updated by Otto Snow

DEDICATION

I dedicate this book to my father: Harry Snow (1921 - 1994)

I am in appreciation of: L. Lewin, E. Späth, A. Heffter, G. Alles, A. Shulgin, C. Naranjo, T. Sargent, D. Nichols, G. Greer, M. Stolaroff, and all those explorers (too numerous to name) who opened a path into the great unknown, unraveling the mysteries of the brain-mind.

I also want to acknowledge those who unravel the mysteries of the galaxies, stars and beyond, namely Carl Sagan, Copernicus and Galileo.

I want to thank the following: National Institute on Drug Abuse for their publications and help in locating specific toxicological studies; Drug Enforcement Administration, Office of Intelligence; U.S. Patent Office; British Patent Office; Eric Sterling of the Criminal Justice Policy Foundation for directing me to look into the Congressional Hearings concerning interpretation of the Analogue Act of 1986; Alexander Shulgin for his insight and words of encouragement.

"(If) every public action which is not customary, either is wrong
or, if it is right, is a dangerous precedent.
It follows that nothing should ever be done for the first time."
Cornford 1908

"Nothing will ever be attempted
if all possible objections must be first overcome."
Samuel Johnson (1709-1784)

"Question: ...the rats are saying it (MDMA) seems to be
amphetamine-like but, in fact, it really is not..."
"Obviously no one knows what the rats are thinking..."
Richard A. Glennon 1988

"Recreation is therapy; at least that's what people tell me."
Otto Snow 1992

"Fill the seats of justice with good men,
not so absolute in goodness as to forget what human frailty is."
Sir Thomas Noon Talfourd

TABLE OF CONTENTS

READER'S NOTICE

This reference guide is a tool for the legal profession and should not be misconstrued as a 'cookbook'. Publisher and author take no responsibility for inaccuracies, omissions, or typographical errors. All reactions are generalized. References are included for those seeking greater detail/descriptions on the construction of any specific molecule. Chemicals and reactions are potentially toxic, explosive & lethal.

This book is for information purposes only. No person is allowed to produce controlled substances without proper permits and authorization. To take/give substances for human consumption whether legal or illegal without a very thorough knowledge of the substance and the health (mental as well as physical) condition/s of the individual is destined to produce catastrophic results and legal ramifications.

Amphetamine Syntheses is a reference guide &
overview on the preparation of:

substituted phenylethylamines, substituted amphetamines,
substituted amino ketones, and other
active & inactive phenylalkylamines,
neurotransmitters, neurotoxins,
immediate precursors, and precursors
obtained from organic sources.

Series and individual reactions are overviewed and extensively referenced. Many different routes are described on altering the molecular structures of known and unknown neurochemicals. The terms and explanations are simplified and interwoven with historical data. Excerpts from the Congressional Hearing, prior to the passage of the Analogue Act of 1986, are included to give the readers a look at the issues of major concern. Chemicals are indexed for quick reference to assist those investigating suspect laboratories to determine probable cause or reviewing cases to determine culpability, criminal activities or innocence of suspect/s.

This guide is an asset and a necessity for:
lawmakers, attorneys, teachers, counselors,
law enforcement and students alike.

Introduction

According to DEA's Special Testing and Research Laboratory, the chemicals and equipment necessary to produce a single kilogram of MDMA can be purchased for as little as $500... The profit margin associated with MDMA trafficking is significant. It costs as little as 25 to 50 cents to manufacture an MDMA tablet, street value can be as high as $40, with a tablet typically selling for between $20 and $30... Hundreds of compounds can be produced by making slight modifications to the phenethylamine molecule. Some of these analogues are pharmacologically active and differ from one another in potency, speed of onset, duration of action, and capacity to modify mood with or without producing overt hallucinations... Many chemical variations of mescaline and amphetamine have been synthesized for their "feel good" effects...

Methamphetamine is, in fact, a very simple drug to produce. A user can go to retail stores and easily purchase the vast majority of the ingredients necessary to manufacture the drug. Items such as rock salt, battery acid, red phosphorous road flares, pool acid, and iodine crystals can be utilized to substitute for some of the necessary chemicals. Precursor chemicals such as pseudoephedrine can be extracted from common, over-the-counter cold medications. A clandestine lab operator can utilize relatively common items such as mason jars, coffee filters, hot plates, pressure cookers, pillowcases, plastic tubing, gas cans, etc., to substitute for sophisticated laboratory equipment. Unlike Fentanyl, LSD, or other types of dangerous drugs, it does not take a college-educated chemist to produce methamphetamine... Nationwide, prices range from $4,000 to $21,000 per pound at the distribution level. Retail prices range from $350 to $3,000 per ounce and $20 to $200 per gram...

Small labs to cook the drug can be set up on tables in kitchens, countertops, garages or just about anywhere.... clandestine labs are not limited to fire, explosion, poison gas, drug abuse, and booby traps; the chemical contamination of the hazardous waste contained in these labs also poses a serious danger to our nation's environment... ... at least five or six methamphetamine producers are now being killed every year from explosions and/or fires in clandestine labs. Many more receive serious burns or develop serious health problems from clandestine laboratory explosions and fires. There have been reports of apartment complexes and a $3,500,000 hotel, which burned down as the result of drug lab "cooks" that turned into chemical bombs. Recent years have seen an increase in the number of injuries to untrained police officers that investigate and/or dismantle clandestine laboratories without utilizing the proper safety equipment. Sources: DEA; Joseph D. Keefe; July 12, 2001

CHAPTER ONE:
AMPHETAMINE LABORATORIES

Amphetamine was first synthesized in 1887 by the German chemist L. Edeleano (Edeleano 1887). During the 1930's, amphetamines were being dispensed by medical practitioners for use as nasal decongestants, in the treatment of hay fever, orthostatic hypotension, epilepsy, parkinsonism, acute and chronic alcoholism, migraine, narcolepsy and as a psychostimulant.

In 1943 the Air Force outlined the use of amphetamine for pilots and ground troops to avoid sleepiness. It was also noted that adequate rest must follow each period of exertion (Air Force 1944). During this time practitioners were dispensing amphetamine as the new panacea for everything that ailed the human condition.

Amphetamine (1-phenyl-2-aminopropane) has long been the focus of study for scientists and organic chemistry students. The uses for amphetamine in the study of brain biochemistry and molecular interactions are endless. To the organic chemistry student it is one of the many psychostimulant drugs that are easily synthesized in the laboratory.

Amphetamine

Although there are numerous molecules which also have psychostimulant effects (Biel 1970), amphetamine has gained the most amount of attention for this effect. The N-methyl (CH3) homolog of amphetamine (N-Methyl-amphetamine) has also received much attention as it is more powerful than its parent substance.

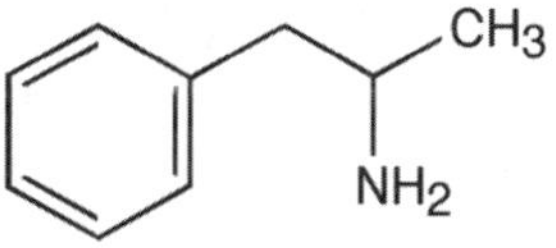

Amphetamine

Methamphetamine

During the 1960's and 1970's it was well known by the 'drug underground' as well as those who studied amphetamines, that speed kills! In 1962, the FDA estimated that 8 billion tablets of amphetamines were being produced legally. Prior to the Controlled Substance Act of 1970 (CSA), over 50% of all amphetamines which appeared on the streets were being diverted from legal sources. Many physicians were knowingly providing prescriptions for profit.

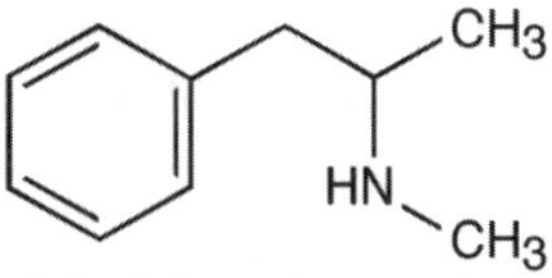

Methamphetamine

There was a decline in the availability of amphetamines following CSA. The response to the decline in availability of amphetamine did not backlash in the increase of clandestine laboratories producing amphetamines. This was because of the increased availability of cocaine (Burton 1991). Another factor was the increased sales of ephedrine tablets and capsules.

In February of 1980, phenyl-2-propanone was placed on schedule 2. Illicit amphetamine manufacturers were producing P-2-P as an immediate precursor. Over seventy-five percent all P-2-P laboratories used a method employing phenyl acetic acid and acetic anhydride as precursors.

In 1978; 63 seizures of methamphetamine laboratories,
    13 seizures of amphetamine laboratories
    3 seizures of MDA laboratories.
In 1979; 121 seizures of methamphetamine laboratories
    20 seizures of amphetamine laboratories,
    5 seizures of MDA laboratories.
In 1980; 121 seizures of methamphetamine laboratories,
    23 seizures of amphetamine laboratories,
    7 seizures of MDA laboratories.
In 1981; 73 seizures of methamphetamine laboratories,
    12 seizures of amphetamine laboratories,
    1 seizure of MDA laboratory. (Frank 1983)

There has been a 600% increase in methamphetamine laboratory seizures from 1981 to 1989. In 1981, there were 88 seizures of laboratories; in 1989, there were 652 laboratory seizures reported to be producing methamphetamine (Irvine 1991).

80% of all drug laboratory seizures were producing methamphetamine. In 1989, fifty-three percent of the laboratories were using a method employing ephedrine, red phosphorus and hydrogen iodide to make d-methamphetamine. Forty-seven percent of the laboratories were producing d,l-methamphetamine from P-2-P. In 1990, ninety percent of methamphetamine laboratories in California were using the ephedrine reduction method to produce methamphetamine (Heischober 1991).

The most commonly used synthesis for amphetamine and methamphetamine uses P-2-P in combination with aluminum amalgam and methylamine (Frank 1983). The Leuckart method is the most popular method used in Norway and the Netherlands (Soine 1989).

In 1988, 50% of methamphetamine laboratories seizures occurred in California, followed by thirteen percent in both Texas and Washington (Irvine 1991) states.

DEA Methamphetamine Laboratory Seizures National Totals

Year	Labs
1973	41
1974	53
1975	53
1976	71
1977	114
1978	143
1979	195
1980	251
1981	184
1982	191
1983	187
1984	198
1985	425
1986	509
1987	682
1988	810
1989	852
1990	549
1991	408
1992	334
1993	286
1994	224
1995	299
1996	734
1997	1321
1998	1627
1999	2155
1999	6782*
2000	6700*
2001	7755*

DEA Domestic Analyzed Methamphetamine Removals (kilograms) *

Year	kg	Year	kg
1990	751.5	1995	960.5
1991	294.0	1996	644.2
1992	357.8	1997	1050.7
1993	499.5	1998	1228.1
1994	709.1	1999	1408.1
		Total	2232.1

*This information represents drug removals that were analyzed in a DEA laboratory and is the net weight after analysis.

Operation Pipeline/Convoy Highway Interdiction Seizures (National totals; kilograms) Methamphetamine

Year	kg
1986	0
1987	20
1988	65
1989	61
1990	18
1991	13
1992	43
1993	46
1994	170
1995	310
1996	449
1997	1100
1998	982
1999	796
Total	4073

DEA Clandestine Laboratrory Training of State and Local Officers

Year	
1991	380
1992	200
1993	80
1994	127
1995	--
1996	100
1997	376
1998	677
1999	1132
2000	1546
2001	1031

Source: DEA Nov. 30, 2001 *Source: EPIC 8/2002

We must take into account that in all seizure statistics, these numbers do not include margins of error or any statistics of non-illegal laboratories that were destroyed and individuals terrorized by law enforcement. It is paramount in any drug case and in any democracy that the enforcers of the law follow the same laws that they are authorized to uphold. A knowledge of drug chemistry is necessary so that law enforcement can protect themselves from toxic chemicals used in drug synthesis. Compensation and restitution to those individuals who are inadvertently terrorized in the war on drugs must be addressed. It is important that America invests and protects scientific curiosity.

A freebase form of *d*-methamphetamine called 'ice' appeared in California. The drug was being imported by organized crime into the US from countries along the Pacific rim (Korea, Taiwan, Philippines) and the distributed in the US by organized crime groups.

"Smoking gives a rapid onset of effect of the drug, comparable in many ways to that from intravenous (IV) administration. The rapid reinforcement also enhances the addicting power of the drug." Cook 1991

In recent years, methamphetamine laboratory seizures have skyrocketed across the nation. Millions of doses of MDMA are being produced in the Netherlands and smuggled into the United States. MDMA has proliferated schools and nightclubs throughout the country.

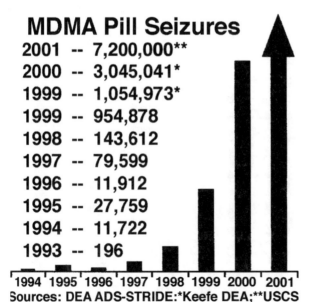

MDMA Pill Seizures

Year	Seizures
2001	7,200,000**
2000	3,045,041*
1999	1,054,973*
1999	954,878
1998	143,612
1997	79,599
1996	11,912
1995	27,759
1994	11,722
1993	196

1994 1995 1996 1997 1998 1999 2000 2001
Sources: DEA ADS-STRIDE:*Keefe DEA;**USCS

Drugs such as MDMA and methamphetamine will remain popular drugs because their large scale synthesis does not involve a knowledge of sophisticated chemical procedures. PMA, a powerful neurotoxin, has also appeared in recent years as it is more easily synthesized than MDMA and precursors are readily available.

MDMA Production

Source	European groups usually based in the Netherlands
Level of processing difficulty	Multistage process requiring a full laboratory setup
Cook proficiency	Typically requires some laboratory experience
Precursor and essential chemicals used	Safrole/isosafrole, MDP2P (3,4-methylenedioxyphenyl-2-propanone), methylamine, piperonal
Availability of chemicals	Regulated List I chemicals
Domestic laboratories seized	Usually fewer than 12 laboratories seized by federal law enforcement each year
Final product	90% tablets or capsules10% powder

Source: National Drug Intelligence Center; Drug Enforcement Administration; United States Customs Service July 2000

Most chemicals used in the synthesis of drugs can be purchased anywhere as they have many uses and are articles of commerce. Chemical suppliers can request End of Use Statements from those purchasing small quantities of suspect chemicals as a deterrent. Large scale diversion of chemicals continues to occur in industry to supply the needs of global organized crime.

Many workers are exposed to hazardous chemicals and toxic environments develope disease/death even years from exposure. Considering there is no national health care system in the US and the staggering cost of health care, workers may consider diverting chemicals for the security of their families. Many illicit drug laboratories are a result of necessity to pay bills in a society that in many cases treats workers like slaves; a second society of indentured servants to Corporate America.

The forensic chemist can look for the trace impurities that occur in a drug sample and determine how the drug was manufactured. Dope chemists manufacture crude drugs which are active, but contain isomers, impurities of incomplete synthesis, etc. Crude distillations of immediate precursors and inadequate purifications of end products leave 'finger prints' for those who investigate drug samples and drug labs.

The book is written for all those who are studying or investigating the syntheses of amphetamine, phenylethylamine and chemical analogs (eg. homologs, and congeners). I would recommend that all readers read PIHKAL for a look into the experiences of a modern explorer. Readers should also read an article written by Dal Cason (1990) for an overview on the syntheses of MDMA.

"During clandestine laboratory investigation the forensic chemist may be asked to illustrate the synthetic route used by the defendant(s). For this reason, the forensic chemist should have a clear understanding of the synthetic routes available to the clandestine chemist." Cooper 1984

To date, I have found no book that describes the synthesis of these molecules in a way in which lawyers, judges, law enforcement and students can easily comprehend. Reaction overviews, precursors, essential chemicals and various molecules are indexed and referenced for easy location of information.

Years ago, chemistry didn't have the impact that it does today. We are all affected by new drug development. The role of the authorities as upholders of justice necessitate a basic understanding of neurochemistry. Although we can have professionals who are more then willing to interpret the law and the science for us; we all must gain a better understanding of drug chemistry to protect our rights and the rights of future generations.

Mr. James N. Hall: *"The name "Designer Drugs," caught the attention of media over the past year and a half as a new trend in America's illicit drug scene. As you are aware the term does not refer to a particular pharmaceutical classification but rather to a method of making new products for the illicit market."* (5/1/86).

The primary objective of drug laws is to stop dangerous drugs from being sold or distributed (dumped on the masses for consumption); yet the Analogue Act does not clarify this problem.

The Analogue Act fails to differentiate between a scientist working on a molecular series and a drug chemist distributing dangerous drugs on the street. The law inadvertently attacks the method of science.

There are many arguments to the Analogue Act which provide a wealth of debate for those who would like to see science move out of the courtroom and back into the laboratory where it belongs. (US vs. Forbes) (Shulgin 1986; 1991) & numerous others.

Science and research are the front lines in war against disease. Pick up a copy of the *Physician's Guide to Rare Diseases*. Suffering and death don't wait for major pharmaceutical monopoly interests to develop drugs. Pain and agony don't wait for big business and Congress to get around to listen to their screams. Injustice and victims of suffering and disease don't wait for laws to allow them to research, develop and take substances to help themselves (this is our right to life).

The Chemist

There are millions of chemists in the United States, yet very few create drugs for distribution. Most chemists are interested in an aspect of molecule that they want to study further. In areas where there are high concentrations of chemical plants or industry there will also be larger concentrations of chemists synthesizing all sorts of molecules for study. Law enforcement in these industrial areas target those who distribute drugs.

The Analogue Act has been used in cases in which psychoactive chemicals, research or experimental, are sold/abused as drugs (eg. XTC-type). in raves and nightclubs. Substances which appear on the street with abuse liability (eg. causes deaths) are emergency scheduled.

American science and technology is very aggressive, sometimes unorthodox, inventive and revolutionary. Research is an adventure, a mystery to be solved; a path to blaze into the unknown; to advance knowledge which in turn our evolutionary society benefits from. The sciences and advanced technologies have always attracted those who are not satisfied with the mundane and question conventional wisdom. There has always been simultaneous attacks against/respect for those who are willing to investigate the unknown in hopes of bringing back something that will change the world; the eureka!

President Kennedy's setting of long term goals for the nation (race to the moon) was a national effort towards a common goal. Industries rose as the exploration of space was promoted. Science is a hands on experience, a reinforcement; an affirmation that all Americans can take part in a national goal. Those technologies that developed were then applied to civilian applications.

Decade of the Brain (Public Law No. 101-58) has appeared to be much different than a national effort in which everyone can take part in. Independent chemists are not publishing their research because of repressive laws and atmosphere. Massive quantities of data have been generated from those who qualify for government grants, but diseases and drug addiction still ravage the nation because of inadequate drug development. Tests to determine defects in neurotransmitter systems have been discovered, yet are not being made available to patients. Complacency in the medical profession allows poor quality medical care. The total disregard of patients' rights and no national health care coverage for the American people is a result of Congress representing medical/pharmaceutical/insurance PACS instead of the American people.

50 Million Americans are effected by mental disease. *"Depression afflicts 5.4 million people. Manic-depressive disorder, a different condition altogether, affects about 900,000. Among anxiety disorders, 14 million people suffer from phobias, 1.8 million from panic disorder, and 2.7 million from obsessive-compulsive disorder."* (Stinson 1990).

Many chemists produce psychopharmaceuticals for their own studies. The Analogue Law has produced an atmosphere of fear that hampers the communication and publication of discoveries. The analogue law is so vague and misleading that it has hampered research, scientific inquiry and progress in the neurosciences. Laws that are passed with good intentions must be followed up with amendments to modify short falls which become apparent later.

Prior to the analogue law, chemists through out the nation were generating new molecules for study. The neurosciences were emerging (and still are) as a new frontier of research. Simultaneously many individuals did not publish in the scientific journals do to prior illegalization of any molecule which may have usefulness in the treatment of the ill. The mediocrity has long made front page news of an issue that can be used as a new sacrifice to feed on like carrion or when politicians need a whipping post to point at as the cause of social problems and unrest.

The object of the analogue law was to stop drug chemists who slightly altered the structure of schedule 1 substances to produce the same effect of the scheduled substance while getting around the law. This is true for some dope chemists who maybe trying to 'get around the law', but dope chemists are not interested in the law, that is why they are criminals.

The neurochemist is not intending to get around the law, the neurochemist is interested in neurochemistry and doing good science. This may also include the testing of a molecule in human subjects to determine its activity or non-activity; to determine what a molecule does or does not do. Applying animal studies to speculate on the activity in humans without testing the molecule on humans remains windmills in the mind of Don Quixote.

The analogue act fails to discriminate the difference between research activities (including self exploration, whether amateur or professional) and the activities of criminals.

The organic chemist that is studying neurochemistry will have hundreds if not thousands of journal articles on a diversified family of psychoactives and neuro-molecules, their synthesis; effects in laboratory animals and human subjects. Dope chemists will generally have notes on the specific synthesis of an illegal substance.

Science is a method. Observation, hypothesize, development of a experiment which will prove or disprove (shed light on what you are looking into) hypothesis, formulation of theory. Continue...

If anything that the analogue law has done is an attack on the method of the development used in the neurosciences. It is safer that a chemist take a molecule themselves than to test (dump) a crude molecule nationally.

The neurochemist has the bug for exploration vs. the hardened dope manufacturer who has a bend towards criminal activities (eg. stealing, violent crime). There is a substantial difference between a chemist having a hobby set up synthesizing small quantities of neurochemicals and the evil hardened 'crank lab' mentality so dramatized by the media.

The dope criminal will dumb large quantities of toxic waste in vacant lots, rivers, poisoning the ground and water or throughout the city sewage system. This can be very dangerous and can blow up an entire neighborhood. Explosions ripping up city blocks have occurred with gasoline vapors escaping from old storage tanks.

If the career criminal were not cooking up some crude drug product (flask gunk) to dump on a city, this person would be doing some other sort of violent felonious act. He or she might be robbing your home or local grocery store, hooking healthy children with addictive drugs; forcing them into the sex trade to sell their bodies for dope that the pusher sells them. Satan lurking in the shadows of the school yard feeding innocent children rat poison.

The neurochemist may produce a small quantity of a neurochemical and share this with close associates for study further. All explorations involve a degree of risk. Yet the Analogue Act makes no difference between the activities of the explorer/scientist and actual criminal activities committed by evil individuals.

At the time that Mr. Rangel introduced H.R. 2014 (April 4, 1985) the bill was primarily designed "*to eliminate the manufacture and distribution of illegal synthetic narcotic analogs.*" When H.R. 2977 was introduced by Mr. Lungren, 'designer drugs' were identified as to "*include, but are not limited to, the following: phenylethylamines, N-substituted piperidines, morphinans, ecgonines, quinazolinones, substituted indoles, and arylcycloalkylamines.*" (July 11, 1985). Passed S.1437. (Dec, 18, 1985).

Phenylethylamines are the building blocks of molecules used in the study of endogenous catecholamines, their isomers and analogs (eg. adrenaline, noradrenaline). The indole family of molecules compose of the serotonergic neurotransmitter system of isomers and analogs (the tryptamine family of endogenous neurochemicals).

Lawrence Smith: "*I don't care which proposal we approve, but I want to see a designer bill enacted into law this session.*" 6/1/86

In hindsight we can see that although the law was intended to curtail the activities of a potential drug menace (narcotics) in the short time, it did not stop illicit drug laboratories in this nation. Dangerous drugs continue to be produced by those who are criminals. While those who want to study neurochemistry are placed in the quagmire of having to defend their inquisitiveness.

Until these short falls are ironed out, it would appear that patenting a molecule, IND, NDA etc. prior to testing, seems like 'the cart before the horse.' Scientists are not going to patent every chemical, or to do rigorous testing on any one specific structure (eg. especially when reviewing several series of structures), with the scrutiny or lack of done for FDA approval. Their objective is scientific inquiry. Those who are ill are not going to be able to develop and go through the FDA approval process for a substance that helps/or might help them, they are already fighting for their lives.

"For the most part, however, if the people who you have annoyed are part of the government, their actions against you will be motivated less by beliefs or philosophies which run counter to your own, than by the simple desire to remind you that they have far more power than you do, and that, even if you don't fear that power, you should at least have a healthy respect for it."   (Shulgin 1997 in TIHKAL)

Einstein : *"(there is) a duty in refusing to cooperate in any under-taking that violates the Constitutional rights of the individual. This holds in particular for inquisitions that are concerned with the private life and the political affiliations of the citizens..."*

Senator Joseph R. McCarthy (Committee for un-American Activities) called Einstein an enemy of America for this statement.

CHAPTER TWO:
METHAMPHETAMINE LABORATORIES

Methamphetamine, in various forms, is available throughout the United States. It is produced illegally in the United States, Mexico, and Asia, but there are no conclusive estimates of the levels of either domestic or international methamphetamine production. Despite an increasingly greater correlation between independent Caucasian laboratory operators and methamphetamine production--which has spread to almost every state--Mexican organizations in Mexico and in the United States probably account for most of the methamphetamine available in the United States. Mexican organizations clearly dominate transportation and wholesale distribution as well, but retail distribution is shared with independent dealers (particularly Caucasians and Hispanics), street gangs, and OMGs (Outlaw Motorcycle Gangs).. Source: NDIC April 2001

Efforts to estimate domestic production are severely hampered by the lack of a universally accepted definition of a clandestine laboratory and the lack of routine reporting of laboratory seizures to the EPIC's National Clandestine Laboratory Database. Information provided to NDIC by the DEA and state and local law enforcement agencies suggests that total laboratory seizures may be underreported.

Methamphetamine laboratory: A clandestine laboratory is an illicit operation with a sufficient combination of apparatus and chemicals that either has produced or could produce methamphetamine. Source: NDIC National Drug Threat Survey, 01/10/2000

Methamphetamine Terms

Dextro-methamphetamine: *d*-methamphetamine is produced using the precursor chemical ephedrine/pseudoephedrine. It is the most potent and widely abused form of methamphetamine and is associated with Mexican drug trafficking organizations.

Dextro, levo-methamphetamine: *d,l*-methamphetamine is produced using the precursor phenyl-2-propanone (P2P). It is only half as potent as *d*-methamphetamine and is associated primarily with outlaw motorcycle gangs.

Ice: Ice is a colorless, odorless form of smokeable *d*-methamphetamine resembling glass fragments or ice shavings. Its production (a process of recrystallizing methamphetamine) and distribution are normally associated with Asian traffickers.

Primary Methamphetamine Production Methods

Ephedrine/pseudoephedrine Method

This method uses the precursors ephedrine/pseudoephedrine, hydriodic acid, and red phosphorus to produce *d*-methamphetamine. It normally results in large quantities of high-quality methamphetamine.

"Nazi" Method

This method uses the primary precursor ephedrine/pseudoephedrine and more exotic secondary chemicals including lithium or sodium metal and anhydrous ammonia. It produces high-quality, low quantity *d*-methamphetamine.

Cold cook Method

This method uses the primary precursor ephedrine and the secondary precursors iodine and red phosphorus. The reaction is typically catalyzed either by using heat from direct sunlight or by burying the chemicals in containers in hot desert sand. It produces high-quality, low-quantity *d*-methamphetamine.

P2P Method

This method uses the precursors phenyl-2-propanone and aluminum to produce lower-quality methamphetamine.

Source: NDIC April 2001

Assessment of the Threat

A combination of factors makes methamphetamine the second greatest drug threat facing the United States. The production, trafficking, and abuse of methamphetamine and the violence associated with all aspects of the illicit methamphetamine trade continue to plague the United States. The methamphetamine problem is moving into urban areas and eastward from the Southwest, Pacific, and West Central Regions into the Great Lakes, New England, Mid-Atlantic, Southeast, and Florida/Caribbean Regions. The illegal methamphetamine trade was limited to relatively low-grade *d,l*-methamphetamine and associated almost exclusively with OMGs. Now, sophisticated Mexican drug trafficking organizations operating large-scale laboratories in Mexico and the United States supply most of the U.S. demand for methamphetamine and dominate wholesale and retail distribution. Thousands of independent laboratory operators, mostly Caucasians, with ready access to precursor chemicals are using a variety of methods to produce *d*-methamphetamine, most of which is intended for personal use or very limited local distribution.

Production Within the United States

The two most frequently practiced methods of methamphetamine production in the United States are the "red phosphorus," or "Mexican," method and the "Nazi" method. Both are capable of producing high potency *d*-methamphetamine. The red phosphorus method is widely used throughout the Southwest and Pacific Regions by most Mexican methamphetamine organizations and by others who acquire the recipe by a variety of means, including the Internet. The red phosphorus method is used most frequently in high-capacity laboratories to produce quantities of methamphetamine of varying purity. The Nazi method is practiced throughout the country by local independent producers and dealers, mostly Caucasians with no affiliation to any criminal organization.

The Nazi method is normally used to produce very high purity methamphetamine in quantities of less than an ounce; it is especially prominent in the West Central Region and in portions of the Southwest Region. Another method, using phenyl-2-propanone (P2P), has been used historically by OMGs to produce the less potent *d,l*-methamphetamine. Its use continues to be reported by agencies in California, Colorado, Delaware, Louisiana, Michigan, Mississippi, Pennsylvania, Texas, and Wyoming, but appears to be most prominent in eastern Pennsylvania, where OMGs still control most of the methamphetamine trafficking.

Operation Backtrack, a DEA Special Enforcement Program initiated in February 1997, was created to target chemical companies and individuals that divert pseudoephedrine, ephedrine, and phenyl-propanolamine to clandestine laboratory operators. Investigations sponsored by Operation Backtrack have helped illustrate the extent and the profitability of the illegal methamphetamine trade. Since its inception, Operation Backtrack has resulted in the following:

The seizure of over $16.5 million in combined assets, over $11 million of which was in cash. The seizure of 152.3 million dosage units of pseudoephedrine--enough to manufacture between 11,500 and 15,000 pounds of methamphetamine. The arrest of 317 individuals on various charges relating to the diversion of precursor chemicals; of those arrested, 46 percent were of Middle Eastern descent and 24 percent were of Mexican descent.

According to DEA's Office of Diversion Control, 152.3 million 60-mg pseudoephedrine tablets at a 60 percent reduction rate would result in 11,562 lbs. of methamphetamine. At the maximum potential reduction rate of 92 percent, the same number of tablets would yield 15,261 lbs. of methamphetamine.

Production Outside the United States

Major methamphetamine producers in Mexico and Asia probably continue to receive bulk ephedrine and pseudoephedrine from the People's Republic of China--the world's largest producer of organic ephedrine--and from India, a supplier of ephedrine for illicit methamphetamine production in Asia. Sophisticated Mexican organizations maintain undisputed control of methamphetamine production in Baja California Norte, Baja California Sur, Jalisco, Michoacan, Sonora, Tamaulipas, and possibly other Mexican states farther south. Although infrequent, laboratory seizures reported by the Mexican Government indicate the possibility of large-scale production of methamphetamine from laboratories located in Mexico. During all of 1999, however, the Mexican Government reported only 12 methamphetamine laboratory seizures, making any effort to quantify methamphetamine production in Mexico very difficult.

Methamphetamine laboratories in Asia supply markets in Southeast and East Asia, where methamphetamine has become the drug of choice, and in Guam, Hawaii, and the Northern Marianas. Southeast Asian methamphetamine is normally produced as a tablet, the preferred form in Asia. Some Asian methamphetamine tablets containing up to 33 percent methamphetamine have been seized on the U.S. West Coast.

Another form produced in Asia, usually referred to as "ice," is preferred in Guam, Hawaii, and the Northern Marianas. Ice is produced in overseas laboratories controlled almost exclusively by Korean criminal organizations and normally is found in powdered or crystalline form at 85 to almost 100 percent purity. Source: NDIC October 2000

A substantial portion of the methamphetamine available in the United States is produced at clandestine laboratories controlled by Mexican organizations based in Mexico and California, which leads the nation in laboratory seizures. Law enforcement agencies throughout the nation mention California most frequently as a source of methamphetamine. Other frequently mentioned sources are Arizona, Florida, Missouri, Oregon, Texas, and Washington. Mexican organizations dominate production in each of these states. Between 1992 and 1998, the number of states in which Mexican nationals were sentenced on methamphetamine-related charges grew from 3 to 30, illustrating the expanding role Mexican organizations are playing in the production and distribution of methamphetamine in the United States.
Source: NDIC National Drug Threat Assessment 2001 - The Domestic Perspective October 2000

METHAMPHETAMINE LABORATORIES
New Hampshire Production

A non-operational, methamphetamine laboratory was seized in an urban multifamily dwelling in Manchester (NH). On June 18, 2000, authorities responded to a reported fire at the home and found what appeared to be several containers of unidentified chemicals. A search warrant was obtained and the laboratory was dismantled. Although non-operational, the laboratory was capable of producing multi-ounce quantities of methamphetamine. The laboratories seized in New Hampshire used the lithium metal "Nazi" reduction manufacturing method, which does not require extensive knowledge of chemistry or sophisticated laboratory equipment. Source: NDIC April 2001

Kansas

September 1998 DEA Kansas City seized a methamphetamine laboratory operated by a non-Mexican group that had the capability to produce more than 100 pounds of methamphetamine.
Source: NDIC National Drug Threat Assessment 2001 - The Domestic Perspective October 2000

Source: INCB 1999

Global Domestic and Entry/Exit Seizures in Table 1

Unit	Ephedrine Kgs.	Isosafrole Liters	3,4-MDP-2-P Liters	1-P-2-P Liters	Piperonal Grams	Pseudoephedrine Kgs.	Safrole Liters
USA							
1994	8997			796	1	478	21
1995	15618		29	81	25000	20528	477
1996	1629			24	10	2673	46
1997	1103			29		8772	9
1998	1778			1049		18635	67
Netherlands							
1994	5500			1035			
1995		3	139			100	2400
1996			4600	3000			
1997		40	1400	10200			40
1998			2	430			3
China							
1995	18025						
1996	10305						
1998	5100						
Thailand							
1994	1519						
1995	38						
1996	45						
Czech Republic							
1995	17		846				
1996	894						
1997	29						
Russian Federation							
1996	8						
1997	3535						
1998	14						

Minnesota Production

Methamphetamine laboratories can be set up virtually anywhere. They have been discovered in settings ranging from farms, homes, and motels to abandoned cars. One was even discovered in an ice-fishing house. Most laboratories are small; the essential chemicals and equipment can be carried in a box. This makes them easily movable and difficult to detect. Using the Nazi method, laboratory operators can in a few hours set up a laboratory, produce methamphetamine, and disassemble the operation.

The Nazi method is popular in agricultural states such as Minnesota because of the availability of anhydrous ammonia, which is used as a fertilizer. Theft of the chemical from farms for methamphetamine production is becoming more common.

Because of the proliferation of Nazi method methamphetamine laboratories in Minnesota, the state legislature enacted a law in August 2000 making it a felony to steal, tamper with, or improperly transport anhydrous ammonia. Maximum penalties are 5 years in prison and a $50,000 fine.

The production of methamphetamine creates public health and environmental hazards. The volatile and toxic chemicals used to manufacture the drug pose a high risk of explosion and fire. Numerous laboratories have been found in Minnesota by officers responding to fire alarms. Some of the chemicals cause burns on contact, and vapors can cause lung damage as well as harm the brain, eyes, and kidneys.

"In July 1999, a container of anhydrous ammonia exploded at a laboratory in a Minneapolis neighborhood. The explosion and resulting toxic fumes injured 10 people including 6 police officers and 3 medics and forced the evacuation of 40 people from their homes." Source: WCCO Channel 4000, July 1999. Source: NDIC August 2001

New Jersey Production

The traditional P2P (1-phenyl-2-propanone) method of producing methamphetamine, also known as phenylacetone, is the most commonly used in New Jersey. OMGs, traditional organized crime groups (e.g., IOC), and teenagers and young adults at raves dominate methamphetamine distribution in New Jersey.

Methamphetamine is commonly distributed in combination with other drugs at raves. Some MDMA users in New Jersey mistakenly purchase methamphetamine believing it is MDMA.

Local independent Caucasian criminal groups, OMGs, and traditional organized crime groups had more P2P available for distribution in New Jersey in 1997 after 1,000 gallons of P2P were successfully transported to the area. Law enforcement officials seized about 130 of the original 1,000 gallons, which ranged in price from $22,000 to $30,000 a gallon. One thousand gallons of P2P can yield 5 tons of methamphetamine.

Crystal Methamphetamine -- "Ice"

In February 1999, DEA Newark arrested two Filipino nationals and seized 4 kilograms of crystal methamphetamine, the largest seizure on the East Coast. Ice is a colorless, odorless form of smokable d-methamphetamine resembling glass fragments or ice shavings. Its production (a process of recrystallizing methamphetamine) and distribution are normally associated with Asian traffickers.

Methamphetamine Production Methods

P2P is the most common method used for producing methamphetamine in New Jersey. The P2P method is also popular in Philadelphia from where some methamphetamine is transported to and distributed in New Jersey.

P2P: This method requires 1-phenyl-2-propanone and aluminum combined in a complex process that produces low-quality d,l-methamphetamine. It is normally associated with OMGs.

"New Jersey-based companies manufacture many of the precursor chemicals used by West Coast distributors to produce methamphetamine. New Jersey, with the largest number of pharmaceutical and chemical companies in the nation, is an ideal location for the exploitation of precursor chemicals. Over 300 New Jersey-based companies are registered in the state as manufacturers, importers, or distributors of regulated chemicals, including controlled substances and precursor chemicals." Source: Association, International Perspective, September 2000.

On February 10, 1999, New Jersey State Police and DEA investigators seized 120 gallons of P2P from a man intending to distribute the precursor to members of the Warlocks OMG. In May 1999, local law enforcement officers arrested a man with ties to the Warlocks and Pagans OMGs for being the lead cooker in a methamphetamine production and distribution operation in South Jersey. In response to the NDIC National Drug Threat Survey 2000, the Warren County Prosecutor's Office reported that methamphetamine laboratories exist in the county but tend to be in remote locations making detection difficult. Source: NDIC May 2001

Ohio Production

The increasing number of methamphetamine laboratories in Ohio is becoming a significant problem. In FY1997, the DEA Detroit Field Division seized 19 methamphetamine laboratories, 8 of which were in Ohio. The number of small methamphetamine laboratories discovered in north central, northeastern, and southeastern Ohio has increased, according to the Ohio BCI&I. These small operations frequently are referred to as "Beavis and Butthead" or "White Boy" laboratories. In north central Ohio, mobile methamphetamine laboratories have been discovered in single-story hotel rooms.

On June 15, 2000, a University of Akron secretary was charged with stealing chemicals from the university and supplying them to a local man who used the chemicals to produce methamphetamine in the basement of his home.   Source: NDIC April 2001

Pennsylvania Production

The introduction of high purity d-methamphetamine to the market is attracting college students, young professionals, minorities, and women in addition to Caucasian, blue-collar workers, who have been the traditional methamphetamine users.

For instance, on April 4, 2000, a Delaware County man pled guilty to selling $72 million worth of P2P on the black market, enough to produce 10 to 13 pounds of methamphetamine*. The individual sold the P2P for $10,000 to $35,000 per gallon. This arrest, which made P2P more difficult to obtain, may have contributed to the decline of P2P methamphetamine production in Philadelphia, thereby opening the market to other forms of methamphetamine. *(HCl salt per gallon?)

Local independent dealers, primarily Caucasians, are responsible for most of the methamphetamine production in western Pennsylvania. Their laboratories typically produce small quantities of high-purity d-methamphetamine for personal use and limited distribution to friends and associates. These low-production laboratories are frequently referred to as "tweaker," "Mom and Pop," or "Beavis and Butthead" laboratories.

The following are some examples of methamphetamine activity in western Pennsylvania:

• In 2000, DEA Philadelphia reported the seizure of a methamphetamine laboratory operating in a mobile trailer in western Pennsylvania that was capable of producing 10 to 12 ounces of methamphetamine per week. The laboratory operator had combined pseudoephedrine extracted from diet capsules with red phosphorus and iodine to produce methamphetamine. He had purchased the diet capsules by the case in Ohio and had ordered the red phosphorus from Louisville, Kentucky.

• On September 15, 2000 an individual arrested in Seattle told authorities he had a methamphetamine laboratory in his apartment in Hampton, a suburb of Pittsburgh. The individual reportedly had purchased precursor chemicals in Oregon and was attempting to transport them back to Pittsburgh by way of Seattle when a bottle of hydrobromic acid broke in his duffel bag and started to smolder and emit fumes. Source: NDIC June 2001

Wisconsin Production

DNE officials indicate that methamphetamine producers, or cookers, from Arkansas came to Wisconsin to teach Wisconsin cookers how to produce methamphetamine. Out-of-state cookers who began production operations in an apartment in Madison, Wisconsin, operated another laboratory seized in 1999 by the Wisconsin DNE. The cookers were arrested, jumped bond, and were again apprehended operating a mobile laboratory from a truck. In another instance, a temporary methamphetamine laboratory seized in 1999 in Milwaukee County was set up in a hotel room; the precursor chemicals found originated in Missouri.

Wisconsin's large national forests and wilderness areas are ideal for clandestine methamphetamine laboratory operations. Wisconsin operates 42 parks, 4 recreation areas, 10 state forests, 13 state trails, as well as 6 million acres of hunting land. The parks range in size from Devil's Lake, with 8,864 acres, to the largest single state recreational facility, the Northern Highland Legion Forest, with 221,946 acres. State trails total 8,928 acres. Limited law enforcement presence makes these areas ideally suited for operating methamphetamine laboratories and disposing of the resulting toxic waste. Furthermore, Wisconsin's proximity to Canada gives local laboratory operators another advantage over law enforcement efforts. Precursors such as ephedrine, pseudoephedrine, and P2P (phenyl-2-propanone) are more readily available in Canada where prices are lower and regulations regarding these chemical precursors are less restrictive.

There are several methamphetamine production methods, but the "Nazi" method is the most popular in Wisconsin. Western Wisconsin is rural and home to hundreds of farms that store anhydrous ammonia, a key ingredient in the Nazi method, as fertilizer. The Wisconsin DNE states there have been increasing anhydrous ammonia thefts from farms and farm supply outlets. A Wisconsin State Representative stated that there have been frequent thefts of 1,000-gallon containers of anhydrous ammonia from farm fields in western Wisconsin.

In February 2000, the Wisconsin State Legislature toughened penalties for stealing farm fertilizers used in methamphetamine production. The Walworth County Sheriff has urged farmers to be aware that methamphetamine production often requires agricultural chemicals and to keep locks on storage tanks. One indication that efforts to curb anhydrous ammonia theft may be working is a report by the Wisconsin DNE that the ephedrine reduction production method, which uses red phosphorus and ephedrine or pseudoephedrine, is becoming more prevalent. The Regional Director of the Eau Claire DNE reports that pseudoephedrine bulk purchases are increasing in the region. The toxic and hazardous waste associated with any methamphetamine production method increases the threat to law enforcement, surrounding communities, and the environment.

Wisconsin law enforcement officials indicate that methamphetamine laboratory operators are pouring toxic waste into thermos bottles, coolers, and other containers and then dumping them into highway ditches. The Lafayette County Sheriff reported that several thermos bottles and water containers containing by-products were found along roads in that southwestern Wisconsin County. State officials report that waste dumped from backwoods laboratories into ditches poses a threat to road crews and volunteers gathering litter along highways.

In February 2000, the Wisconsin State Legislature toughened penalties for dumping the hazardous waste associated with methamphetamine production. DNE officials report that it takes significant time, physical effort, and money to clean a dump-site. Remediation costs are between $3,000 and $10,000 per site. The Regional Director of the Eau Claire DNE reports that money for laboratory cleanup is nonexistent, forcing the DNE to coordinate with the Wisconsin Department of Natural Resources to continue laboratory cleanup. The Regional Director also reports a significant increase in the number and size of toxic dumps in southwestern Wisconsin.   Source: NDIC May 2001

Hazardous Waste

Profound environmental damage results from methamphetamine production, much of which occurs within the United States, and the costs of remediating laboratory sites are daunting. In 1998 and 1999 combined, law enforcement agencies seized clandestine laboratories in every state except Connecticut, Rhode Island, and Vermont. In 1998, the DEA seized 70 "superlabs," those capable of producing 10 or more pounds of methamphetamine in a single cook. Of those 70 laboratories, 56 were seized in California, 4 in Colorado, 3 in Pennsylvania, and 1 each in Arizona, Delaware, Michigan, Missouri, Montana, Nevada, and Washington.

Information from the U.S. Forest Service documents a significant increase in the use of public lands for methamphetamine production. Seizures of methamphetamine laboratories on lands administered by the U.S. Forest Service have increased from 28 in 1995 to 105 in 1998. The identification of dump sites in National Forests and on National Grasslands has shown a corresponding increase over the same period.

The proliferation of methamphetamine laboratories in the United States poses a threat to the safety of citizens, especially children, in areas near those laboratories and to law enforcement personnel called upon to remove those laboratories. According to EPIC, law enforcement agencies seized almost 7,200 clandestine methamphetamine laboratories in 1999, although the DEA acknowledges that a significant number of laboratory seizures are not reported to EPIC or Regional Intelligence Sharing Systems. In the course of these seizures, law enforcement agencies noted the presence of nearly 870 children at the sites--180 of the children were exposed to toxic chemicals, and 12 were injured by toxic chemicals. Explosions occurred at 111 of the laboratories seized, and explosives or booby traps were found at 81. Comparing data from the California Drug Endangered Children (DEC) office suggests that like laboratory seizures in general, the effect of methamphetamine production on children may be underreported. DEC reports that in 1999, over 1,000 children were present at 482 methamphetamine laboratories in only seven counties. Preliminary data from DEC for 2000 indicate similar numbers.

The average methamphetamine laboratory produces 5 to 7 pounds of toxic waste for every pound of methamphetamine produced. The cost of cleaning laboratory sites places a heavy financial responsibility on law enforcement agencies and governments at all levels. Law enforcement personnel are required by federal law to be trained and certified to participate in a laboratory cleanup operation. According to state and local law enforcement agencies, the costs of remediating a methamphetamine laboratory range from $2,500 for the smallest laboratories to over $250,000 for the largest. While some remediation costs are borne by the DEA, the expense of removing methamphetamine laboratories is prohibitive for most law enforcement agencies, especially smaller, rural departments with limited staffing, limited funds, and an abundance of local laboratories. Increasing laboratory seizures nationwide have depleted available remediation funds; one department has reported that it "cannot afford to seize any more meth labs." Source: NDIC 2000

Hazardous Waste Cleanup

Whenever a Federal, State or local agency seizes a clandestine methamphetamine laboratory, Environmental Protection Agency (EPA) regulations require that agency to ensure that all hazardous waste materials are safely removed from the site in accordance with 40 CFR 262.

With regard to environmentally sound cleanup of clandestine drug laboratories, DEA has established hazardous waste cleanup and disposal contracts. There are currently 27 contract areas, served by ten contractors. These companies provide removal and disposal services to DEA, as well as State and local law enforcement agencies. As DEA has heightened its enforcement efforts concerning methamphetamine in recent years, there has been a corresponding focus on methamphetamine from State and local law enforcement agencies, resulting in a dramatic increase in the number of clandestine laboratories seized. In fiscal year (FY) 1998, DEA was provided $14.6 million ($9.6 million in Asset Forfeiture Funds (AFF) and $5.0 million from the Community Oriented Policing Service (COPS)) to pay for clandestine laboratory cleanups. In FY 1999, DEA was provided $16 million ($6.9 million AFF, $5.0 million COPS and $4.1 million DEA Appropriated Funds) to pay for clandestine laboratory cleanups.

In FY 2000, DEA was initially provided $9.9 million ($5.8 million AFF and $4.1 million in DEA Appropriated Funds) to pay for clandestine laboratory cleanups. DEA did not receive any direct COPS funding in FY 2000. The FY 2000 COPS funding was earmarked to 16 "HOT SPOTS" areas. (Eventually, 12 "HOT SPOTS" grantees set aside funding totaling $3.8 million to fund cleanups within their respective areas. However, DEA did not receive the set aside funds until FY 2001.) In March 2000, funding for state and local cleanup was exhausted. As a result, DEA ceased State and local cleanups. State and local cleanups resumed in June 2000 upon receipt of $5.0 million in Supplemental Funding from DOJ. DEA subsequently reimbursed ten State and local organizations for cleanups performed between March and June of 2000. Source: DEA 7/12/2001

CHAPTER THREE:
CHEMICALS AND THE LAW
Principal Provisions of the
Chemical Diversion Control Laws and Regulations

The Chemical Diversion and Trafficking Act of 1988 (CDTA), the Domestic Chemical Diversion Control Act of 1993 (DCDCA), and the Comprehensive Methamphetamine Control Act of 1996 (MCA) are the legislative acts which are the foundation of the government's program to prevent chemical diversion. These laws and the implementing regulations seek to strike a balance between allowing the chemical handler to pursue legitimate business while limiting the availability of chemicals for illicit drug production.

The laws and regulations require regulated persons (manufacturers, distributors, importers, and exporters of listed chemicals) to implement measures which prevent diversion by:
• obtaining proof of identity from their customers (21 U.S.C. § 830 (a)(3) and 21 CFR §1310.07) • maintaining retrievable receipt and distribution records (21 U.S.C. § 830 (a) and 21 CFR Part 1310), and
• reporting to the Drug Enforcement Administration (DEA) any suspicious orders 1 (21 U.S.C. § 830 (b)(1) and 21 CFR §1310.05 (a)(1)).

Manufacturers who distribute or export, distributors, importers, and exporters of List I chemicals are also required to:
• register with DEA (21 U.S.C. § 822 (a)(1) and 21 CFR §1309.21), and
• provide controls and procedures to guard against theft and diversion. (21 U.S.C. § 823 (h) and 21 CFR §1309.71-73).

Regulated persons (importers, exporters, brokers and traders in international transactions and transshippers) are required to notify DEA at least 15 days prior to the date of the transaction (21 U.S.C. § 971 (a) and 21 CFR Part 1313). The notification may be provided to DEA on or before the date of importation or exportation under certain conditions. The conditions are specified in the sections titled "Waiver of 15-Day Advance Notification Requirement" and "Criteria for Waiver of Advance Notification Requirement."

Some manufacturers of List I and List II chemicals are required to report annual production data (21 U.S.C. § 830 (b)(2) and 21 CFR §1310.05 (d)).

Inspection Authority 21 U.S.C. § 822 (f) and 21 CFR § 1316.03

DEA has the authority to enter and conduct an inspection of places, including factories, warehouses, or other establishments and con-

veyances, where persons registered under the CSA, or exempted from registration under the CSA, or regulated persons may lawfully hold, manufacture, or distribute, dispense, administer, or otherwise dispose of controlled substances or listed chemicals or where records relating to those activities are maintained. Inspectors are authorized to:
   • enter controlled premises and conduct administrative inspections for the purpose of inspecting, copying, and verifying the correctness of records, reports, or other required documents;
   • inspect within reasonable limits and to a reasonable manner equipment, finished and unfinished controlled substances, listed chemicals, and related materials and containers;
   • make a physical inventory of all controlled substances and listed chemicals on-hand at the premises;
   • collect samples of controlled substances or listed chemicals.

Who Must Register

Every person (unless specifically exempted below) who engages or proposes to engage in any of the following activities is required to register annually with DEA:
• manufacturing a List I chemical for distribution • distribution of a List I chemical • importation of a List I chemical • exportation of a List I chemical

Proof of Identity 21 U.S.C. § 830 (a)(3) and 21 CFR § 1310.07
The CSA requires that a regulated person engaging in a regulated transaction must identify the other party to the transaction. The regulated person must verify the existence and apparent validity of a business entity ordering a listed chemical, tableting or encapsulating machine and maintain customer files. If the regulated person is unable to establish the identity or legitimacy of a customer, sound practice requires the handler to postpone opening an account with this customer until such information is satisfactorily established. Regulated persons should maintain customer files which may be reviewed for adequacy by DEA during on-site visits. For domestic transactions, this may be accomplished at the time the order is placed by having the other party present documents to verify their identity and registration status if a registrant. Verification of documents may be accomplished through the following sources: telephone directory, local credit bureau, local Chamber of Commerce, or the local Better Business Bureau. DEA registration may be verified by DEA. When transacting business with a new representative of a firm, the regulated person must verify the agency status of the representative.

Thresholds for Regulated Transactions in List 1 Chemicals

List 1 Chemical	Threshold by base weight
Benzaldehyde	4 kilograms
Benzyl cyanide	1 kilogram
Ephedrine and *	regulated
Ethylamine and its salts	1 kilogram
Hydriodic acid (57%)	1.7 kilograms (or 1 liter by volume)
Hypophosphorous acid and its salts	regulated
Isosafrole	4 kilograms
Methylamine and its salts	1 kilogram
3, 4-Methylenedioxyphenyl-2-propanone	4 kilograms
N-Methylephedrine	1 kilogram
N-Methylpseudoephedrine and *	1 kilogram
Nitroethane	2.5 kilograms
Phenylacetic acid and its salts and esters	1 kilogram
Phenylpropanolamine and *	2.5 kilograms
Piperidine and its salts	500 grams
Piperonal	4 kilograms
Pseudoephedrine and *	1 kilogram
Red phosphorus	regulated
Safrole	4 kilograms
White phosphorus (Other names: yellow phosphorus)	regulated

* its salts, optical isomers, and salts of optical isomers; Source: DEA

For cash sales or sales to individuals, the proof of identity must consist of at least the signature of the purchaser, a driver's license and one other form of identification. It is recommended that the second form of identification should corroborate the first and should be valid in its own right. If an individual presents an identification card issued by an appropriate state authority in lieu of a driver's license, such identification is acceptable provided that it contains the individual's name, address, a unique identification number, and the individual's photograph. A record, preferably a photocopy, should be kept of proof of identity information.

For new customers that are not individuals or cash customers, the regulated person must establish the identity of the authorized purchasing agent(s) and have on file that person's signature, electronic password or other identification. Once the authorized identity has been established the agent list may be updated annually rather than on each order.

For electronic orders, the identity of the purchaser shall consist of a computer password, identification number or some other means of identification consistent with electronic orders.

Each regulated person who engages in a regulated transaction involving a listed chemical, a tableting machine, or an encapsulating machine must keep a readily retrievable record of the transaction. Distribution records are required if the cumulative amount for multiple transactions to a person within a calendar month exceeds the threshold. Thresholds can be found in Appendix B and Appendix C. 21 U.S.C. § 830 and 21 CFR Part 1310

Contents of Regulated Transaction Records 21 CFR § 1310.06

Each record for a domestic transaction must contain the following information:

1. The name, address, and if required, the DEA registration number of each party to the regulated transaction. 2. The date of the transaction. 3. The name, quantity, and form of packaging of the listed chemical, or a description of the tableting machine or encapsulating machine (including make, model and serial number). 4. The method of transfer (company truck, picked up by the customer, etc.). 5. The type of identification used by the purchaser and any unique number of that identification.

Thresholds for Regulated Transactions in List 2 Chemicals

List 2 Chemicals	Domestic Sales		Imports and Exports	
	by volume	by weight	by volume	by weight
Acetic anhydride	250 gallons	1023 kgs	250 gallons	1023 kgs
Acetone (2-Propanone; Dimethyl ketone)	50 gallons [1]	150 kgs [1]	500 gallons	1500 kgs
Benzyl chloride	not applicable	1 kg	not applicable	4 kgs
Ethyl ether	50 gallons	135.8 kgs	500 gallons	1364 kgs
Hydrochloric acid [2]	not regulated	not regulated	50 gallons [2]	not applicable
Hydrogen chloride [2] (anhydrous)	not applicable	0.0 kgs	not applicable	27 kgs [2]
Iodine	not applicable	0.4 kgs	not regulated	not regulated
Methyl ethyl ketone (2-Butanone)	50 gallons [1]	145 kgs [1]	500 gallons	1455 kgs
Methyl isobutyl ketone	not regulated	not regulated	500 gallons [2]	1523 kgs [2]
Sulfuric acid	not regulated	not regulated	50 gallons [2]	not applicable
Toluene	50 gallons [1]	159 kgs [1]	500 gallons	1591 kgs

[1] The cumulative threshold is not applicable to domestic sales of Acetone, Methyl ethyl ketone, and Toluene.

[2] Threshold applies to exports, transshipments, and international transactions to western hemisphere except Canada. Imports are not regulated.

Source: DEA 02/2001

Maintenance of Records 21 CFR § 1310.04

A record must be kept for two years from the date of transaction.

Types of Required Reports

In addition to periodic written reports required of bulk manufacturers and certain mail order distributors, there are four events that require prompt oral reporting to DEA.

Oral Reports 21 CFR § 1310.05

There are four types of transactions specified in the CSA which require a regulated person to make oral notification to the Special Agent in Charge, or a designee, of the local DEA Division Office whenever possible. The oral report must be made as soon as possible, and as far in advance of the conclusion of the regulated transaction, as possible. A written report of a transaction listed in paragraphs 1, 3, and 4 below is required to be sent to that office within 15 days after the regulated person becomes aware of the circumstances of the event. The four circumstances are: 1. Any regulated transaction involving an extraordinary quantity of a listed chemical, an uncommon method of payment or delivery, or any other circumstance that the regulated person believes may indicate that the listed chemical will be used in violation of the law. 2. Any proposed regulated transaction with a person whose description or other identifying characteristic has been previously furnished by DEA to the regulated person. Such a transaction may not be completed unless the transaction is approved by DEA. 3. Any unusual or excessive loss or disappearance of a listed chemical that is under the control of the regulated person. The regulated person responsible for reporting a loss in transit is the supplier. 4. Any regulated transaction involving a tableting or encapsulating machine.

Special Surveillance List of Chemicals, Products, Materials and Equipment Used in the Clandestine Production of Controlled Substances or Listed Chemicals

Appendix G : Background

The Comprehensive Methamphetamine Control Act of 1996 (MCA) makes it unlawful for any person to distribute a laboratory supply to a person who uses, or attempts to use, that laboratory supply to manufacture a controlled substance or a listed chemical, with reckless disregard for the illegal uses to which such laboratory supply will be put. Individuals who violate this provision are subject to a civil penalty of not more than $25,000; businesses which violate this provision are subject to a civil penalty of not more than $250,000. The term "laboratory supply" is defined as "a listed chemical or any chemical,substance, or item on a special surveillance list published by the Attorney General, which contains chemicals, products, materials, or equipment used in the manufacture of controlled substances and listed chemicals."

Special Surveillance List Chemicals

All listed chemicals as specified in 21 CFR § 1310.02 (a) or (b) or 21 U.S.C. § 802 (34) or (35). This includes all chemical mixtures and all over-the-counter (OTC) products and dietary supplements which contain a listed chemical, regardless of their dosage form or packaging and regardless of whether the chemical mixture, drug product or dietary supplement is exempt from regulatory controls.

Chemicals: Ammonia Gas; Ammonium Formate; Bromobenzene; 1,1-Carbonyldiimidazole; Cyclohexanone; 1,1-Dichloro-1-fluoroethane (e.g., Freon 141B); Diethylamine and its salts; 2,5-Dimethoxy-phenethylamine and its salts; Formamide; Formic Acid; Lithium Metal; Lithium Aluminum Hydride; Magnesium Metal (Turnings); Mercuric Chloride; N-Methylformamide; Organomagnesium Halides (Grignard Reagents); (e.g., ethylmagnesium bromide and phenyl-magnesium bromide); Phenylethanolamine and its salts; Phosphorus Pentachloride; Potassium Dichromate; Pyridine and its salts; Sodium Dichromate; Sodium Metal; Thionyl Chloride; ortho-Toluidine; Trichloromonofluoromethane (e.g., Freon-11, Carrene-2); Trichlorotrifluoroethane (e.g., Freon 113)

Equipment: Hydrogenators; Tableting Machines; Encapsulating Machines; 22 Liter Heating Mantels

Additional Information

The Special Surveillance List appeared as a Final Notice in the Federal Register on May 13, 1999. A Correction to the Final Notice appeared in the Federal Register on September 17, 1999.

"Any person who possesses or distributes a listed chemical knowing, or having reasonable cause to believe that the listed chemical will be used to manufacture a controlled substance except, as authorized by this title, shall be fined in accordance with Title 18, or imprisoned not more than 10 years, or both." ....Title 21 U.S.C. § 841 (d)(2).

CHAPTER FOUR:
PSYCHOPHARMACEUTICAL TRADE

In 1914 the Harrison Drug Act was passed by Congress to stop the adulteration of over the counter medicinals and food products with narcotics. This act placed the responsibility of narcotic distribution in the hands of the pharmaceutical-medical community.

The face of mass addiction has changed but the name of game remains the same. All drugs are accommodated by the biochemistry of the body and or brain (Gaday 1965). The degree of accommodation could be viewed as a dependence scale. The screening of a drug's dependence potential in laboratory animals is called reinforcement testing. Some drugs produce more habituation and or addiction (reinforcement) than others. Some drugs produce habituation-addiction more rapidly than others. The primary ability to produce addiction depends on how the molecule interferes and interacts with an individual's normal biochemistry.

All psychotropic-psychoactive drugs produce biochemical changes in brain chemistry (neurochemistry) (Maas 1977) (Meadows 1982). All psychotropic (psychiatric) drugs produce withdrawal (Gardos 1978). The types of withdrawal symptoms depend on the drug's actions in the body and the body's and brain's biochemical adjustment to non-drug biochemistry. The severity of the withdrawal symptoms increases with the length of time that a person has been taking the drug. All drugs which have been taken chronically will produce withdrawal.

Some drugs (e.g. benzodiazepines) have been reported to produce withdrawal symptoms that can last for a year after discontinuation of the medication (Higgitt 1985). Benzodiazepines are reinforcement drugs, this class of drugs is addictive. Benzodiazepine tranquilizers can produce addiction in individuals in a short a period as four weeks. Most individuals who become addicted to benzodiazepines will remain addicted for the rest of their lives.

The withdrawal symptoms of most psychotropic (psychiatric) drugs resemble the same condition-symptoms that the drug is approved (by FDA) to treat.

Barbituric acid was first synthesized by A. Bayer in 1863. Substituted barbiturates were first synthesized by Conrad and Gutzeit in 1882. In 1904 barbituric acid was first used as a sedative. In 1936, three hundred suicides were reported to have taken place with the use of barbiturates (Hambourger 1939). In the same year approximately 80 thousand kilos (80 metric tons) of barbiturates were dispensed in

America for drug use. 2 Million doses of barbiturates were being consumed daily.

In the 1930's an insecticide called phenothiazine was used in agriculture. It was also used as a urinary antiseptic and as a treatment for pin worm infestation. A French Navy Doctor, Henri Labori discovered that chlorpromazine possessed powerful sedative effects. In 1951, this effect was exploited; phenothiazines were used on mental patients.

Asylums were closed down as sedated mental patients were sent home or into the streets. Elderly individuals in nursing homes were drugged to produce less work for attendants and medical staff.

Once heralded as the 'new miracle drugs;' today the phenothiazines are considered no less then chemical straight jackets (Beers 1988; Garrard 1991; Sloane 1991). Analogs of the phenothiazine class of drugs continued to be patented, manufactured, and dispensed to mental patients, the elderly and the public. Phenothiazines and analogs are a class of drugs known as antipsychotics, major tranquilizers and neuroleptics. Their action is not a cure for mental illness or old age, but to shut down the limbic system of the patient. The limbic system is a part of the brain that controls decision making, reasoning, reality, personality; those behaviors and emotions critical for survival and self preservation.

A class of antidepressants was accidentally discovered in the 1950's. These drugs inhibit enzymes (monoamine oxidase) which break down neurotransmitters. Their abbreviation is MAOI.
Pharmaceutical firms patent new drug analogs to:

1) reduce the toxic effects (referred to as side effects, adverse effects).
2) alter the activity of a previous drug of the same class.
3) get around a competitor's previously patented drug.
4) get a monopoly on the distribution of a new drug
5) make a major profit; big business.

Another class of drugs was created, patented and dispensed by pharmaceutical firms, they are known as iminodibenzyl drugs, commonly referred to as tricyclic antidepressants. Imipramine was the first to be marketed in 1958. It is closely related to chlorpromazine. Their actions are like that of cocaine and amphetamine (Scheel-Krüger 1972) (Pacholczyl 1991). Amitriptyline, and nortriptyline, both have a high affinity to d-LSD binding sights in the brain and reduce serotonin activity (Ogren 1979). Imipramine, desipramine, chlorimipramine and mianserine reduce d-LSD binding in the brains of rats (Ogren 1979).

During the 1960's another class of drugs called the benzodiazepines began being marketed as tranquilizers and sleep aids. They were touted as being safe, effective and non-addictive. Pharmaceutical firms began designing, patenting and marketing numerous analogs of benzodiazepine drugs. According to government statistics, in 1981, pharmacies dispensed 65 million prescriptions of benzodiazepine drugs. In 1985, retail pharmacies dispensed 81 million prescriptions of benzodiazepine drugs (61 million prescriptions for tranquilizers and 20 million prescriptions for sedative-hypnotics). In 1987, pharmacies dispensed more than 85 million prescriptions for benzodiazepine drugs (NADI). These statistics do not include the millions of free samples given by practitioners.

Psychiatric drugs, known as psychotropic drugs, neither cure disease, rebuild the body or mind and can actually create disease.

See: A Killing Cure, Confessions of a Medical Heretic, Dr. Caligari's Psychiatric Drugs, Drug Interactions in Psychiatry, The Neuroleptic Malignant Syndrome and Related Conditions, Neuropsychiatric Side-Effects of Drugs in the Elderly, Psychiatric Drugs, Hazards to the Brain, Toxic Psychiatry, You Must Be Dreaming.

Neuroleptics cause tardive dyskinesia, drug induced parkinsonism and increase the severity of schizophrenic symptoms in patients who stop taking them. They also produce ocular, liver, and cardiac damage. Although these drugs are classified as antipsychotics they induce hallucinations, severe depression, confusion, and memory problems in many patients. Anticholinergic syndrome, neuroleptic malignant syndrome and serotonin syndrome (Sternbach 1991) are toxic psychotic reactions produced by these drugs. All syndromes can cripple or kill the patient by paralytic ileus and cardiac arrest.

The benzodiazepines have been determined by the government and scientific studies to only be affective sleep aids for 14 days.

Benzodiazepines reduce sleep stages 3 and 4. Both sleep states are necessary for the proper functioning of the brain (Willis) (Hecht).

Tricyclic antidepressants have been dispensed as a panacea to patients for any symptoms which in one way or another may qualify under the symptoms of depression. These drugs produce severe dryness of mucous membranes leading to respiratory infections, ocular problems and disease, constipation, candidia infections, mood-swings, memory problems, sleep problems (insomnia, reduction of REM sleep) and a long list of miscellaneous symptoms.

In recent years there has been more public awareness to the increasing statistics of suicides and violence occurring in individuals who are being prescribed these drugs.

Serotonin (5-Hydroxy-tryptamine) (Neurotransmitter)

Tricyclic antidepressants (amitriptyline, nortriptyline, mianserine) do not increase serotonin (a neurotransmitter) neurotransmission in the brains of patients (Aghajanian 1978) (Murphy 1978)(Coppen 1976)(see also Sussaman 1995). These drugs block both presynatic and post synaptic receptors (Ogren 1979). Drugs such as zimelidine primarily act by blocking presynaptic receptors, but also block post synaptic receptors and reduce serotonin neuron firing with chronic use. Tricyclic antidepressants (amitriptyline and nortriptyline) also decrease a serotonin metabolite in the spinal fluid called 5-hydroxy-indole acetic acid (Maas 1977). See also: Serotonin Syndrome.

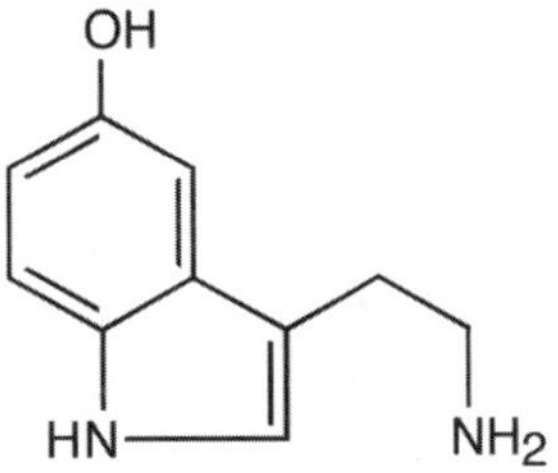

Serotonin

Reduced levels of 5-hydroxyindoleacetic acid (biochemical marker) have been found in suicide victims (*Biology of Suicide*). A reduction of serotonin levels also reduces levels of 5-HIAA. Laboratory animals have been fed diets missing L-tryptophan to cause serotonin depletion. The depletion of serotonin resulted in sleep loss, aggression and violence in the laboratory animals (Brown 1986) (Messing, 1976, 1978) and depression in humans (Beitman 1982) (Coppen 1976). Pretreatment of laboratory animals with 5-hydroxy-tryptophan (Pradhan 1978) (Taylor 1977) blocks the stimulation induced by cocaine.

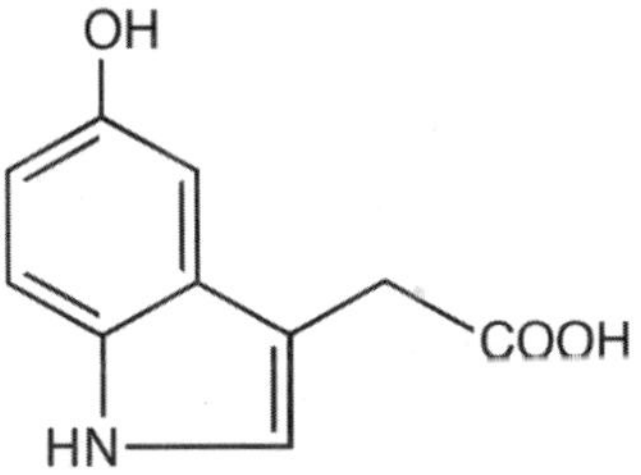

5-Hydroxyindoleacetic Acid

L-tryptophan is an essential amino acid necessary for the production of serotonin in our body and brain. L-Tryptophan is absorbed from the food we consume. L-Tryptophan is bound to other proteins in our food. Some individuals can not absorb proteins such as L-tryptophan unless they are bound to dipeptides (Fleischmajor 1961).

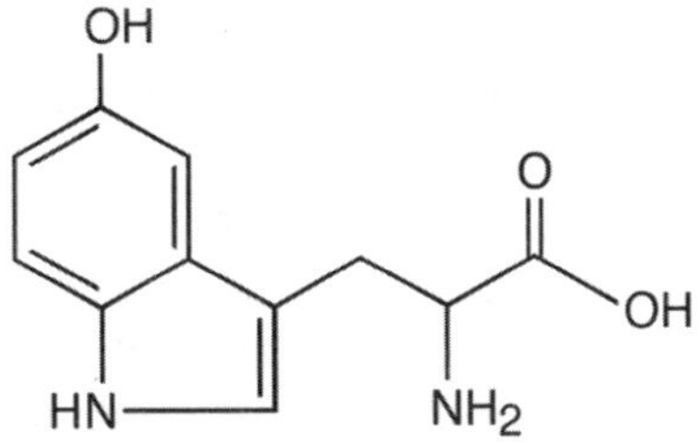

5-Hydroxytryptophan

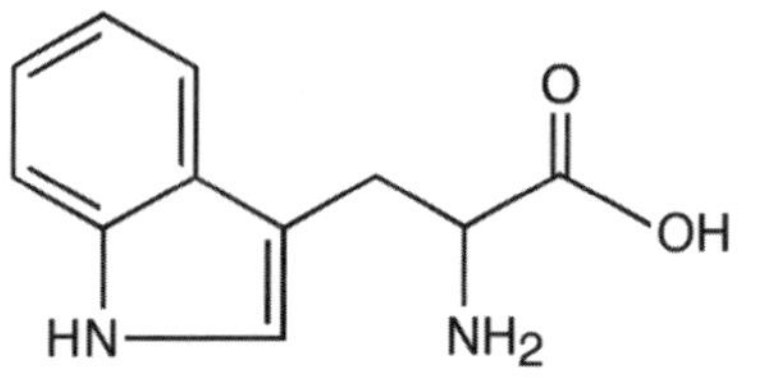

L-Tryptophan (Essential Amino Acid) (Serotonin Precursor)

Tryptophan

L-Tryptophan increases both serotonin in the brain and 5-hydroxy-indole acetic acid in the spinal fluid.

All drugs are potentially dangerous. Whether obtained over the counter (OTC), by prescription or from the street does not change the deadly potential of drugs.

Psychotropic (psychiatric) drugs are generally prescribed for short periods, to insure that the patient is closely monitored for therapeutic effect, toxic effects and behavioral disturbances. In all long term drug treatment there must be medication management and communication with psychotherapist.

Psychotherapy is done concurrently by someone independent of the prescribing physician; a patient may then be evaluated to determine therapeutic usefulness of a psychotropic medication.

When drugs are dispensed with no regard for the safety, health and welfare of the individual and no psychotherapy is done, then, the risk out ways the benefit; hence the drugs become toxic, life threatening and deadly.

Psychedelic Amphetamines

Louis Lewin used the term phantastic (meaning drugs of illusion) to describe the class of drugs which have the effects of mescaline. This class of drugs has been referred to as hallucinogens (drugs which produce delusions), psychotomimetics (means induces psychosis), psychedelics (mind-manifesting) and numerous new terms to describe/clarify the specific effects of these phantastic drugs.

Most scientists working on these types of materials describe them in more defined/refined terms. The term entheogen (awakens the God within) is used to describe the actions drugs or botanicals which have been extensively used as religious sacraments and provoke religious enlightenment. These drugs include mescaline, LSD-25 and psilocybin.

The term stimulant is used to describe psychostimulant drugs such as cocaine, amphetamine, methamphetamine, and to a lesser extent ephedrine and phenylpropanolamine. Tricyclic drugs such as amitriptyline and imipramine also cause stimulation in some individuals and sedation in others. All psychostimulant drugs will produce hallucinations if taken in large dosages or for extended periods of time. Amphetamine psychosis produces symptoms which closely resemble schizophrenia (Giffith 1970) (Jönsson 1970).

The substituted amphetamines have many different effects, high doses generally will produce visual activity, where as low dosages produce mood elevation. Most studies (human testing) done on these molecules involved administering large doses to patients, which would naturally produce effects outside therapeutic window and increase adverse effects. The dosages, listed for the molecules described, are the tested dosages noted in the literature and should not be misconstrued as an excepted or 'safe' dosage within any therapeutic window.

3,4,5-Trimethoxyamphetamine (TMA) is hallucinogenic; so is 4-methyl-2,5-dimethoxyamphetamine (DOM). Yet there are also differences between the effects of both of these drugs. DOM has been reported to produce more physical awareness (concern for physical health) in subjects and is longer acting then other amphetamine psychoactives (14-20 hours).

MDMA (3,4-methylenedioxy-N-methylamphetamine), and MDEA (3,4-methylenedioxy-N-ethylamphetamine) are termed entactogens. These substances produce feelings of empathy and bonding in subjects. These drugs are not considered hallucinogenic at therapeutic dosages. MDMA's effects are shorter acting than that of MDA. The 3,4-methylenedioxy class of drugs is unique in its effects, differing from both hallucinogens and stimulants.

Another series of phenylalkylamines has been found to be non-hallucinogenic and may have psychotherapeutic usefulness. One member of this family of molecules called N-methyl-1-(1,3-benzodioxol-5-yl)-2-butanamine has been tested in humans (Nichols 1986). This molecule remains undeveloped.

Hofmann's synthesis of LSD-25 and subsequent discovery of its effects in 1943 catalyzed research and studies in neurochemistry and the neurosciences. Before Hofmann's serendipity, the primary psychotomimetic of study was mescaline.

Mescaline's effects were known throughout the world during the first half of the 20th century. It was used in the scientific community, the medical community and by those who wanted to know more about the brain-mind sciences. Aldous Huxley took 400 mg. of mescaline and opened the world to the novel The Doors of Perception.

With every new discovery in science there is a new innovation, and with it was a new way of looking at the world; a new paradigm. The 1950's and 1960's were the dawn of the techno-revolution, a revolution in art, in forms of media, expression and concern for the rights of individuals and the environment. The world turned on, scientifically, technologically, intellectually and spiritually.

During the 1960's and 1970's, many new psychoactives were synthesized and studied. These materials primarily remained in the hands of scientists, psychologists and chemists. Only sporadically would these psychoactives appear on the street, until the 1980's.

In the 1980's, the DEA placed ads in Popular Science for formulas on preparing controlled substances and also placed ads offering precursors and immediate precursors used in these formulas (NY Times, 1983). Chemists throughout the country began ordering and selling precursors and immediate precursors. These precursors and immediate precursors were used by chemists to construct new uncontrolled psychoactives for research and psychotherapy. One of the many psychotherapeutic drugs which appeared on the street was MDMA, then MDEA and 2CB.

Many psychoactive substances appear in Schedule 1 meaning:

1) The drug or other substance has a high potential for abuse.

2) The drug or other substance has no currently accepted medical use in treatment in the United States.

3) There is a lack of accepted safety for use of the drug or other substance under medical supervision.

Some substances which have little potential for abuse are still included in Schedule 1. A botanical called *Tabernanthe iboga* appears in Schedule 1. Its effects resemble *Datura*, which is a deliriant, and is not considered 'user friendly.' N,N-dimethyltryptamine (DMT), a neurotransmitter in the brain, is excreted in the urine of all individuals and is a controlled substance.

According to the Federal Code of Regulations the following phenylalkylamine chemicals, their isomers (optical, geometric, positional) and their salts are currently listed under Schedule 1 as hallucinogenic or stimulant substances:

    aminorex
    4-bromo-2,5-dimethoxyamphetamine
    4-bromo-2,5-dimethoxyphenylethylamine
    cathinone
    2,5-dimethoxyamphetamine (not psychoactive)*
    *should be listed under CII or C III as an immediate precursor.
    2,5-dimethoxy-4-(n)-propylthiophenethylamine (2C-T-7)
    N-ethylamphetamine

methcathinone
4-methoxyamphetamine
5-methoxy-3,4-methylenedioxyamphetamine
4-methylaminorex
4-methyl-2,5-dimethoxyamphetamine
3,4-methylenedioxyamphetamine
3,4,5-trimethoxyamphetamine
3,4,5-trimethoxyphenylethylamine
3,4-methylenedioxy-N-methylamphetamine
3,4-methylenedioxy-N-ethylamphetamine
3,4-methylenedioxy-N-hydroxyamphetamine

Dr. Greer states: *"The single best use of MDMA is to facilitate more direct communication between people involved in a significant emotional relationship. Not only is communication enhanced during the session, but afterward as well. Once a therapeutically motivated person has experienced the lack of true risk involved in direct and open communication, it can be practiced with out the assistance of MDMA."*

The media publicized the use of MDMA as an adjunct with psychotherapy to save failing marriages, relationships and families. A DEA spokesperson, Frank Sapienza, said to Chemical & Engineering News (10/9/85):

"I think the different views of MDMA are compatible. They might not call that abuse. They might call it recreational use. Must go through accepted procedures to prove that it is safe, that can be produced in pure form, and it treats some condition. MDMA may be able to fit into that category, but the studies have not been done to show that. Therefore, we have to say that it has no accepted medical use, and it has to go into Schedule 1."

The National Institute on Drug Abuse stated that MDMA is a nationwide problem and serious health risk. They further stated the adverse effects are much like amphetamines and cocaine. They cited, psychological difficulties, including confusion, depression, sleep problems, drug craving, severe anxiety and paranoia.

These adverse symptoms are commonplace reactions of psychotropic drugs such as amitriptyline, promethazine, flurazepam, diazepam and thioridazine. Most psychotropic drugs are not controlled.

The DEA's stand on MDMA was that it was neurotoxic to serotonergic neurons. The neurotoxic effect of amphetamine and fenfluramine towards serotonergic neurons has been demonstrated and known in the scientific community for two decades. Fenfluramine has been taken off the market (FDA) because it causes heart disease.

Amphetamine and methamphetamine are listed under Schedule 2 meaning:

1) The drug or other substance has a high potential for abuse.

2) The drug or other substance has a currently accepted medical use in treatment in the United States or a currently accepted medical use with severe restrictions.

3) Abuse of the drug or other substance may lead to severe psychological or physical dependence.

Schedule 2 also includes P-2-P which is one of many immediate precursors to amphetamine and methamphetamine.

P-2-P also appears under the chemical names benzylmethylketone or phenyl-2-propanone.

Benzphetamine and Chlorphentermine are listed under Schedule 3 which means:

1) The drug or other substance has a potential for abuse less than the drugs or other substances in Schedules I and II.

2) The drug or other substance has a currently accepted medical use in treatment in the United States.

3) Abuse of the drug or other substance may lead to moderate or low physical dependence or high psychological dependence.

The following substances are listed under schedule 4:

Fenfluramine
Cathine ((+)-norpseudoephedrine)
Diethylpropion
Phentermine

1) The drug or substance has a low potential for abuse relative to the drug or other substances in Schedule 3.

2) The drug or other substance has a currently accepted medical use in treatment in the United States.

3) Abuse of the drug or other substance may lead to limited physical dependence or psychological dependence relative to the drugs or other substances in Schedule 3.

Mr. Sapienza (DEA) also stated that MDMA's abuse potential was demonstrated by the fact that a lot of the drug is being synthesized and sold on the street.

It is a known fact that many people use drugs in personal psychotherapy. Many individuals are seeking alternative forms of psychotherapy and adjuncts to psychotherapy because of the short falls of conventional psychotropic drugs:

1) psychotropic drugs do not cure mental and emotional afflictions.

2) the toxic effects of psychotropic drugs make them ineffective for many people to tolerate.

3) the addictive nature of many psychotropic drugs. Drug addiction effects the lives of all those around them.

4) psychotropics can mimic mental illness, especially on withdrawal. Drugs should be discontinued with the assistance of those who have a very thorough understanding of drug mechanisms and patient biochemistry. Rapid discontinuing of some medications can cause serious reactions. Some drugs must be tapered.

5) chronic drug treatment is not a solution for mental or emotional afflictions. Psychotherapy is necessary to gain coping skills.

6) the high cost of psychotropic drugs. Price gouging is no good.

7) psychotropics can cause violence & rage reactions in some patients.

8) conventional psychotropic medications are not effective in all biochemical disorders (eg. the use of marijuana to help PTSD victims).

9) there are few, if any, protections for patients who are abused by psychiatry in the United States.

It is important that patients find psychiatrists who have a strong understanding of brain biochemistry and drug interactions. There are many very knowledgeable psychiatrists in this country. Patients must be treated with compassion, understanding and empathy or psychiatry becomes a pill mill. This country needs more research and faster drug development.

Psychiatric drugs will remain the arsenal against what afflicts the human condition; until a better understanding of disease mechanisms is achieved; until governments, states, agencies, associations, institutions and communities recognize the needs of and protect the rights of the individual and families.

Many psychologists and psychotherapists were caught off guard with the DEA's emergency scheduling of MDMA under Schedule 1 in July 1985. Psychotherapists requested that MDMA should be placed on Schedule 3 meaning that the drug has a low potential for abuse and that it has accepted medical use.

Frank Sapienza (DEA) commented: *"We didn't know that it was being used in therapy sessions."*

CHAPTER 5: DESIGNER DRUGS

The term 'designer drugs' used in The Analogue Act of 1986, is so vague and misleading that its interpretation has been subject to much debate; and I speculate will continue until a more clarified law is written. The term analog used in chemistry is so infinite; it may include homologs, congeners etc. in reference to a parent substance. The term analog, in chemistry, differs from the term analogue, in the Analogue Act, by the fact that the legalese term, analogue, lacks a scienter.

On May, 1, 1986, a hearing was held before the Subcommittee on Crime of the Committee on the Judiciary House of Representatives, to review the problem of 'designer drugs.'

Hon. William J. Hughes was presiding. Present were Representatives Hughes, Smith, Staggers, McCollum, Lungren, Shaw, and Gekas. Staff Present were: Hayden Gregory, counsel; Eric E. Sterling and Edward O'Connell, assistant counsel; Charlene Vanlier Heydinger, associate counsel; Phyllis Henderson, clerk.

I will take various excerpts from the transcripts (except where noted) to give the reader some insight into what went into the creation of the Analogue Act of 1986.

Hon. William J. Hughes: *"Today the Subcommittee on Crime is continuing its examination of the problem of designer drugs. Two years ago, in the course of our examination of the diversion of controlled substances from medical purposes to the black market, we looked at the problem of designer drugs such as the fentanyl analogs, and MPPP, which were causing death and paralysis, particularly on the west coast.*

In conjunction with the DEA, we developed an approach to the problem that allows the Drug Enforcement Administration to schedule these substances on a very short time frame on an emergency basis. This process for temporary scheduling freed DEA from the usual time-consuming requirement of scientific study that is the basis for determining what drugs ought to be controlled and in what schedule they can most approximately be controlled.

Since the law became effective, as part of the Comprehensive Crime control Act of 1984, DEA has used the authority 5 times to control some 13 substances....

A neurologist in San Jose, California, says that working with the Centers for Disease Control they have identified 400 persons who have been exposed to MPTP which causes Parkinsonism, and irreversible form of brain damage that is appearing. This doctor says that its is the tip of the iceberg. Seven of those persons, almost 2 percent of those known who are so severely ill, are permanently crippled and in danger of dying of the disease. Twenty of these persons were exposed, another 5 percent have mild symptoms of the disease. All of the young people exposed are at risk for developing Parkinson's symptoms. They are, as an investigator of the National Institutes of Health says, "walking time bombs." And now we are seeing people who have used the drug 2 years ago beginning to exhibit symptoms. We are facing a potential public health crisis that may make our current drug abuse problems look mild." pg. 2

Rudy M. Baum: *"The fentanyl analogs make up one of three classes of drugs that generally have been lumped together as designer drugs. Analogs of another, chemically distinct narcotic - meperidine - make up a second class. The third class contains a single member, 3,4-methylene-dioxymethamphetamine (MDMA), which for a number of reasons, probably should not be designated a designer drug."*

(Baum 1985, page 8)

Rudy M. Baum: *"Henderson coined the term "designer drugs" specifically in reference to the fentanyl analogs he was analyzing... For a variety of reasons, Henderson believes that a single "world class medicinal chemist" has been responsible for the various fentanyl analogs that have appeared... Henderson bases his assessment that a single, highly sophisticated chemist has been responsible for all the fentanyl analogs that have appeared..."* (Baum 1985, page 8 & 10)

Henderson: *"the quality control is really remarkable. These aren't garbage drugs. They are well made, with very few impurities, and the doses are uniform."* (Baum 1985, page 11)

"In a DEA investigation begun about a year ago (1985), Kenneth Baker, a California chemist operating a clandestine laboratory, was identified as a manufacturer and distributor of 3-methylfentanyl, a drug which was scheduled pursuant to the emergency scheduling process. By the time the laboratory search took place (only six weeks after the start of the investigation), Baker had discontinued his production of 3-methylfentanyl but had produced substantial quantities of eight other fentanyl analogs. Unfortunately, however, not one these analogs had been scheduled under the Controlled Substances Act. The search revealed that Baker had obtained information on the scheduling of drugs by the Drug Enforcement Administration, presumably so that he could tailor his production to stay ahead of the scheduling process.

When it was learned that the drugs found in Baker's laboratory were not controlled substances and that charges could not be brought under the Controlled Substances Act, prosecutors determined that some means should, never less, be found to prosecute Baker and his co-con-spirators. The Federal Food, Drug, and Cosmetic Act was reviewed for relevant provisions. In a multi-count indictment filed on March 20, 1986, Baker and others were charged with violating provisions of the Federal Food, Drug, and Cosmetic Act, including manufacturing a drug without registering drugs, with intent to defraud."   (p. 31)

Letter from John C. Lawn to Edwin Messe III: *"In one instance, a Ph.D. chemist employed by DuPont Chemical Company prepared substantial quantities of fentanyl analogs in that company's laboratories. He attempted to locate distributors for these substances and was apprehended by DEA agents after he attempted to pick up payment for fentanyl analogs delivered to an undercover agent."* (p. 146)

3-Methyl-fentanyl

Mr. Lungren: *"At the same time, I don't wish to suggest that we should rely solely on a death count as a measure of the threat that these drugs pose to our society. Mere statistics fail to express that misery perpetrated by contemporary Dr. Frankensteins who are transforming human beings into chemical zombies."*   (p. 3)

Mr. Lungren's statement specifically refers to deaths related to overdoses from high doses of narcotic analogs and contaminated 1-methyl-4-phenyl-4-propionoxy-piperidine (MPPP) (a narcotic analgesic) with the neurotoxic 1-methyl-4-phenyl-1,2,3,6-tetahydropyridine (MPTP). This accidental contamination resulted in a new and better understanding of Parkinson's Disease mechanisms for the scientific community. In rat tests this contaminant was not neurotoxic. It is unfortunate that narcotic addicts could not obtain legal narcotics with rehabilitation which is the true cause of their deaths (*Opiods in Mental Illness* 1981; *OXY* 2001).

Mr. Lungren's concern is that we should not rely solely on a death count as a measure of the threat. Hundreds of thousands of Americans are injured each year by FDA approved drugs. Elderly people and the mentally ill continue to be abused, and tortured with dangerous psychiatric drugs. Families continue to suffer the consequences of unsafe FDA approved drugs, as authorities turn their backs to this epidemic in our country. Society pays the price for both dangerous (FDA approved and unapproved) drugs and inadequate drug development in this nation.

With the passage of the analogue law no further development of medications to help the mentally ill has taken place which has shown promise or relief without high cost and adverse effects. The passage of the Analogue Act has locked pharmaceutical development into the hands of those who have the most to gain from addiction, toxic reactions to substantiate continued drugging of the ill.

Drugs and nutrients which have been found to be helpful to those afflicted are unpatentable (orphan status) hence remain undeveloped and, in many cases, out of reach for those who are most in need.

Larry Smith: *"We need to be proactive rather than reactive. That is why I support legislation to change the definition of the crime being committed. The legislation which I have introduced would change the illegality from the substance itself to the effect this substance has on an individual."*   (pg. 7)

The Analogue Act must not interfere with the method of science. The practice of neurochemistry is analogous to the practice of law. Both build on the earlier precedents of others, in the case of neurochemistry, it is to build on previously known active and inactive molecules, this also includes human testing. Anything less than that would seriously hamper scientific advancements in the understanding of the mind/brain.

Dr. Schuster: *"Over the past decade, the illicit use of meperidine has increased when heroin became scarce. Two other designer drugs with pharmacological effects similar to heroin have been identified and found to be similar in structure to meperidine. These two analogs, 1-methyl-4-phenyl-4-propionoxy-piperidine (MPPP) and 1-(2-phenyl-ethyl)-4-acetyloxypiperidine (PEPAP), have been shown in analgesic tests by NIDA to be many times more potent than meperidine....*

The abuse of MPPP was first reported in the Washington, D.C. area in 1976, when a 23 year old man was referred to the NIMH for evaluation after exhibiting symptoms of Parkinson's Disease. A known drug user, he had used the meperidine analogue MPPP which he himself had manufactured. Since he was able to provide the chemical formula and procedures he had followed to produce the MPPP, it was discovered through subsequent analysis that he had inadvertently created the substance MPTP (1-Methyl-4-phenyl-1,2,3,6-tetahydro-pyridine) as a side product in the synthesis. Only the most stringent chemical controls would prevent some production of MPTP during the intended production of MPPP."

"(1-(2-phenylethyl)-4-phenyl-4-acetoxy-piperidine), (PEPAP), is a recent addition to the street scene, having been identified by the DEA in confiscations in California in 1985, and in the form of a precursor in a lab arrested in Texas in 1984. Its action is substantially similar to that of MPPP and, just as MPTP results from the production of MPPP, PEPTP from the production of PEPAP although preliminary research   indicates it does not have the devastating neurotoxic properties of MPTP." (p. 43-44)

MPPP

Charles B. Rangel: *"Designer drugs are subject to no quality controls on potency or purity, thus exposing users to unknown dangers... The clandestine manufacture of controlled substance analogs was first encountered in the late 1960's, with several hallucinogenic drugs similar to LSD. In the 1970's, chemical analogs of PCP were prevalent. However, it was in the 1980's, with the creation of extremely potent analogs similar to heroin, or "synthetic heroin," that the real crisis developed."*
(pgs. 12-13)

Although analogs of controlled substances have always been used in research, few entered the illicit market. Many of the analogs were not controlled as their appearance was sporadic. The PCP congeners that Mr. Rangel is discussing were not popular and were considered dangerous by many drug users. The drug was being sprayed on marijuana and also tableted and sold on the street. I was talking with a DEA agent concerning a PCP type molecule that had appeared on the street. I had received several reports of toxic reactions from individuals expecting pleasurable effects. I stressed that these molecules should be scheduled as they were dangerous especially at the dosage that was being distributed. The agent mentioned that these molecules would be scheduled soon. He also mentioned that every time that they scheduled one analog another would appear and were causing problems for law enforcement and dangerous to anyone who took these drugs.

It has been theorized that PCP congeners that bind to *mu* opiod receptors may have creativity enhancing effects. The major obstacle with phencyclidine type molecules is that elevated dosages have effects which can be dangerously sedating and hallucinogenic, resembling psychosis inducing 'chemical straight jackets' (neuroleptics).

Lawton Chiles: *"It is interesting to note that some of the labs for designer drugs in California were broken up not by law enforcement people, but by organized crime people, because they felt it was interrupt-*

ing their sales and distribution that had been set up for heroin, for the illegal drugs that come in. Now at what stage do those same organized crime people decide hey, wait a minute, we don't need to break up their labs, we will merge with them, so to speak. Will buy the small company. We will take it on and we will put it into our operation. That is where I think the real potential danger is." (p. 24)

Organized crime is always interested in recruiting chemists to 'cook up bathtub drugs' for them, generally these groups are not interested in 'designer molecules'. Organized crime syndicates have unlimited pipelines for narcotics from international smuggling groups.

John White: *"The National Association of Retail Druggists (NARD) represents owners of more than 30,000 independent pharmacies, where over 75,000 pharmacies dispense more than 70 percent of the nation's prescription drugs. Together they serve 18 million persons daily.*

We were concerned that the emergency scheduling authority, as originally drafted, was far too broad, and we were pleased when the Chairman and his colleagues agreed to a modification... ... which could in no way deny due process to the retail pharmacists we represent, who have numerous controlled substances with approved medical usefulness in their inventory." (p. 197-198)

Mr. Hughes: *"If you look at the data, the Dawn reports, upward of 75 percent of the overdoses and deaths are caused by prescription drugs- the diversion of prescription drugs into the illicit markets. It is big business in this country."*

"A few years ago we had diversion investigative units. They were phased out in that 1981-82 round, as you well know." (p. 20)

The enforcement of laws against drug diversion by physicians, pharmacists, and detail men was made a responsibility of the states. Law enforcement at the state level (in most states) are not trained, equipped, or even want to be bothered with investigating script doctors. Funding to investigate script doctors was cut from the DEA (1983). One third of street drugs come from practitioners, yet the DEA's hands are tied by political agendas, which are backed by campaign contributions from pharmaceutical firms, medical associations and all those who benefit from the drugging of America.

The following law went into effect in 1986 primarily to curb the barrage of homologs and analogs of the synthetic narcotics, meperidine, fentanyl that was being distributed by illicit networks as a replacement for street heroin. The most serious problem with a law controlling 'analogues' is that it inadvertently placed a blanket repression on the development, synthesis and study of research neurochemicals by private individuals, students and small businesses.

Controlled Substance Analogue Act of 1986
Treatment of Controlled Substance Analogues

"A controlled substance analogue shall, to the extent intended for human consumption, be treated, for the purposes of this title and title 3 as a controlled substance in schedule 1."

Definition

Section 102 of the Controlled Substances Act (21 U.S.C. 802) is amended by adding at the end thereof the following:
"(32)(A) Except as provided in subparagraph (B), the term 'controlled substance analogue' means a substance-

"(i) the chemical structure of which is substantially similar to the chemical structure of a controlled substance in schedule 1 or 2;
"(ii) which has a stimulant, depressant, or hallucinogenic effect on the central nervous system that is substantially similar to or greater than the stimulant, depressant, or hallucinogenic effect on the central nervous system of a controlled substance in schedule 1 or 2; or
"(iii) with respect to a particular person, which such person represents or intends to have a stimulant, depressant, or hallucinogenic effect on the central nervous system that is substantially similar to or greater than the stimulant, depressant, or hallucinogenic effect on the central nervous system of a controlled substance in schedule 1 or 2.
"(B) Such term does not include-
"(i) a controlled substance;
"(ii) any substance for which there is a an approved new drug application;
"(iii) with respect to a particular person any substance, if an exemption is in effect for investigational use, for that person, under section 505 of the Federal Food , Drug, and Cosmetic Act (21 U.S.C. 355) to the extent conduct with respect to such substance is pursuant to such exemption; or
"(iv) any substance to the extent not intended for human consumption before such an exemption takes effect with respect to that substance".

CHAPTER 6:
THE REPRESSION OF NEUROCHEMISTRY
THE TWO PRONG ATTACK

The first prong:
"the chemical structure of which is
substantially similar to the chemical structure
of a controlled substance in schedule 1 or 2."

Dr. Hawks: *"If I understand what you are getting at, if you mean can two compounds differ very slightly in structure and have quite different pharmacological properties--*
Mr. Hughes: *Yes.*
Dr. Hawks: (continuing). *Yes, that is very true. One primary example being the discovery some years ago of narcotic antagonists, where you can take the morphine molecule, make a small structural change to one position on it and have a morphine antagonist, so it has the opposite pharmacological effect...*
Mr. Hughes: *What determines the effect of a chemical compound?*
Dr. Hawks: *Its structure. As we have said, small structural changes can have, in some cases... can have tremendous effects on the pharmacology, or the pharmacological effect of that drug. And this is primarily based on structural changes, so structure is the main thing that causes the activity of the chemical.*
Mr. Hughes: *Do all chemicals in a particular chemical class have similar psychopharmacological effects?*
Dr. Hawks: *No."* (pgs. 52-53)

U.S. Patent Office will not grant a patent on a chemical described as 'substantially similar.' Chemicals indexed in chemical and scientific journals are not listed under headings of 'substantially similar,' because no such term exists in chemistry.

A Change in Structure; A Change in Activity.

In the phenylethylamine class of chemicals, a slight change in the structure will dramatically change the activity of a molecule. Examples: 3,4,5-Trimethoxyphenylethylamine (mescaline) is active. 3,4,5-Trimethoxy-N-methyl-phenylethylamine (an inactive molecule) is created when a methyl (CH_3) group is added to the amino group (NH_2) on the mescaline molecule.

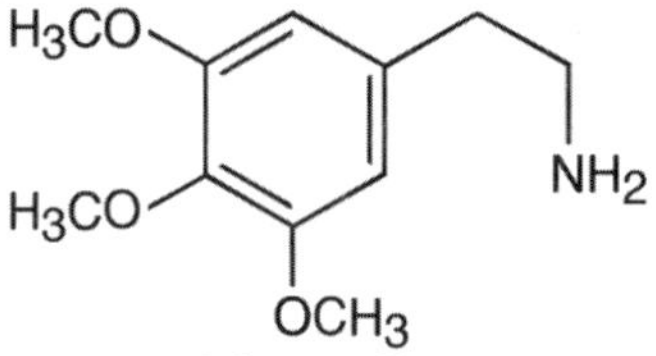

Mescaline

3,4,5-Trimethoxyphenylethylamine (mescaline)

M.F. C11H17NO3   M.W. 211.25

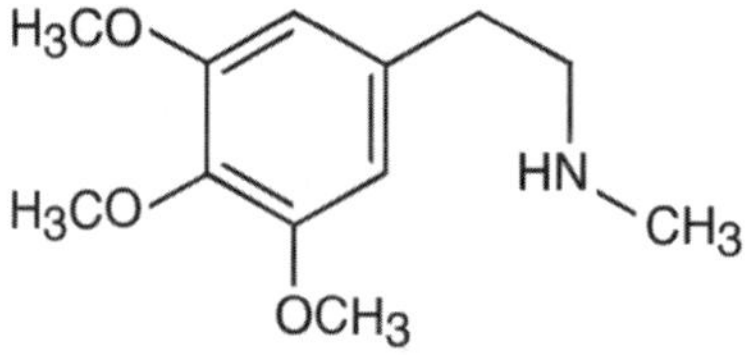

N-Methyl-mescaline

3,4,5-Trimethoxy-N-methyl-phenylethylamine

M.F. C12H19NO3   M.W. 225.28

Substantial Differences in Amphetamines
A Change in Structure; A Change in Activity.

Here are a few more examples showing slight alterations in the molecular structure which produce substantially different biological and psychological effects.

para-Methoxyamphetamine

para-Methoxyamphetamine; (PMA)
4-Methoxyamphetamine

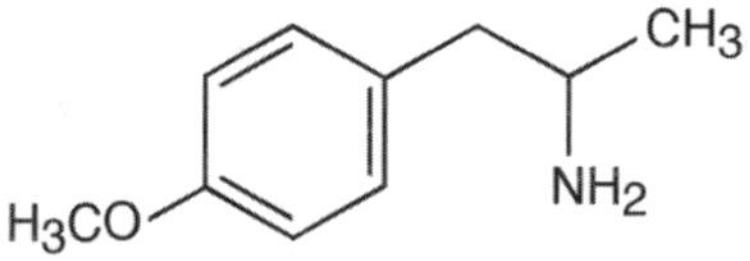

M.F. C10H15NO   M.W. 165.23

para-Methoxyamphetamine is a hallucinogen; which was hypothesized to be endogenously formed during amphetamine psychosis (Smythies 1967).Testing concluded that this metabolic reaction did not occur (Angrist 1970).

2-Methoxy-N-methylamphetamine
(Methoxyphenamine)

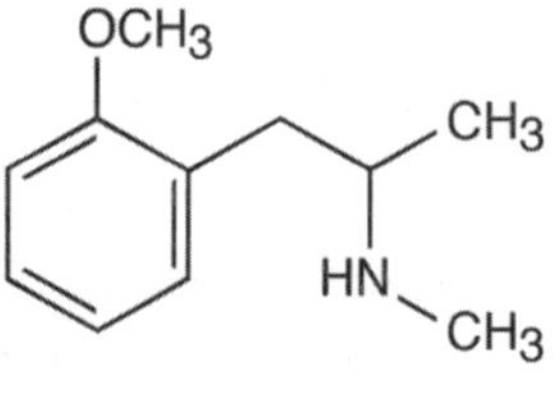

M.F. C11H17NO   M.W. 179.25

Moving the methoxy group (OCH3) from the 4th carbon to the 2nd carbon on the phenyl group of PMA and adding a methyl (CH3) group to the amino group (NH2) results in a totally different chemical with a different molecular formula and a different molecular weight. 2-Methoxy-N-methylamphetamine is called methoxyphenamine.

Methoxyphenamine is a vasopressor. Without laboratory animal and human testing, its usefulness as a vasopressor would not have been discovered.

para-Methoxy-N-methylamphetamine
M.F. C11H17NO M.W. 179.25

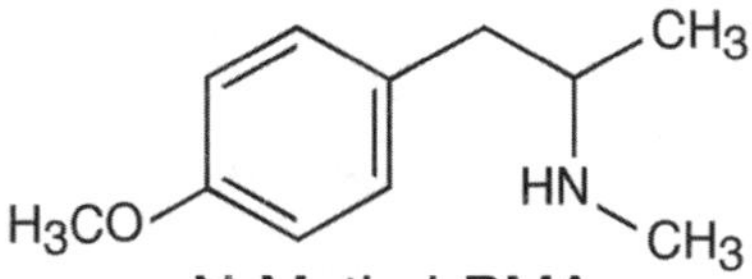

N-Methyl-PMA

para-Methoxy-N-methylamphetamine is an active substance. Its effects are reported to be unlike DOM (4-methyl-2,5-dimethoxy-amphetamine) and amphetamine. It has the same molecular weight, the same chemical formula, but not the same molecular structure as methoxy-phenamine.

Prior to testing a chemical (of a specific molecular structure) on laboratory animals and humans, we can not scientifically or accurately determine, (without a substantial degree of uncertainty), assume or imply anything about the activity or non-activity of a molecule.

The Same Molecule, Different Species, Different Activity

3,4-Dimethoxyphenylethylamine

3,4-Dimethoxyphenylethylamine
M.F. C10H15NO2   M.W. 181.24

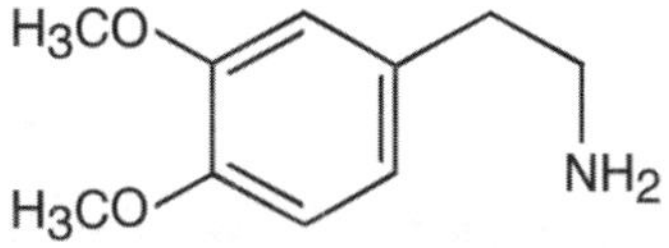

This molecule has been found in the urine of some schizophrenics. It was weakly active when tested in laboratory rats and inactive when tested in humans (Shulgin 1969). Meaning, if no humans would have tested this chemical it may have been assumed to be hallucinogenic and then assumed to be the endogenous cause of schizophrenia; which it is not. 3,4-Dimethoxy-phenylethylamine is a neurochemical metabolite, not a biochemical marker in individuals with schizophrenia.

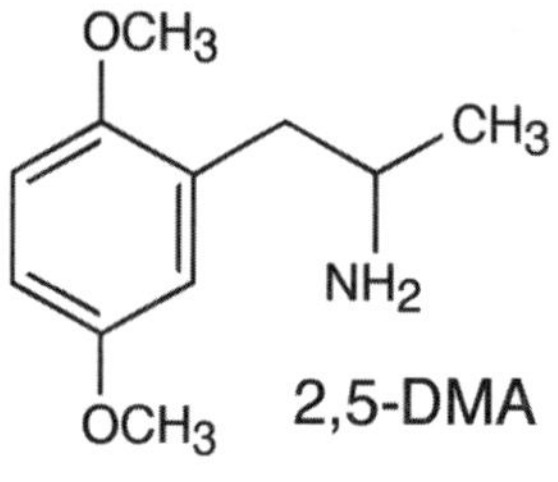

OCH3
CH3
NH2
OCH3   2,5-DMA

2,5-Dimethoxyamphetamine
M.F. C11H17NO2 M.W. 195.25
2,5-Dimethoxyamphetamine, also called DMA, is inactive in laboratory rats (Smythies 1970) and also non-hallucinogenic in humans (Shulgin 1991). Rats metabolize many drugs differently than humans (Beckett 1970; Boissier; Smith 1970).

2,3,4-Trimethoxyphenylethylamine
M F. C11H17NO3   M.W. 211.25 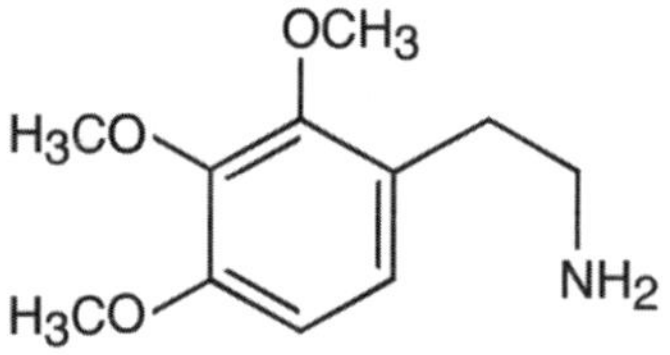
2,3,4-Trimethoxyphenylethylamine is a positional isomer of mescaline (3,4,5-Trimethoxyphenylethylamine). It is inactive in normal subjects, but is hallucinogenic in schizophrenic patients (Slotta 1936) and is 'mescaline like' in rats. (Winter 1973)

OCH3
H3CO
H3CO
NH2

"If you are familiar with the drug discrimination literature, you can get false-positives, and perhaps Professor Glennon will correct me if I am wrong, but I am not aware of false negatives."
(Nichols 1989).

A misinterpretation of a molecule's activity can occur when tests are applied to inappropriate species.

The second prong: "effect on the central nervous system that is substantially similar to"

"*3,4-Methylenedioxyamphetamine (MDA) is recognized as both d-amphetamine-like and DOM-like by rats trained to discriminate these drugs from saline.*
3,4-Methylenedioxymethamphetamine (MDMA), is recognized only as d-amphetamine-like in the same tests.

3,4-Methylenedioxy-N-ethylamphetamine (MDE) and 3,4-Methyl-enedioxy-N-hydroxy-amphetamine, (N-hydroxy-MDA) in rodent drug discrimination studies with d-amphetamine and DOM as training drugs, do not generalize to either d-amphetamine or DOM. Based on this information alone it would appear that MDE and N-hydroxy-MDA are neither amphetamine-like stimulants nor DOM-like hallucinogens. These studies alone would further suggest that MDA, MDMA, MDE, and N-hydroxy-MDA have different abuse potentials."

(McClain 1989, pg. 31)

"Some phenyl-substituted phenylisopropylamines, such as MDA, PMA and MDMA, have pharmacological properties distinct from those of amphetamine or DOM. Therefore, prediction about the abuse liability of these compounds based on their similarities to or differences from classic stimulants (such as cocaine or amphetamine) or hallucinogens (such as LSD or DOM) may provide inappropriate results."

(Sannerud 1989)

"INTENDED FOR HUMAN CONSUMPTION"
"A controlled substance analogue shall, to the extent intended for human consumption..."

Dr. Grinspoon: *"Under the provisions of this law, a chemist who synthesized a new drug might actually be committing a crime by taking it. Self experimentation of this kind is the way in which most new drugs with valuable medical and scientific properties have been discovered. It is true not only of synthetic drugs, but of drugs found naturally in plants. If the federal government makes it a crime to work with any new substance thought to have some undefined resemblance to a controlled drug, entire fields of therapeutic pharmacology may go undiscovered.*

Many of the discoveries of new medicines and therapies have been made by scientists who try one thing and fail, and then try something else. The controlled development of analogs -- in effect, designer drugs -- is essential to the advance of pharmacology. Many of the antipsychotic and antidepressant drug discoveries of recent years are minor variations on a common molecular theme with similar effects. However, it is precisely the differences that are medically significant -- different potencies, different side effects, and most important, different therapeutic uses.

The same is true of analogs that do not belong to class of drugs with presently accepted therapeutic uses. One drug that has recently received some publicity is MDMA (3,4-methylenedioxy-methamphetamine). It is chemically related to several controlled substances. A number of researchers also take seriously its potential as an aid to insight and communication in psychotherapy, and they are interested mainly because its effects are not identical with those of the chemically related drugs.

When MDMA first appeared on the American scene in the early 1970's, it was known only to a few scientific and medical researchers; there was no significant illicit street use. It could not be patented, and no drug company was interest in it. If the proposed legislation had been in effect at that time, all research could have been brought to a hold. Since reputable physicians and scientists would not have been willing to become outlaws to work with MDMA, we would never have learned about its therapeutic potential. The small illicit market, on the other hand, would have been affected very little. Under the new law, if there are any therapeutically useful analogs of currently controlled drugs, we many never come to know of their existence.

The proposed "designer drug" legislation needs to be redesigned. Its language must be clarified or the exemption for scientific and medical research rewritten to protect the public against opportunist illicit drug profiteers without discouraging research on pharmacology in areas where early commercial application is unlikely."   (pgs. 83-85)

26 Year old female school teacher (rape victim): *"Adam (MDMA) has helped me look at this suffering, to see my life as a whole and to understand it better. It has given me the courage to face the fears instead of ignoring them, to know that the most important thing is to struggle to trust myself. I don't know what my life will be like now, or how much I want to live, but I do know that the experiences I have gone through, even though painful, have also been full of tenderness and trust, and there is no longer this feeling of emptiness. I am not leaving a hospital with a prescription in my hand for anti-depressants. Rather, I'm leaving... with the courage to try to face my fears and to face life."*

Ralph Metzer, Ph.D.: *"One therapist has estimated that in five hours of one MDMA session clients could activate and process psychic material that would normally require five months of weekly therapy sessions."*   (*Through The Gateway of the Heart*; 1985, pgs. 51 & 2)

Angarola, Esq.: *"It is also possible that some legitimate researchers could inadvertently violate the law by producing and investigating substances which may meet the criteria of the proposed amendments. As an example, there are substantial questions as to the interpretation of the term "intended for human consumption." Virtually every time a pharmaceutical company researcher synthesizes a compound, he or she is looking for something the will eventually be intended for human consumption after FDA approval. Would that researcher violate the law because of his long-term intention?"* (pgs. 93-94)

Angarola, Esq.: *"One representative testified to the fact that her company would not go forward in investigating a schedule 1 controlled substance unless the condition which was to be treated was life-threatening. The controlled substance analog legislation could have a similar chilling effect."* (pg. 87)

Dr. Grinspoon: *"Well, I am not a lawyer, but in fact, in the real world a drug company does not - you see if you're dealing with a drug let's say for the treatment of congestive heart failure and you can put an animal into congestive heart failure and you can see if this new digitalis or this digitalis analog improves the congestive heart failure. If you are dealing with a psychoactive drug, animals don't tell you that they feel less anxiety or feel less depression or what have you. And a drug company is not going to go ahead and put the thousands and thousands of dollars involved in getting an IND because in the real world some people in that drug company have tried that drug themselves.*

Now I am sure these people are very experienced researchers. They know a lot about the chemical from which this analog arrived. They do it under very careful circumstances, take it in tiny doses at first, and so forth. But in the real world drug companies don't deal with psychoactive drugs unless they have some pretty good idea that let's say Valium is going to be a good antianxiety drug. That is the real world."
(pg. 109)

Mr. Lungen: *"You have a specific complaint about the bill in which you say, first of all, criminal penalties are imposed without a requirement for evidence that anyone has been injured by a new analog or even that anyone has abused it... Some of these drugs that have been discovered in recent years have helped me get through pain, so I understand it like everyone else does. I don't want to stop the quest toward more science. My father is a doctor and I greatly respect the medical profession. In fact, I was in it until I ran into organic chemistry in premed, so I became a lawyer. [Laughter.]"* (pgs. 112, 114, 115.)

Dr. Tocus: *"I can understand that if someone wants to know what the effect maybe, is it going to cause him to hallucinate, going to cause them to feel something, the investigator may take it one time to to see what is going to happen to his patients."* (pg. 116)

Hon. William Hughes: *"I think that I am pretty much persuaded by the argument that is made that if you are talking about psychoactive drugs in particular that the only way you are going to find out just what impact they have upon humans is to try it."*   (pg. 117)

Common Sense vs. Legalese

Many proteins are composed of phenylethylamine and tryptamine structures. Milk contains phenylalanine which is the carboxylic acid analogue of phenylethylamine. Phenylalanine could also be described as the des-methyl-carboxylic acid analog of amphetamine. When phenylalanine is decarboxylated it becomes phenylethylamine which is the des-methyl analog of amphetamine.

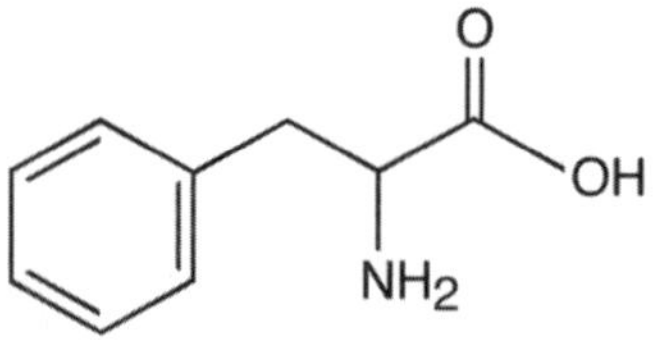

Phenylalanine
M.F. C9H11NO2 M.W. 165.19

Phenylethylamine; (des-methyl-amphetamine)
    M.F. C8H11N   M.W. 121.18
Phenylethylamine is in chocolate. Chocolate is psychoactive. The effects are powerful enough that feeding a small dog too much chocolate can kill the animal. Phenylethylamine is responsible for some of the mood elevating effects of chocolate.

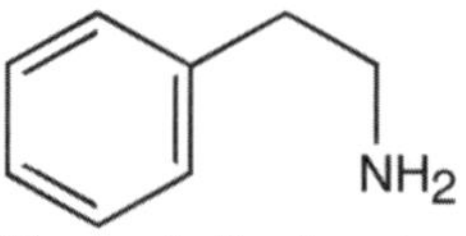

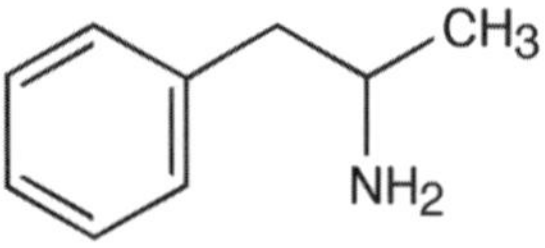

Phenylethylamine

Amphetamine
(*alpha*-Methyl-phenylethylamine)
MF. C9H13N   MW. 135.20

Amphetamine

Many people give loved ones chocolate or to those who are sad to boost their spirits. Although individuals may say that they enjoy chocolate, that it brings pleasure to their lives; under the current law; (in strict accordance with the law); is "intending" or "treating" someone with a piece of chocolate illegal?   Would mixing chocolate milk for the purpose of a "pick me up" or a mood elevator (eg. "I feel energetic/good when I have chocolate.") be manufacture?

Mr. Trott: "*A statute must also protect legitimate scientific research. That is, chemists should be free to conduct legitimate experimentation without fear of committing a serious federal felony.*" (p. 34)

The prohibitionist atmosphere has overloaded the courts as more serious crimes are not given the investigative attention and assets that they desperately need. The free reign given to law enforcement in many parts of the country under a guise of a 'drug war,' has undermined the foundations of civil liberties. Illegal drug money has corrupted many courts. Minimum mandatories have tied the hands of judges seeking the best possible solutions for those appearing before them. Impure & hazardous illegal drugs continue to be 'churned out' of make shift labs by criminals, as scientists are not permitted to study or develop safer substitutes.

From a business standpoint, intent is to produce a profit. From a scientific point of view, there is no intent, a scientist can not apply any preconceived ideas on a structure of an unknown non-existent molecule.

Scientists can not intent on the activity of any molecule as the molecule it self exhibits activity or non-activity regardless of what anyone thinks, wishes or contrives it will do, or could do.

The structural activity relationships of molecules are not precise, much is unknown. Chemists (psychopharmacologists) intend on creating better substances, with increased potency, less side effects (toxic effects), longer or shorter action, new therapeutic actions and/or new research applications: totally new chemicals. In simple terms, a scientist hopes and wishes for the best, (e.g. end human suffering, help to alleviate depression, disease, pain, etc.), but only the testing of a molecule in laboratory animals and humans will tell what the molecule actually does.

If chemists could predict what the effects of a contrived chemical structure would be, then drug companies would not be spending billions of dollars synthesizing, researching and developing new drugs. If chemists in chemical companies were so successful in their intent at 'designing' drugs and chemicals, is killing of the planet with toxic waste part of their intention? Everyone knows that you can't market products to a dead world.

The primary purpose of a scientist is to question, test, and continue researching; no action has any one specific purpose except that of seeking to transcend the unknown into the known. The most a scientist can do is hope to find something which will advance scientific knowledge which in turn will benefit the human race.

The very nature of neurochemistry involves the purchase of drug precursors as they are the precursors of many neurochemicals. Many chemicals that are used in the construction of neurochemicals are also used in clandestine laboratories, the only differences being the end products and their distribution. The very action of purchasing precursors places neurochemists under suspicion.

In all laboratory raids, a forensic chemist must be present to evaluate the chemicals and paperwork. A chemist is also necessary to identify chemicals which may be hazardous and to shut down reactions. Most laboratories have many chemicals. All individuals (law enforcement officers and suspects) are at risk of exposure to toxic chemicals if they are not contained; safety is paramount. Chemicals are safe as long as they are handled/stored and disposed of properly.

Mere suspicion is not a valid reason/grounds for the issuance of search warrants as this blocks scientific study, inquiry and advancement. 'Good intentions' as a reason for home invasions and confiscating of all scientific and technical paperwork as evidence is also not valid when there is a disregard for the scientific facts. The end does not justify the means to allow violation of 6th amendment rights.

Independent and law abiding neurochemists have been forced to purchase chemicals in a stealth matter to avoid suspicion and harassment from the state and federal government. These purchases are no different in the clandestine ways in which illegal drug chemists use to avoid detection by authorities.

The overbearing paranoia placed on neuroscientists is not conducive to a scientific atmosphere and hampers scientific inquiry and neurochemical development.

A Functional Knowledge of Chemicals & Chemistry

Society itself is primarily composed of those who are functionally ignorant of chemistry and research. Most individuals would not know the difference between dihydrogen oxide and deuterium oxide or the uses of either of these chemicals never mind more complex and unfamiliar chemical structures. This lack of scientific skills by average individuals is serious considering that technology is common place and is part of everything in our modern society. Those who are ignorant of science and technology are most likely to perceive it as a threat and repress development.

Most individuals are not fortunate enough to have a university library next door, wealthy enough to afford a modem, computer and be able to pay for access on multi data bases. All of this hinders the education of the individual, society and the evolution of science. A national toll-free data base access to all encompassing libraries of scientific and medical journals is necessary to foster independent study and to generate progressive development in the sciences. Large user accessibility, cross reference capabilities to vast amounts of information and rapid transfer of information are necessary.

When science is dynamic, students are attracted by curiosity, develop interest, get involved and want to learn more. Societies and national policies that invest in the sciences, reap profit from the advancement of technology. When governments and societies nurture, support and expedite public access to information and knowledge, the end result is a nation that can compete and is not handicapped in the world marketplace.

An exam was given to students world wide. The scores of American students were in the bottom third. Students in America are doing very poorly in sciences. Even Cuba has more literate individuals per capita than the United States.

Here are a few responses, (Parade Magazine 6/2/1991), from a 10th grade class when shown the poor test results (spelling, grammar and punctuation appear this way in the original letters):

"Not a Americans are stupid. We just rank lower in school big deal."

"And if other countries are doing better what does it matter, their most likely going to come over the U.S. anyway?"

"Maybe that's good that we are not as smart as the other countries. So then we can just import all of our products and then we don't have spend all of our money on the parts for the goods."

"I am studying to be a lawyer and frankly I do agree with my parents when they say I have an attitude problem toward science."

When individuals are not educated enough to make decisions for themselves, they rely on the opinion of those who have the most to gain by representing their own interests instead.

"We don't know one millionth of one percent about anything."
Thomas Edison

"The universe belongs to those who, at least to some degree, have figured it out."
Sagan 1974

There are no lists of controlled substance analogues that are subject to control. Sapienza (DEA) and McClain (DEA) state: *"The responsibility falls on DEA to advise attorneys whether or not a particular substance falls within the definition of a controlled substance analogue. Subsequently DEA staff or others may provide expert testimony regarding these matters."*   (McClain 1989)

The DEA are enforcers of the law. It would be dangerous to allow them to also interpret the law; this is an area for experts in science, research, law and a society based on individual liberties to develop, define and interpret.

The term analog to a chemist is a way of describing the relationship of a molecule's structure in comparison to another molecule's structure. This differs from the term used in the Controlled Substances 'Analogue' Act.

Analog does not mean that a molecule is inherently active or inactive; this is determined by testing the molecule in laboratory animals and in human subjects. An analog of a specific chemical does not inherently mean that the analog has an effect which is 'substantially similar' to the specific chemical or any other molecule for that matter. All the structural activity relationships that have been done to help predict the activity of theoretical molecules have proven to scientists how little is known and how much less can be predicted.

The transformation of technical terms to suit legalese is non-scientific and results in misinformation. A common example is lumping non-narcotic substances (e.g. marijuana) under a guise of narcotic. Narcotics are analgesic drugs (e.g. morphine, heroin, fentanyl, etc.) that are highly addictive. Classifying and portraying substances contrary to their actual effects on humans distorts their implications, if any, on society.

A misrepresentation of a drug's actions and effects is a non-factual foundation from which only further distortions and misconceptions will result.

Dr. Grinspoon: "*Although the aim of the Senate bill and related House measures is a worthy one, I believe in its present form the legislation is seriously deficient in several ways that may be easily overlooked but are bound to have unfortunate effects on medical research. First of all, criminal penalties are imposed without a requirement for evidence that anyone has been injured by a new analog or even that anyone has abused it. Instead, the law relies on Justice Department officials and the courts to evaluate the molecular structure of a chemical or read the mind of its manufacturer. Even if the Justice Department and the courts were scientific authorities, they could not properly do that. No one can know in advance the specific effects of a substance that has not yet been created, and the term "substantially similar" as used in the proposed law is both vague and unscientific. What may seem to be a small change in the chemical structure of a drug sometimes leads to a large difference in pharmacological effect.*" (pgs. 81 & 82)

Dr. Ellinwood: "*...we (Research Council of the American Psychiatric Association) are aware of the difficulty in steering legislation in order to avoid after-the-fact legal action directed only piecemeal at a series on new compounds and at the same time avert an over inclusive, presumptive scheduling based on no facts other than the intent to distribute to humans. In more parabolic language, we understand your desire to avoid closing the barn door after the horses are out, yet hesitate to count your chicks before they hatch...*

Points that we would like to have considered in developing the law and its interpretation:

... Means of establishing positive FDA and NIDA advocate procedures for facilitating appropriate legitimate human research on these drugs in order to balance the effects of needed restrictive legislation. These advocate procedures for establishment of a separate independent science-legal-ethics panel to expeditiously review procedures and to process proposal requests for research with drugs addressed in schedule 1 under the new law.

... Allow leeway for expediting significant, rigorous investigations on psychedelic drugs especially their therapeutic utility in certain mental disorders, and the nature of their potential for adverse mind altering effects. Research in this area has been so severely constricted that we have only limited knowledge of the parameters mediating the balance between a therapeutic and adverse outcome.

Means for allowing the expeditious approval of human research on psychedelic drug responses in appropriate research settings need to be facilitated by:

a) Establishment of a separate FDA panel of individuals from several science disciplines and persons concerned with legal and ethical aspects of drug research;

b) Psychedelic drug manufacture for research under the auspices of NIDA or other appropriate agencies.

c) An approval for research on a time limited basis with extensions available only after appropriate feedback and progress reports."

(pgs. 102-104)

A scientist: *"What does 'substantially similar' mean? To me, that is almost a meaningless phrase."* (Baum 1985)

Dr. Hawks: *"One could think of words such as establishing credentials for people who might not have an IND and who have been doing research on certain kinds of compounds or for certain kinds of purposes, but you very quickly get into the kinds of things that people would bring up if they were taken to court to prove their innocence, or from the other side, to provide their lack of innocence. It almost seems like those kinds of subtleties are going to have to be worked out when this bill starts being used for enforcement and from interpretations from the courts and in the policy that results from that."* (pg. 65)

Hon. William Hughes: *"We are a Nation of entrepreneurs. You would be surprised the number of experts I have in my congressional district on a myriad of subjects."* (pg. 58)

Paul De Kruif: ... *"great new medical things are rarely found in hospitals specifically endowed and designed to discover them; and great new medical things are rarely brought to light by scientists especially trained to uncover them."* (A Man Against Insanity, p.11)

Hon. William Hughes: *"We want to make sure that we custom tailor the statute to reach those individuals who are creating designer drugs that end up on the marketplace being harmful to people.*

We don't intend to chill the research that takes place in laboratories or universities that is legitimate research. Or in private homes, if some entrepreneur is interested some aspect of life, human life or animal life. Frankly, I have a hard time understanding how we could determine, you know, what really intent is unless there has been distribution."

(pg. 59)

CHAPTER 7: THE CHEMISTRY

Organic and brain chemistry are far more exciting than inorganic and high school chemistry. Organic chemistry is dynamic, exciting and the 'juice' of the earth and brain.

People who enjoy mystery, magic and quests usually enjoy organic chemistry. It is very easy once an individual understands the rules and learns how to look at molecules. It is much like a puzzle; an adventure.

Molecules are composed of elements. Each element bonds to a defined number of elements or functional groups. Bonds are drawn as a line from one element to another.

-C- Carbon 4 bonds	H- Hydrogen 1 bond	-O- Oxygen 2 bonds
-N- Nitrogen 3 bonds	Br- Bromine 1 bond	Cl- Chlorine 1 bond

Alkanes are a type of carbon-hydrogen chain.

Alkyl Group	Alkyl Chain
Methyl	-CH3
Ethyl	-CH2-CH3
Propyl	-CH2-CH2-CH3
Butyl	-CH2-CH2-CH2-CH3

Chemical	Structure	Alkane Chain	Formula
Methane (Marsh gas)	H H-C-H H	CH_4	CH_4
Ethane	H H H-C-C-H H H	CH_3CH_3	C_2H_6
Propane (Natural gas)	H H H H-C-C-C-H H H H	$CH_3CH_2CH_3$	C_3H_8

Benzene is a chemical that is found in the distillation of oil and of coal tar. It is used in chemical synthesis and also as a solvent. Like all molecules, benzene, can be looked at described and drawn in many ways.

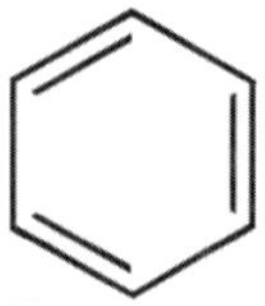

Benzene

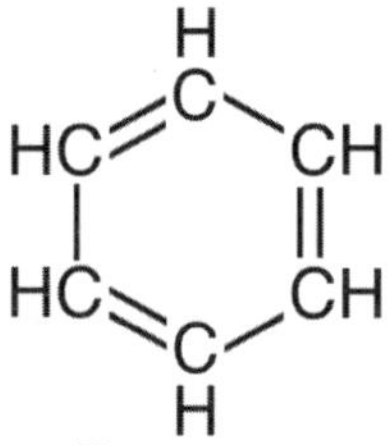

Benzene

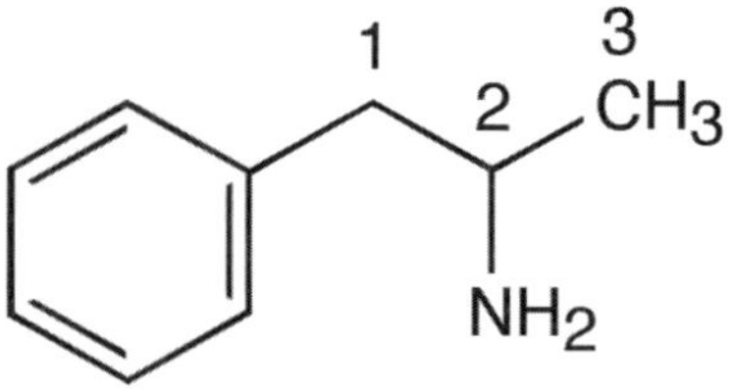

Carbon atoms are numbered: 1   2   3

$$CH_3-CH_2-CH_3$$

so that we can describe what groups are attached where.

The phenyl group may also have substitutions and the carbon atoms are also numbered:

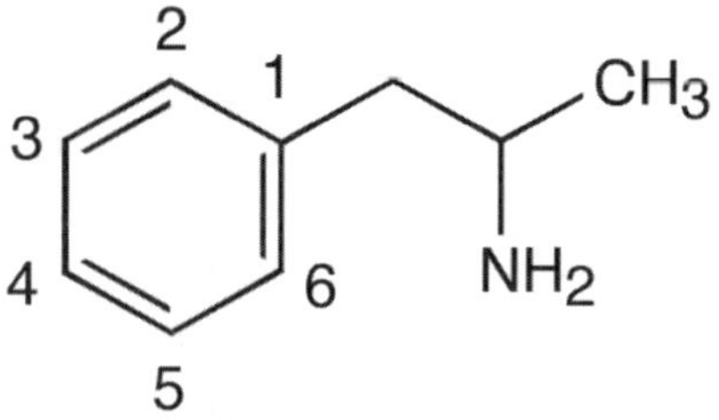

Chemical Names:

d,l-phenyl-2-aminopropane
d,l-phenylisopropylamine
d,l-desoxy-norephedrine
d,l-ß-aminopropylamine

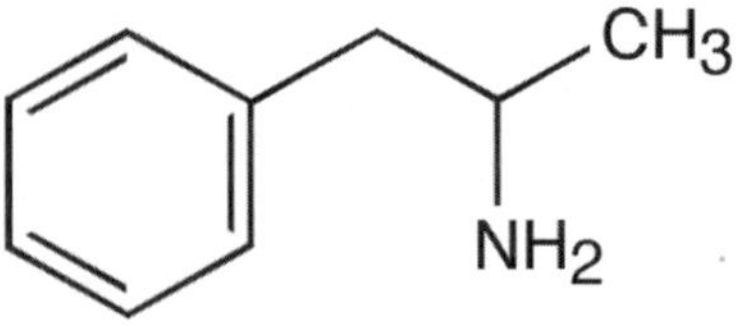

Generic Name: *d,l*-Amphetamine

Trade Name: Benzedrine

Functional (e.g. amino group; NH2) groups are groups of elements that make up many molecules and are manipulated by the chemist in the construction of molecules. Functional groups that contain oxygen:

HO– Alcohol	–C=O O–H Acid	–C=O H Aldehyde
RO– Ether	–C=O O–R Ester	–C=O R Ketone

Molecular Weights; (Moles) Keys of Chemistry

The molecular weight of a molecule is calculated by adding the atomic weights (from the periodic chart of the elements) of all the elements in the molecule.

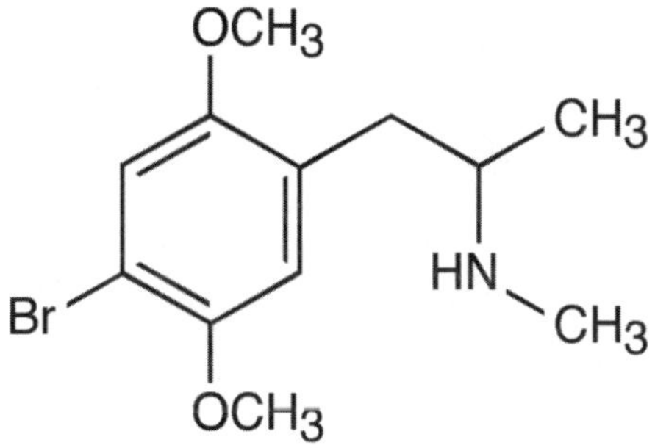

4-Bromo-2,5-dimethoxy-
N-methylamphetamine

M.F. $C_{12}H_{18}O_2NBr$
M.W. 288.18

Element	Atomic Weight	x	No. of Atoms	=	
Carbon	12.011	x	12	=	144.132
Hydrogen	1.0079	x	18	=	18.1422
Oxygen	15.9994	x	2	=	31.9988
Nitrogen	14.0067	x	1	=	14.0067
Bromine	79.904	x	1	=	79.904
			Molecular Weight = Total = 288.1837		

The molecular formula of 4-bromo-2,5-dimethoxy-N-methyl-amphetamine is $C_{12}H_{18}O_2N_1Br_1$ Its molecular weight (one mole) is 288.1837 grams. Chemistry uses the metric system; weights are in grams; temperatures are in Centigrade.

References: *Handbook of Chemistry and Physics*; *Merck Index*.

The Reactions

The following text contains an overview of many reactions that are used in producing psychoactives, inactives, neurotransmitters, neurotoxins, unknowns and precursors to research chemicals.

Chemical reactions have specific as well as non-specific attack sites on a molecule or element. By products of reactions are distilled or extracted from trailings and recycled. Depending on what is run through a specific reaction will determine what will be the product or products. Theoretical yields can be achieved in some chemical reactions. In many reactions, yields are significantly lower and isomers are produced.

It is important to have a analytical testing laboratory analyze chemicals every step of the way in the construction of the final end product. This is necessary to determine:

1)   completeness of the reactions.
2)   by products which are being created and can be recycled. Controlled substance by products must be destroyed as described under CFR 21 § 1307.22
3)   identification and purity of the end product.

Chemistry is a lot of fun. It is a pure science and has predictable results that can be duplicated. Chemistry must be given the respect that it deserves. Like anything, safety precautions must be followed when working with chemicals. Those that do not follow appropriate safety precautions will quickly learn respect when a reaction goes haywire.

The prankster that envisions haphazardly mixing chemicals together like a mad scientist will learn respect through fear. Improper ventilation will result in the asphyxiation of the chemist. Improper preparation techniques will result in an impure mush of unknowns, exothermic reactions, fire and explosions. Common sense has a lot to do with safety in the laboratory setting. You wouldn't pump gas into your car with a cigarette hanging out of your mouth. A simple mistake such as unplugging an electric plug in a room that contains a solvent vapor can result in explosion.

Safety smocks, gloves and proper face shields should always be worn in the laboratory whether working on a reaction or in the presence of someone who is. A safety shower should be tested before doing a reaction to make sure that it is running properly. A safety shower is a necessary protection for someone who has spilled chemicals on themselves.

Although I have mentioned a few safety precautions, there are many more, too numerous to cover because of the variabilities with any experiment. I would strongly suggest to anyone, who is interested in learning proper chemical procedures, to take a course in inorganic chemistry. There is nothing that can replace the hands on experience gained through the help of a patient and experienced instructor.

I describe the synthesis of molecular series in a generalized scope because of the versatility of reactions. I strongly recommend that any one interested in a particular reaction read all references cited in book. Journal articles contain specific reagent quantities and a more detailed description of syntheses. Those interested in studying the preparation of any specific molecule must also continue with a thorough search of the periodicals.

Laboratory setups are not described. This reference guide provides an over view of various syntheses and should not be misconstrued as a treatise or instruction manual. Information on organic laboratory setups and chemical syntheses can be obtained from several books included in the suggested reading section.

Legal as well as illegal chemicals are produced from the same precursors and many of the same immediate precursors. The primary reactions may only differ in the amount of chemicals added, temperatures and reaction times; and yet the end products may be very different. This is a problem for independent chemists in America who are currently researching brain chemistry.

"On July 17, 1990 President Bush issued a Decade of the Brain Proclamation, calling upon all public officials and the people of the United States to observe the decade with appropriate programs and activities. (from Decade of the Brain 1990 - 2000; Maximizing Human Potential; Subcommittee on Brain and Behavioral Sciences; pub. April 1991):

Several developments have converged to make the goals of the Decade of the Brain attainable in the 1990's:

1) The science essential to an understanding of the brain has matured dramatically in the past few decades, permitting greater transfer of basic laboratory knowledge to practical applications.

2) The methodologies and research tools to examine the processes at work in the healthy and unhealthy brain are rapidly maturing.

3) Medical, research and other professional institutions and organizations in the United States and countries around the world are strongly committed to advancing our understanding of the human brain.

To pursue all possible leads about the brain in health and disease, the United States supports and works with scientists in institutions throughout the world. International programs take many forms:

1)   joint research conducted under country-to-country agreement,
2)   efforts involving multinational organizations,
3)   research grants and training programs,
4)   collaborative research projects uniting individual
        U.S. scientists and foreign colleagues, and
5)   international meetings to share knowledge.

Investigators will build on the growing foundation of information about brain-drug interactions to develop medications, techniques and approaches that can be utilized to:

1)   block the effects of abused drugs,
2)   reduce the craving for abused drugs,
3)   reduce the withdrawal effects of drug addiction,
4)   reverse the toxic effects of abused drugs,
5)   develop substitutes for abused drugs with less
        toxic effects, and
6)   prevent the initiation of drug use."

CHAPTER 8:
AMPHETAMINE, METHAMPHETAMINE EPHEDRINE, AMINOREX, AMINO KETONES, AND SUBSTITUTED PHENYLISOPROPYLAMINES

Amphetamine is a central nervous system stimulant (Kefalas). It is used to increase alertness and as an anorexic. It is prescribed for exhaustion, narcolepsy and to hyperactive children. Amphetamine is also called phenylisopropylamine. It is active at 5 mg.

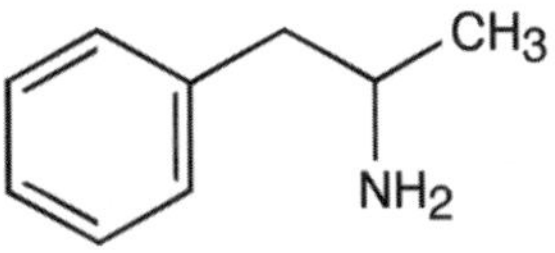

Amphetamine

Methamphetamine (N-methyl-amphetamine) is a more powerful central nervous system stimulant than amphetamine. Ethamphetamine (N-ethyl-amphetamine) is also a central nervous system stimulant. Its actions are less stimulating than that of amphetamine.

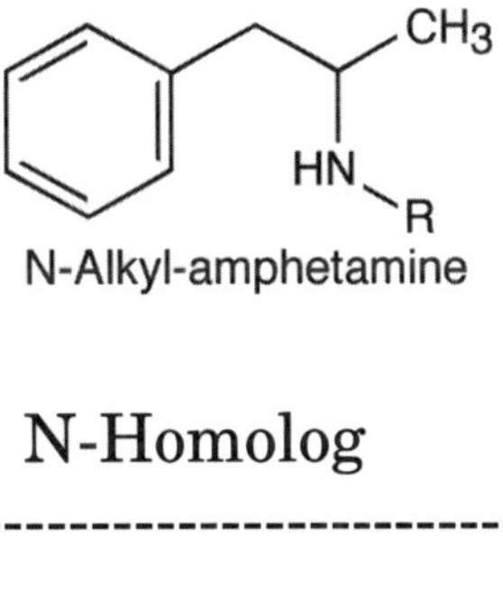

N-Alkyl-amphetamine

Chemical Name	R	N-Homolog
Amphetamine	R = H	
Methamphetamine	R = CH3	N-methyl
Ethamphetamine	R = CH2CH3	N-ethyl

MDA is the abbreviated name for a substituted amphetamine psychoactive called 3,4-methylenedioxy-amphetamine. It has been abbreviated as EA-1299 by the Edgewood Arsenal, U.S. Army Chemical Warfare Service. MDA is a stimulant empathogenic drug. The reported dosage

MDA

is between 50 to 200 mg. It produces mood elevation, bonding and empathy. The drug's actions last from 6 to 8 hours. MDA's actions are non-hallucinogenic in low dosages. This differs from most of the other substituted amphetamines which are hallucinogenic. L-MDA maintains self injection in monkeys (Beardsley 1986) (Lamb 1987).

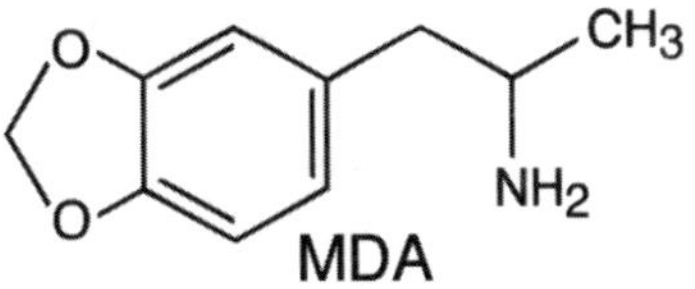

MDMA

3,4-Methylenedioxy-N-methylamphetmaine

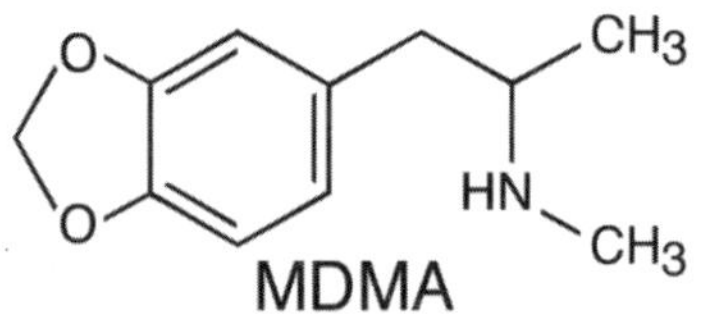

MDMA

MDMA is the abbreviation for 3,4-methylenedioxy-methamphetamine. It is the N-methyl homolog of MDA. It has been abbreviated in literature as MDMA, MDM and also EA-1475. The reported dosage for MDMA is between 50 to 250 mg. The average dosage is 125 mg. The drug's duration of action is 4 to 6 hours. It has less stimulating side effects compared to MDA. Both MDA and MDMA have been extensively used as adjuncts in psychotherapy (Bakalar 1990) (Greer 1983, 1986, 1990) (Naranjo 1967) (Smith 1985) (Turek 1974) (*Through The Gateway of the Heart* 1985) (Yensen 1976).

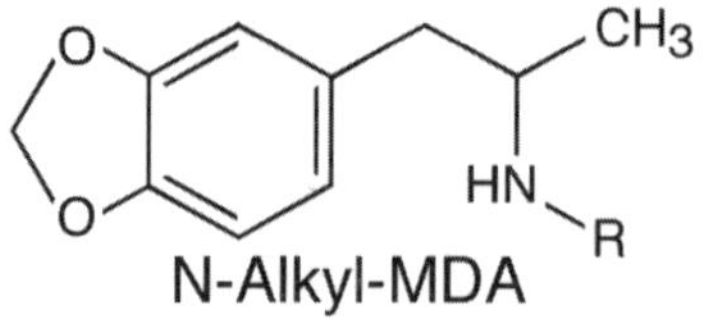

MDMA was patented in 1912 by E. Merck (Merck 1912). The Army Chemical Center performed toxicological and behavioral studies of this drug during the 1950's. The report was declassified in 1967 and published six years later. The N-ethyl homolog of MDA is called MDEA. N-hydroxy-MDA is also active.

N-Alkyl-MDA

3,4-Methylenedioxy-N-alkylamphetamines

Abbreviated Name   R =   Homolog =

Abbreviated Name	R =	Homolog =
MDA	R = H	
MDMA	R = CH3	N-methyl
MDEA	R = CH2CH3	N-ethyl
N-hydroxy-MDA	R = OH	N-hydroxy

MDMA Story

MDMA (3,4-methylenedioxymethamphetamine) is a stimulant and low-level hallucinogen. During the 1980s, growing recreational use began in Europe and spread to the United States. The Drug Enforcement Administration (DEA) controlled MDMA as a Schedule I drug on the Controlled Substances List in 1985 and the MDMA precursor chemicals safrole, isosafrole, and piperonal as List I regulated chemicals in 1990. While the number of domestic MDMA laboratories has remained relatively low, traffickers in Western Europe—primarily in the Benelux countries of Belgium, the Netherlands, and Luxembourg—greatly increased production throughout the 1990s. In the Benelux countries, drug trafficking organizations (DTOs) have easy access to precursor chemicals and multimodal commercial transportation hubs to transport the MDMA to consumer countries. Seizure statistics indicate that the amount of MDMA smuggled into the United States has greatly increased through the 1990s and that the amount of MDMA smuggled in individual shipments has been increasing within the past year.

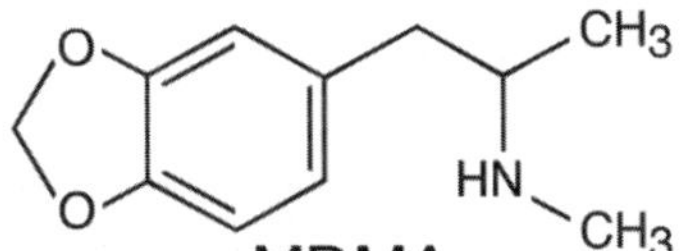

Since the mid-1990s, Israeli and Russian DTOs have dominated the importation of MDMA into the United States. The strength of these DTOs rests largely in organizational discipline and access to European commercial transportation hubs; the small number of dogs trained to detect MDMA at airports also gives them an advantage. Israeli and Russian DTOs rely on express mail services, couriers, and sea containers to smuggle MDMA from Europe to the United States.

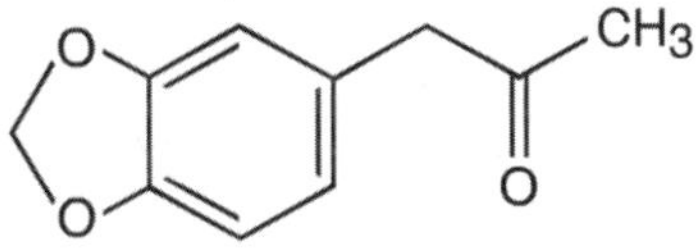

Production

MDMA production is more complicated than methamphetamine production when the laboratory operators use safrole, isosafrole, or piperonal as starting methods. Although safrole (the primary constituent of sassafras oil), isosafrole, and piperonal are the three primary MDMA precursor chemicals, many production groups are able to acquire MDP2P (3,4-methylenedioxyphenyl-2-propanone), and produce MDMA in a simple conversion process rather than starting the process with one of the precursor chemicals.

MDMA Precursor Chemicals

Precursor Chemical	Hazards	Form	Process	Comments
Safrole			Purification requires acetic acid and ethanol	Many MDMA production groups begin the process with safrole, an extract from sassafras oil
acetic acid	Corrosive to tissue	Liquid		
ethanol	Flammable, toxic	Liquid		
Isosafrole			Isomerized from safrole using strong bases such as potassium hydroxide and calcium oxide	Used to wash away impurities
potassium hydroxide	Caustic	Solid or liquid		
calcium oxide	Caustic	Solid		
10% hydrochloric acid (muriatic acid)	Corrosive	Liquid		
Piperonal		Powder or liquid	Conversion of piperonal to 3,4 MDP2P and then to MDMA (does not use any form of safrole)	Yield will be around 50% pure
Bromosafrole	Flammable, toxic	liquid		
Safrole	Corrosive	Liquid		
66% hydrobromic acid	Corrosive	Liquid		
sulfuric acid	Corrosive	Liquid		
DMSO	Readily absorbed	Liquid		
MDP2P			Conversion of safrole to MDP2P using sulfuric acid, sodium hydroxide, and solvents; conversion from isosafrole using hydrogen peroxide and formic acid results in reduced yields	Most common route for production of MDMA; palladium bromide catalyst method results in higher yields
sulfuric acid	Corrosive	Liquid		
sodium hydroxide	Caustic (lye)	Liquid or solid		
dichloromethane	Flammable, toxic, carcinogen (solvent)	Liquid		

Note: MDMA can be made with any of the precursor chemicals listed in the Precursor Chemicals column. The essential chemicals listed under each precursor often are used with that precursor chemical in the cooking process. Source: NDIC, DEA, USCS

MDP2P is a commercial product made overseas and imported for use by the flavoring and fragrance industry. Groups that produce MDMA by starting with MDP2P considerably reduce production time and complexity. Although there are more than 20 chemical recipes for MDMA production, clandestine laboratory operators commonly use only seven methods. Six of the seven common methods use either safrole or isosafrole; one uses piperonal. In the methods using safrole or isosafrole, the cook usually produces MDP2P which is then converted into the final product, MDMA. When using piperonal, an intermediate product is initially produced that is then converted into MDP2P; this is then converted into MDMA.

In a successful production process, the resulting MDMA is a nearly 100 percent pure powder with a distinctive licorice scent. The powder is pressed into pills with identifying designs or symbols. DEA estimates that over 90 percent of all MDMA smuggled into the United States is in capsule or pill form; the remainder is in powder form. MDMA powder is pressed into tablets that contain adulterants, diluents, and approximately 100 milligrams of MDMA. Although presses vary greatly in speed and quality, the best are capable of processing as much as 50 kilograms of MDMA powder into 500,000 tablets per hour. As the pills or powder dry, the odor of the solvents used in the production process diminishes to a slightly sweet scent. According to DEA's Special Testing and Research Laboratory, the chemicals and equipment necessary to produce a single kilogram of MDMA can be purchased for as little as $500, depending on the method used and the fluctuating prices of illegally diverted precursor chemicals.

DEA Special Agents in the Netherlands and Germany report that most MDMA production organizations are able to produce MDMA for as little as 20–25 cents per pill. These pills are then sold to a wholesale group for approximately $1 to $2 per pill. Throughout the 1990s, production of MDMA in the United States remained relatively low according to the DEA, while production groups in many other countries greatly increased their output. Although clandestine laboratories have been seized in Africa, Asia, North America, and South America, Western Europe is now recognized as the primary source of the world's MDMA. Driven primarily by the availability of precursor and essential chemicals and international multi-modal commercial transportation hubs, most of the large, well-organized MDMA production groups have established operations in rural regions of the Benelux countries— Belgium, the Netherlands, and Luxembourg.

During most of the 1980s, illicit domestic production of MDMA was able to meet the low demand of the U.S. user population. As the drug gained in popularity in the late 1980s and the number of domestic MDMA laboratories increased, the United States regulated MDMA's primary precursor chemicals, safrole, isosafrole, and piperonal as List I regulated chemicals in 1990, making it illegal to purchase or possess these chemicals without a permit. After the regulation of these precursors, the number of laboratory seizures dropped to approximately 10–12 each year throughout the 1990s. Although most of the domestic laboratories seized were relatively small, some were capable of significant production.

For example, one laboratory seized in Westport, Massachusetts, in 1998 could have produced up to 25 pounds of MDMA with the amount of chemicals seized. In addition, an MDMA laboratory seized in October 1999 outside Vancouver, British Columbia, was the largest MDMA laboratory ever seized in North America, which raised concerns by Canadian authorities regarding a possible increase in MDMA production in Canada.

Clandestine laboratories in rural areas of the Netherlands and Belgium now produce approximately 80 percent of the MDMA consumed worldwide, according to DEA estimates. Laboratories are also located in Australia, Canada, Germany, Luxembourg, and Eastern European countries such as the Czech Republic, Hungary, Latvia, and Poland. The Benelux region is attractive to clandestine drug manufacturers and has become the center of MDMA production largely because of well-established precursor chemical routes and easy access to international air and rail transportation hubs. According to the DEA Office of Diversion Control, the most common MDMA precursor chemicals—safrole, isosafrole, MDP2P, and piperonal—are produced in China, India, Poland, and Germany.

DEA case information shows that in the late 1980s methamphetamine production organizations established ephedrine smuggling routes to move bulk shipments of ephedrine from chemical plants in China, India, Poland, and Germany through the Netherlands and on to North America. Those established chemical supply routes through the Netherlands were still in use as recently as 1996, when MDMA production in the Netherlands was rapidly increasing. Today, MDMA production groups may be capitalizing on those existing chemical supply routes to move MDMA precursor chemicals from China, India, Poland, and Germany into the Netherlands.

MDMA production groups supplying users throughout Europe, Canada, and the United States are most effective in areas that offer high-volume commercial transportation to major market areas. The Netherlands and Belgium, because of their multiple air, sea, and rail connections to countries throughout Europe and to the United States, are ideal locations for moving MDMA to markets.

DTOs (Drug Trafficking Organization) in countries other than the Benelux countries now appear to be developing an MDMA production capability. Analysts and Special Agents at DEA's Special Operations Division who watch for emerging trends in MDMA production warn that recent, first-time MDMA laboratory seizures in China and Colombia and methamphetamine production in Mexico during the 1990s mark traffickers in these countries as potential sources of supply. In contrast to some other countries where MDMA laboratories have been discovered, China, Colombia, and Mexico offer advantages similar to those of the Netherlands and Belgium: access to international multimodal (air, sea, and rail) transportation and established precursor chemical supplies. If DTOs exploit these advantages, the production dominance of traffickers in Belgium and the Netherlands could be challenged.

As MDMA popularity increased in the 1990s, a distinctive division of labor evolved. Groups have specialized in acquiring precursor chemicals, producing MDMA powder, pressing powder into pills, or smuggling MDMA into consumer countries. It appears that no single organization currently controls all aspects of production, wholesale, midlevel wholesale, or retail sales. Today, the wholesale groups smuggling MDMA into the United States usually pass the pills on to separate midlevel wholesale distribution groups that in turn pass them to retail-level distributors.   Source: NDIC October 2000

MDMA use can sometimes result in severe dehydration or exhaustion, or other adverse effects such as nausea, hallucinations, chills, sweating, increases in body temperature, tremors, involuntary teeth clenching, muscle cramping, and blurred vision.

MDMA users have also reported after-effects such as anxiety, paranoia, and depression. An MDMA overdose is characterized by high blood pressure, faintness, panic attacks, and, in more severe cases, loss of consciousness, seizures, and a drastic rise in body temperatures to 105-106 degrees Fahrenheit. MDMA overdoses can be fatal, as they may result in heart failure or extreme heat stroke.

MDMA is manufactured clandestinely in western Europe, primarily in The Netherlands and Belgium, which produce 90% of the MDMA consumed worldwide. A typical clandestine laboratory is capable of producing 20 - 30 kilograms of MDMA per day, with one kilogram of MDMA consisting of approximately 3,500 tablets. Dutch Police reported the seizure of one laboratory capable of producing approximately 100 kilograms (350,000 tablets) of MDMA per day.

Drug Abuse Warning Network (DAWN) estimates reveal that nationwide hospital emergency room mentions for MDMA rose dramatically from 1,143 in 1998 to 2,850 in 1999 and 4,511 in 2000. Seizures of MDMA have also increased drastically. Seizures of MDMA tablets submitted to DEA laboratories have risen from a total of 1,054,973 in 1999 to 3,045,041 in 2000. DEA arrests for MDMA violations also increased from 681 in 1999 to 1,456 in 2000.Similarly, the number of DEA initiated cases targeting MDMA violators increased from 278 in 1999 to 670 in 2000. Source: Joseph D. Keefe Chief of Operations DEA Before the Senate Governmental Affairs Committee Date: July 30, 2001

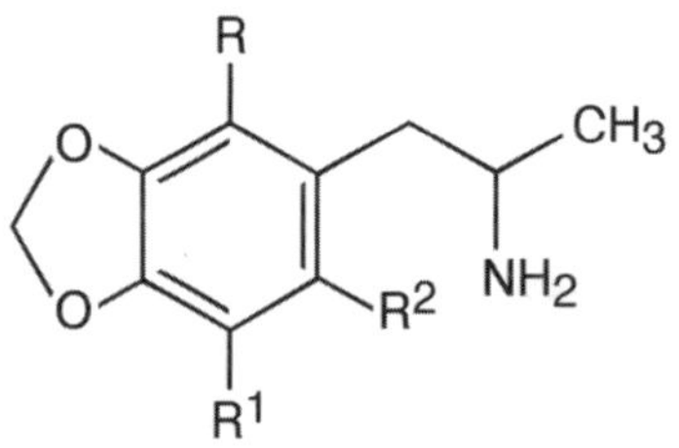

Substituted-3,4-methylenedioxyamphetamines

Abbreviated Name	R =	R1 =	R2 =
DMMDA	CH3O	CH3O	H
DMMDA - 2	H	CH3O	CH3O
MMDA - 2	H	H	CH3O
MMDA - 3a	CH3O	H	H
MMDA	H	CH3O	H

2,5-Dimethoxy-3,4-methylenedioxyamphetamine is active in humans, at 30 to 75 mg. (abbreviated: DMMDA).

2,3-Dimethoxy-4,5-methylenedioxyamphetamine is active in humans, at 50 mg. (abbreviated: DMMDA-2).

2-Methoxy-4,5-methylenedioxyamphetamine is active at 25 to 50 mg. in humans (abbreviated: MMDA-2).

2-Methoxy-3,4-methylenedioxyamphetamine is active at 20 to 80 mg. in humans (abbreviated: MMDA-3a).

3-Methoxy-4,5-methylenedioxyamphetamine is active at 100 to 250 mg. in humans (abbreviated: MMDA). These substances produce euphoria, bonding, mood elevation and empathy (Shulgin 1967).

Amphetamine, methamphetamine, MDA, MDMA, *p*-chloro-amphetamine, *p*-chloromethamphetamine and fenfluramine are all neurotoxic to serotonin axons in laboratory animals (Costa 1971) (Ricaurte 1989). Methamphetamine causes long lasting dopamine nerve terminal and nerve fiber destruction in rat brains. Pretreatment or post treatment with fluoxetine blocks neurotoxicity to serotonin axions (Battaglia 1988a) (Schmidt 1987). GABA-transaminase inhibitors also block neurotoxicity (Stone 1987).

The 2,4,5-substituted amphetamines possess powerful psychoactivity. 2,4,5-Trimethoxy-amphetamine (abbreviated TMA-2) is hallucinogenic at a reported dosage of approximately 20 mg. in humans. 4-Ethoxy-2,5-dimethoxyamphetamine is called MEM. Its effects are empathogenic.

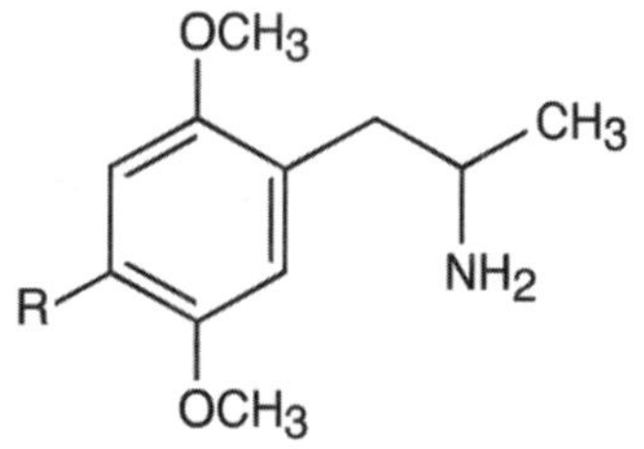

DOM is the abbreviation for a long acting hallucinogen called 4-methyl-2,5-dimethoxyamphetamine. It does not cause self-injection reinforcement behavior in monkeys (Hoffmeister 1975). The primary effects of DOET are MDA like. 2,5-DMA (see literature) is not psychoactive in both humans and in rats.

4-Substituted-2,5-dimethoxyamphetamines

Abbreviated Name   R =   Tested Human Dosage

Abbreviated Name	R =	Tested Human Dosage
2,5-DMA	R = H	80 to 160 mg.
TMA-2	R = OCH3	20 to 40 mg.
MEM	R = OCH2CH3	20 to 50 mg.
DOM	R = CH3	3 to 10 mg.
DOET	R = CH2CH3	2 to 6 mg.
DOI	R = Iodine	1.5 to 3 mg.

4-Bromo-2,5-dimethoxyphenylalkylamines

4-Bromo-2,5-dimethoxyphenylethylamine (abbreviated names are 2C-B and also described as alpha-des methyl DOB) has an approx. dosage of 10 mg. in humans. It has an empathogenic effect in humans.

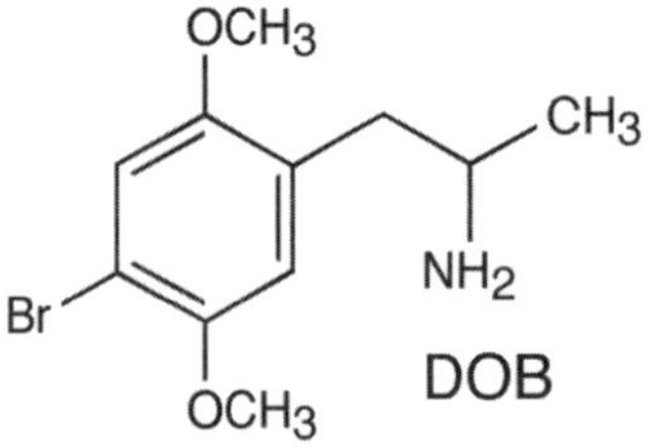

4-Bromo-2,5-dimethoxy-amphetamine (abbreviated as DOB) has a reported dosage of 0.5 to 1.0 mg. in humans. It has an empathogenic effect in humans.

4-Bromo-2,5-dimethoxy-N-methyl-amphetamine has a reported dosage of approximately 5 to 10 mgs in humans. It is also empathogenic.

4-Bromo-2,5-dimethoxy-N-ethyl-amphetamine may also be active.

4-Bromo-2,5-dimethoxy-N,N-dimethylamphetamine is inactive in humans.

The primary action of 4-bromo and 4-chloro 2,5-dimethoxy-phenylalkylamines is described as MDA like. The effects of DOB are long acting, six to twelve hours. Restlessness is the major side effect. At low dosages they produce euphoria, mood elevation and empathy (empathogenic). References: (Baltzly 1940a, 1940b, 1950) (Barfknecht 1971, 1978) (Knoll 1970).

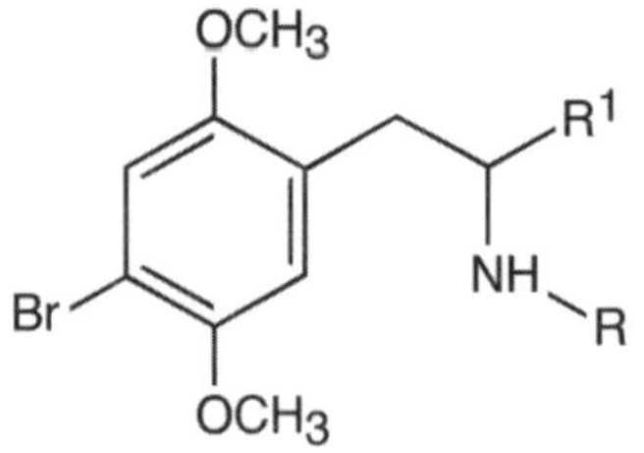

4-Bromo-2,5-Dimethoxy
Substituted N-Alkylphenylalkylamines

Abbreviated Name	R=	R1=
2C-B	R = H	R1= H
DOB	R = H	R1= CH3
N-Methyl-DOB	R = CH3	R1= CH3

ortho-Methoxy-N-methylamphetamine is called methoxy-phenamine. Methoxyphenamine is used as a vasopressor.

para-Chloroamphetamine and *para*-chloro-N-methyl-amphet-amine are both neurotoxic to serotonin axons, reduce both serotonin in the brain and 5-hydroxy-indole acetic acid in spinal fluid. They are used in research.

para-Chloro and *para*-bromomethamphetamine have been reported to be anorexic without an increase in motor activity (Kefalas 1962). *meta*-Trifluoro-N-ethylamphetamine is called fenfluramine. It is used as an anorexic (Beregi 1970). It is neurotoxic. It does not cause significant self-injection reinforcement in monkeys. Fenfluramine (Primetime Live 5/8/96) has been linked to primary pulmonary hypertension (incurable) causing death within 3 years. Fenfluramine was taken off the market (FDA) as it causes serious heart disease in approximately one in three patients (news sources).

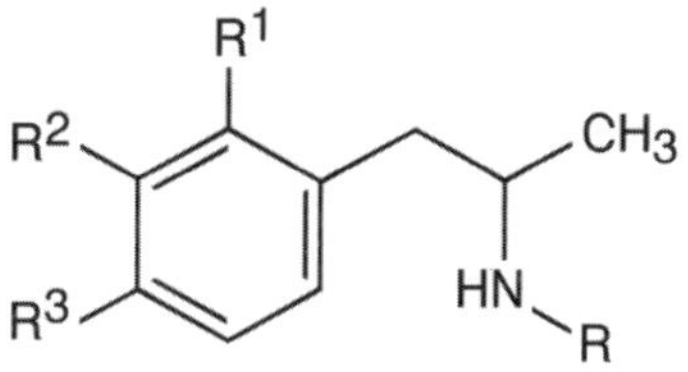

The effects of *para*-methoxy-N-methyl-amphetamine, in rats, are unlike DOM and amphetamine.

Amphetamine	R	R1	R2	R3
o-Methoxy	H	OCH3	H	H
p-Methoxy	H	H	H	OCII3
p-Methoxy-N-methyl	CH3	H	H	OCH3
p-Methoxy-N-ethyl	CH2CH3	H	H	OCH3
p-Methoxy-N-hydroxy	OH	H	H	OCH3
p-Chloro	H	H	H	Cl
p-Chloro-N-methyl	CH3	H	H	Cl
m-Trifluoro-N-ethyl	CH2CH3	H	CF3	H

On PMA: *"Extraordinarily sensual, it enhanced physical experience so that whatever turned you on - dancing, bathing, dressing up in silks and satins - gave you almost orgasmic pleasure. Making love on PMA gave you orgasms that were out of this world,"* Angela Bowie

"The initial effects of a low dose of PMA might feel a little bit like MDMA, but PMA takes more than half an hour longer to come on. This may cause some people to take another pill thinking that they got "weak Ecstasy." By this time the person may have taken a lethal dose," Dancesafe.org

PMA

para-Methoxyamphetamine (PMA), also known as 4-methoxy-amphetamine, is an illicit, synthetic hallucinogen that has stimulant effects similar to other clandestinely manufactured amphetamine derivatives like MDMA (Ecstasy). Until recently, illicit abuse of PMA was briefly encountered during the early 1970s in the United States and Canada. However, since February 2000, PMA has re-emerged in Florida, Illinois, Michigan, Virginia, and Canada. Moreover, since May 2000, PMA ingestion has been associated with three deaths in Chicago, Illinois, and seven deaths in central Florida.

Effects: PMA is a potent and potentially lethal synthetic hallucinogen, which was placed into Schedule I of the Controlled Substances Act in 1973. The drug has been sold in tablet, capsule, and powder form, and its appearance and cost are comparable to MDMA. Common street names for PMA are "Death" and "Mitsubishi Double-Stack."

The effects associated with PMA vary depending on the dose and whether other drugs are present. PMA typically is administered orally in pill or capsule form. PMA powder, although uncommon, may be inhaled or injected to accelerate the response. Ingesting a dose of less than 50 milligrams–usually one pill or capsule–without other drugs or alcohol, induces symptoms reminiscent of MDMA. Such effects include increased pulse rate and blood pressure, increased and labored respiration, elevated body temperature, erratic eye movements, muscle spasms, nausea, and heightened visual stimulation.

Doses over 50 milligrams are considered potentially lethal, especially when taken with other drugs, such as amphetamine derivatives, cannabis, cocaine, prescription medications like fluoxetine (Prozac), and alcohol. Higher doses can produce cardiac arrhythmia and arrest, breathing problems, pulmonary congestion, renal failure, hyperthermia, vomiting, convulsions, coma, and death.

Abuse/Availability

In 1973, PMA was produced by clandestine laboratory facilities in Canada. PMA manufactured by these operations appeared in limited areas of Canada and the United States. During that time, three deaths were suspected and two deaths were determined to be associated with PMA abuse in the United States. Eight deaths in Canada were attributed to PMA abuse. Federal, state, and local forensic laboratories in Georgia, Kansas, Missouri, and the Centre of Forensic Science in Toronto, Canada, confirmed that PMA contributed to those deaths.

From 1974 to early 2000, no deaths attributed to PMA abuse were reported in Canada or the United States. Since May 2000, however, three deaths in the cities of Lisle, McHenry, and Naperville, Illinois, and seven deaths in central Florida were associated with PMA ingestion.

Since mid-2000, PMA also has been associated with four deaths in Europe. Austria, Denmark, and Germany reported that the victims died after consuming what they believed to be Ecstasy, but was later identified as PMA. In 1994, the use of PMA emerged in isolated areas of the Australian drug-abusing population. Currently, the drug is still available illicitly in Australia at nightclubs and rave parties where it is generally sold as MDMA. In fact, dealers and purchasers may be unaware that they are selling or buying PMA. Since PMA appeared in 1994 it has been associated with approximately 12 deaths there. Forensic science centers in Australia confirmed that most of the overdose victims ingested toxic amounts of PMA.

PMA Production

Currently, PMA is produced legally in the United States for limited commercial applications. A small quantity also is allocated for Schedule I scientific research. The illicit form of PMA is produced in clandestine laboratories. Although PMA can be manufactured by several methods, the method used depends largely upon the availability of certain precursors. The exact synthesis procedure recently used to manufacture the PMA found in Florida, Illinois, Michigan, Virginia, and Canada is still unknown. Contrary to initial newspaper reports from Australia, the likelihood that PMA is inadvertently produced during the manufacture of MDMA is highly unlikely. To date, four clandestine PMA laboratories have been seized worldwide: in Toronto, Canada, in 1973; in Worms, Germany, in 1991; and, in 1999, two laboratories in northern Germany, one located in Brandenburg.

PMA: Cause for Concern: The increasing popularity associated with designer drugs increases the risk that users may inadvertently ingest substances such as PMA, which is similar in appearance to MDMA but is more toxic. The continued presence of PMA in Australia and the recent appearance in Canada, Europe, and the United States are causes for concern that PMA will be associated with additional overdoses and deaths. The DEA is actively conducting investigations in order to identify the source of production and distribution networks.

Source: DEA; Intelligence Division; Office of Diversion Control, Drug and Chemical Evaluation Section; October 2000

Ephedrine Alkaloids

Ephedrine alkaloids are used throughout the world for their symptomatic actions. They have a wide variety of actions depending on their molecular structure and various substitutions. These molecules possess nasal decongestant, vasopressor (increase blood pressure), anorexic (appetite suppressant) and CNS (central nervous system) actions such as CNS stimulation (Chen 1929).

The Chinese herb Ma Hung (*Ephedra vulgaris*, *Ephedra sinica*, *Ephedra equisetina*) has been used for thousands of years as a symptomatic in China. It is the first natural source in which ephedrines were discovered. In 1887, a Japanese chemist by the name of Nagai isolated ephedrine from Ma Hung. Several isomers and analogs have been extracted from Ephedra species (Kanao 1927; 1930) (Nagai 1928). Ephedrine also occurs in the leaves of yew (Taxus baccata), in *Roemeria refracta* D.C. *papaveracoe* and also *Aconitum napellus*.

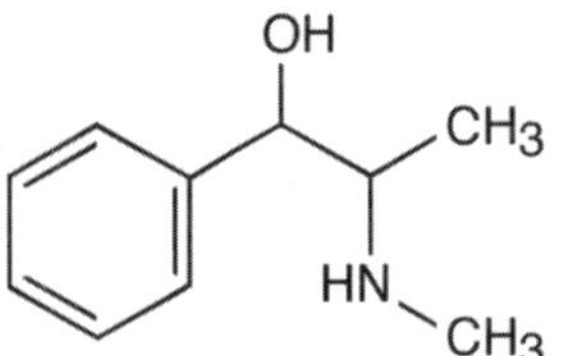

Many isomers (e.g. pseudoephedrine), homologs and analogs of ephedrine occur naturally as trace alkaloids in plants. These materials are produced synthetically (Manske 1929) (Wilbert) because it is more economical than extraction from natural sources. Pseudoephedrine is used as a nasal decongestant (Besson 1936). Pseudoephedrine may cause birth defects (gastroschisis) if taken by pregnant women during their first trimester (Fackelmann 1995).

Racemic phenylpropanolamine is also called *dl*-nor-ephedrine. Phenylpropanolamine was taken off the market as it caused strokes in some individuals. When taking any ephedrine type medication, it is best only to take a very small dosage (eg. quarter tablet) to check for sensitivity as some people are very sensitive (eg. causes weakness, lethargy).

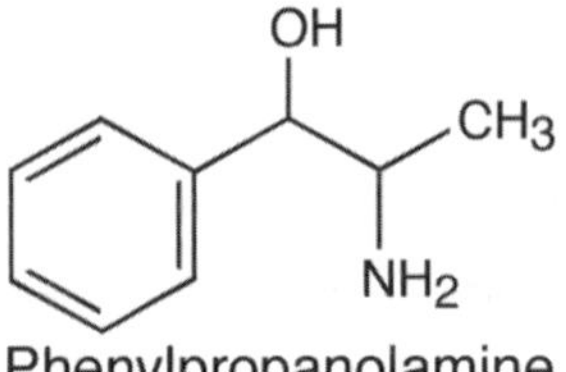

Ephedrine alkaloids are relatively safe when used in accordance with dosage guide lines for short periods. Individuals with heart conditions, liver disorders or kidney disorders should not take these materials (Wilbert).

Cathine

Cathine, also called kathine (*d*-nor-pseudo-ephedrine), occurs (0.1 %) in the Arabian plant, *Catha edulis* (Alles 1961). The leaves of this plant have been used (chewed for its stimulating affect) for thousands of years by the Arabs (Brucke 1941). Kathine has been identified in a South American tree called *Maytenus krukovii*. *d,l*-Norpseudo-ephedrine is used as an anorexic and CNS stimulant (Hofmann 1955; 1/6th as potent as *d,l*-amphetamine) (Horst-Myer 1959) (Kanao 1928). The dextro isomer has 6 times the stimulant action of the levo isomer (Hofmann 1955). Kathine is also an isomer of phenylpropanolamine.

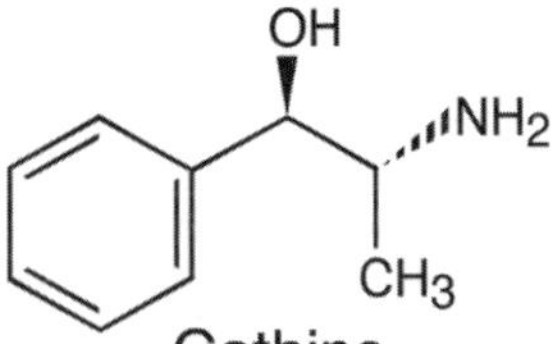

3,4-Methylenedioxy-norpseudoephedrine

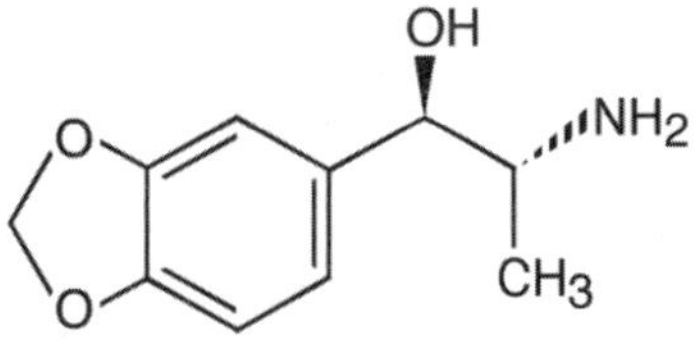

3,4,5-Trimethoxy-norpseudoephedrine

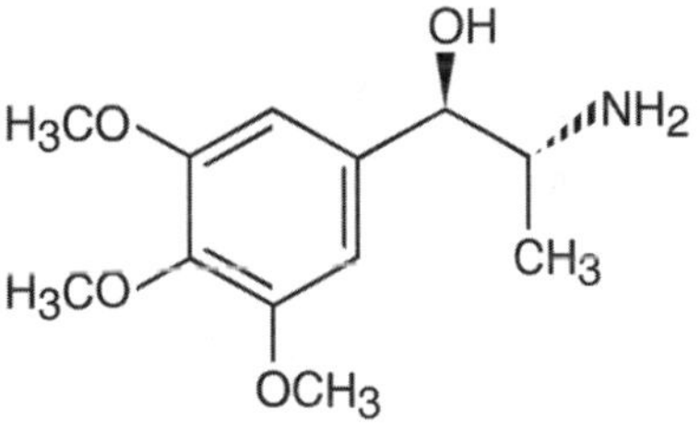

Methoxamine is the generic name for 2,5-dimethoxy-phenylpropanolamine. It is used as a vasopressor (Morishita 1961).

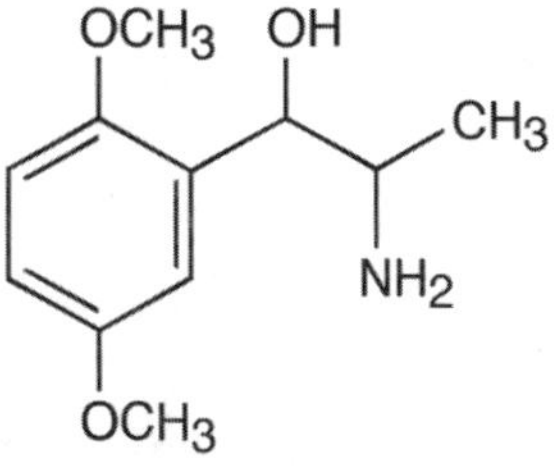

p-Chloro-norephedrine has been reported not to be neurotoxic (Smith, 1974). In preclinical reinforcement studies, phenyl-propanolamine was not self administered by baboons.

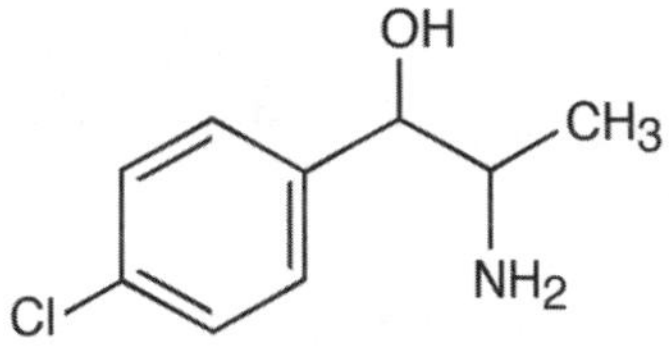

Aminoketones

Cathinone

(S)-2-Amino-1-phenyl-1-propanone also called Cathinone, occurs in the Arabian plant, *Catha edulis* (Peterson 1980). The leaves are chewed for recreation and anti-fatigue properties (Nencini 1986). Cathinone has been found to have anorexic and stimulating effects in humans. It is equal in potency to amphetamine (Glennon 1987). It is prepared by the oxidation of phenylpropanolamine (Parke 1957).

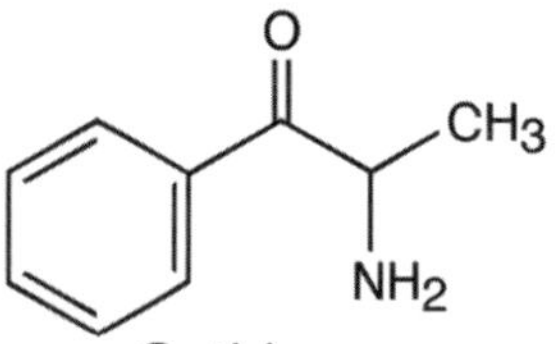

Cathinone

Methcathinone

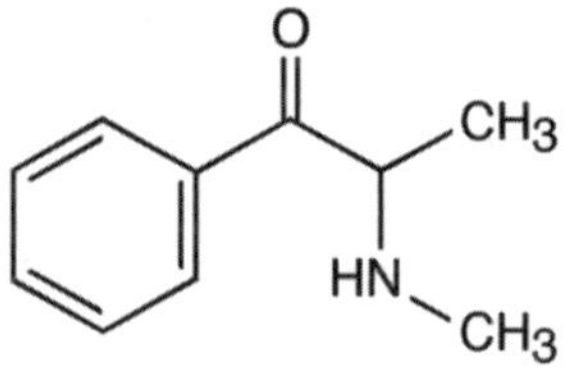

2-Methamino-1-phenyl-propanone (ephedrone) is a molecule that has not been tested in human subjects, but appears to be a psycho-stimulant in animal testing. It is a drug of abuse in USA, Russia, the Ukraine, and Europe. It maybe neurotoxic. Ephedrone is a homolog of 2-(dimethylamino)propiophenone. References: (Goldstone 1993) (Young 1993) (Zingel 1991)

Ethcathinone

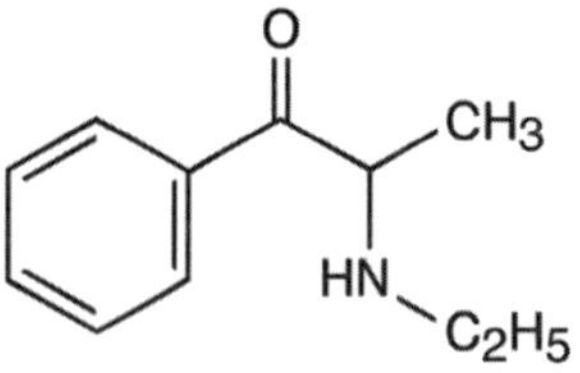

No studies have been conducted on cathinone, methcathinone, ethcathinone in the treatment of hyperkinetic children, narcoleptics, or the obese.

2,5-Dimethoxycathinone

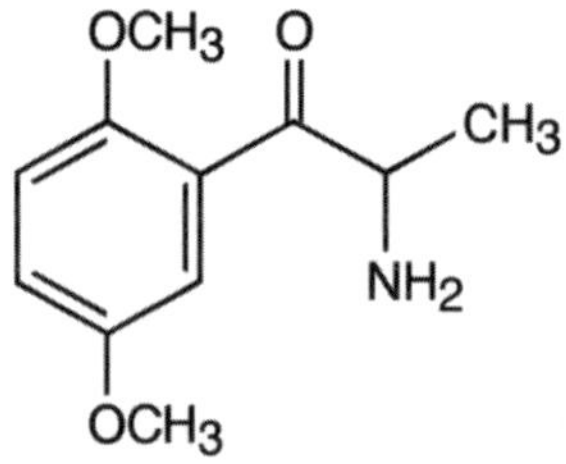

2,5-Dimethoxy-cathinone is a peripheral blood-vessel contractor (Morishita 1961).

Phentermine

Phentermine is an anorexic drug used for weight reduction in the obese and in attention deficit disorder.   It is marketed in 30 mg. tablets/capsules for use. It is available in most night clubs and high schools throughout the nation.

3,4-Methylenedioxy-phentermine

In the exploration of potential non-neurotoxic entactogenic medications, this drug was tested and found not to be active (Nichols 1989).

3,4,-Methylenedioxy-N-methyl-phentermine

In the exploration of potential non-neurotoxic entactogenic medications, this drug was tested and found not to be active (Nichols 1989).

3,4,5-Trimethoxy-phentermine

3,4,5-Trimethoxy-N-methyl-phentermine

2-Amino-5-aryloxazolines

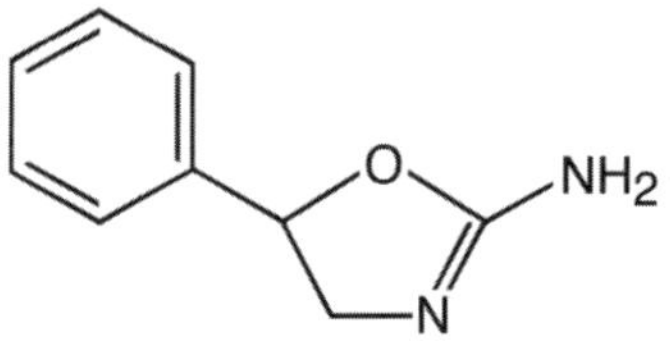

Aminorex

Aminorex is a potent anorexic psychostimulant.

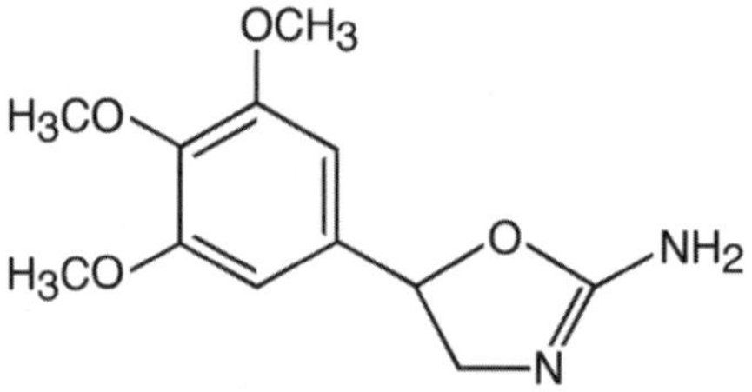

3,4,5-Trimethoxy-aminorex

2-amino-5-(3,4,5,-trimethoxyphenyl)oxazoline

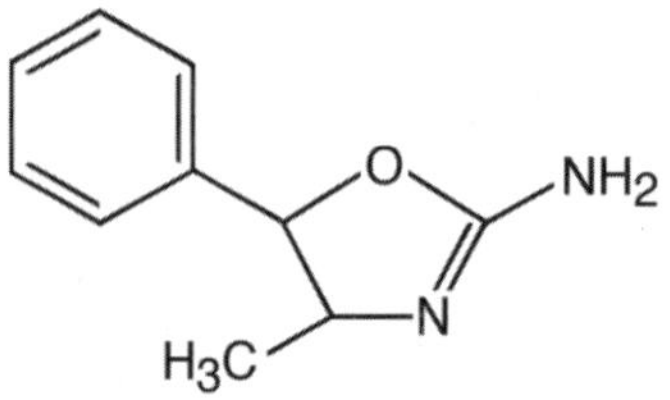

4-Methylaminorex

4-Methylaminorex is a powerful psychostimulant and anorexic. The reported dosage is 5mg. to 20mg.; duration 12 to 16 hours.

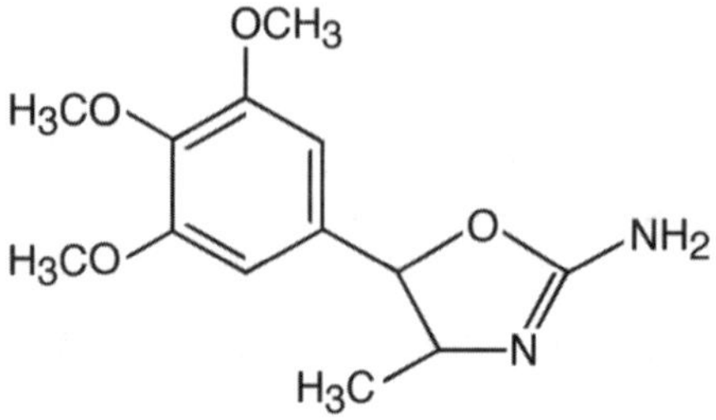

3,4,5-Trimethoxy-(4-methyl-aminorex)

2-amino-4-methyl-5-(3,4,5,-trimethoxyphenyl)oxazoline

CHAPTER 9: REDUCTIONS USING METALS

Reductions (also called hydrogenations) can be dangerous. Chemists have been injured in explosions from mishanding a chemical. Explosions resulting from the use of powerful reducing agents (eg. contacting water) have involved the use of, but not limited to, reducing agents such as lithium aluminum hydride, sodium borohydride, sodium, potassium, etc. Hydrogen gas is evolved during reductions. Appropriate precautions must be taken (e.g. ventilation with a sparkless fan) to avoid explosion as hydrogen gas is flammable.

"*Activated aluminum is aluminum which has been superficially amalgamated with mercury. When it contacts with water, it liberates hydrogen and an insoluble aluminum hydroxide is formed. Activated aluminum thus serves as the source of hydrogen for the reaction,*" Gustav Hildebrandt.

Aluminum amalgam is a commonly used reducing agent because of its availability, low cost and ease of preparation. It can be produced on location which alleviates the hazard of storing the reducing agent. Keep in mind that the decanted aluminum amalgam may be pyrophoric!

Allen and Cantrell did an excellent review of reductions used in clandestine laboratories, see (Allen 1989).

Preparatation of Aluminum Amalgam
by Chinoin Gyogyszer

3.5 grams of fine aluminum shavings are washed with ethanol, and 1 gram of mercuric chloride and 30 mL. of an aqueous solution of 15 grams of sodium chloride are added. The mixture is warmed and gas evolution occurs. 6 - 8 minutes later the solution is decanted and the aluminum shavings are washed with water. Source: (Gyogyszer 1963)

Preparation of Aluminum Amalgam from Foil

20 grams of aluminum foil are sliced into 0.5 x 0.5 inch squares and washed with naphtha (lighter fluid) to degrease the metal. The metal is then covered with 2% sodium hydroxide solution. When the hydrogen evolution sets in, the solution is decanted from the metal, washed quickly and repeatedly with water. 150 mL. of a 0.5% solution of mercuric bichloride is poured on the metal and allowed to sit for 2 minutes. At this time the metal is quickly washed several times with water and 95% alcohol. References: Augustine (1968) in *Reductions*.

Journal of Organic Chemistry (1946) 11: 823

Aluminum Amalgam Preparation
by Robert G Briody and Ephraim A. Cuevas

As shown in the Figure, a pool of mercury 2 is located in the bottom of a flask 1, which is surrounded in its lower half by an electric

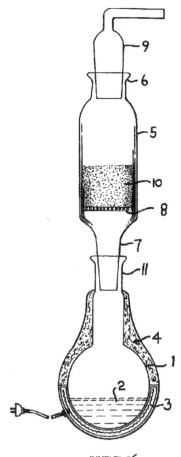

INVENTORS

ROBERT G. BRIODY
EPHRAIM A. CUEVAS

heating mantle 3. The flask is insulated on he upper portion of the bottom with glass wool 4 to a point slightly below the neck of the flask. The reaction vessel 5 is fitted with a fritted glass disc 8 and a bed of aluminum particles 10 placed on the fritted glass disc. The reaction chamber 5 is provided with a tapered end 7 open at the bottom and a neck member 6. The tapered end section 7 is inserted in the neck of the flask 1. A glass elution tube 9 is placed in the upper neck 6 of reaction vessel 5 and is connected to a vacuum pump and cold trap (not shown).

In the operation of the above device, the hating mantle is plugged into an appropriate socket and heated to a temperature sufficient to cause vaporization of the mercury 2 contained in the bottom of flask 1. As the mercury evaporates, it pumps up through the fritted glass disc 8 and the bed 10 of aluminum particles contained in the reaction vessel 5. Excess mercury vapors are removed via line 9 to the cold trap and are collected at that point. When a sufficient period of time has passed to produce saturation of the aluminum powders contained in the bed 10, the heating mantle is disconnected. The aluminum powders are then removed, washed with methanol and the aluminum amalgam analyzed for mercury content.

Fifty grams of aluminum powder was placed on the fritted glass disk of a reactor such as that depicted in the drawing. Reactor vessel 5 consisted of a 5-inch high glass reactor. A 250 millimeter round bottom flask containing a pool of mercury about half full was connected to the reaction vessel. At the top of the reactor, tube 9 led to a trap connected to a vacuum pump. The pump was maintaining 674 millimeters of mercury continuous vacuum on the reaction system. The mercury was heated in the bottom of the flask until it refluxed at temperature of approximately 250° C. The mercury vapors rose through the bed of particles and condensed above the aluminum powder. After 12 hours of constant vaporization of the mercury, the reactor was cooled and three samples of the powder were removed in a nitrogen atmosphere for analysis of the mercury content. After the analyses of the particles was completed, the remainder of the sample was recombined an slurried with methanol in a separtory funnel. This allowed the removal of any free liquid mercury which collected at the bottom. The powder was then filtered, dried and reanalyzed in the duplicate. A second batch of aluminum powder was treated in the same equipment and at about 155° C. and with a vacuum of 649 millimeters of mercury maintained on the reaction zone for 12 hours. The free mercury was removed this time using a benzene slurry, after which the powder was filtered and dried. Separate mercury analyses were made on riffled portions of the powder. A portion of the product was examined through a microscope and compared with the starting material. All handling and sampling of the powders before and after treatment with the mercury was done in a nitrogen atmosphere. Source: Briody 1971

Reduction of P-2-P Using Amalgamated Aluminum Turnings
by Gustav Hildebrandt

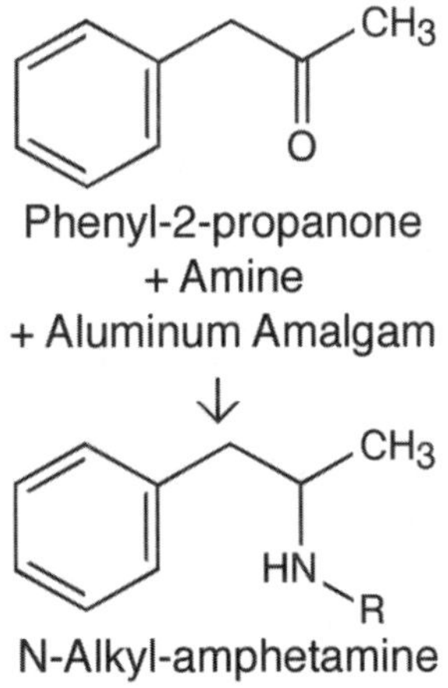

Phenyl-2-propanone
+ Amine
+ Aluminum Amalgam

N-Alkyl-amphetamine

0.2 moles of methyl-benzylketone, 350 ccs. of 85% alcohol, 30 grams of activated aluminum tunings and 40 ccs. of 40% aqueous methylamine solution are refluxed for 16 hours. After separating from aluminum sludge and washing with alcohol, the solution is acidified with hydrochloric acid and evaporated to dryness....

Yield 30.6 grams: 93% theory.

Source: Hildebrandt 1939 Ref.: Gyogyszer 1963, Wassink 1971

Starting Molecules: *p*-Methoxyphenyl-2-propanone & ammonia
Product: *p*-Methoxyamphetamine   Reference: (Fusco 1948)

Starting Molecules: *p*-Methoxyphenyl-2-propanone & methylamine
Product: *p*-Methoxy-N-methamphetamine   Reference: (Fusco 1948)

Starting Molecules: *p*-Methoxyphenyl-2-propanone & ethylamine
Product: *p*-Methoxy-N-ethamphetamine   Reference: (Fusco 1948)

Methamphetamine; P-2-P + Aluminum Foil
by József Knoll et al.

0.1 moles of (phenyl-2-propanone) are dissolved in 100 mL. of ethanol, whereupon 0.105 moles of methylamine are added. 3.5 grams of aluminum foil are degreased with ethanol and thereafter activated with a solution of 1 gram of mercuric chloride and 15 grams of sodium chloride in 30 mL. of water. The activating solution is decanted after 6 to 8 minutes and the activated aluminum foil is washed with cold water and added to the alcoholic solution previously prepared under stirring. An exothermic reaction takes place and the temperature is kept at 15° to 30° C. by cooling. The reaction mixture is stirred for 24 hours, whereupon 30 mL. of 40% sodium hydroxide are added. The two phases are separated, the lower aqueous phase is extracted three-times with benzene. The benzene solutions are united with the previously separated alcoholic phase and evaporated. The residue consists of an organic oily layer and an aqueous phase which is extracted with benzene and the benzene solution is dried over potassium carbonate. The benzene is removed and the residue is distilled off in a vacuo leaving the methamphetamine.

Phenyl-2-propanone
+ Amine
+ Aluminum Foil
+ Mercuric Bichloride
↓
N-Alkyl-amphetamine

Source: Knoll 1979 Reference: Laboratories Amido 1963

Starting Moles: 1-(1,3-Benzodioxol-5-yl)butan-2-one & methylamine HCl or methylamine
Product: N-Methyl-1-(1,3-benzodioxol-5-yl)-2-butanamine
References: (Nichols 1986) (Wassink 1971)

St. Moles.: 1-(3,4-Methylenedioxyphenyl)-2-propanone & methylamine HCl or methylamine
Product: 3,4-Methylenedioxy-N-methylamphetamine
References: (PIHKAL 1991): ethyl-K; methyl-K; Adam; Eden; Eve; MDMC

Reduction of P-2-P Using Aluminum Turnings (Amalgamated) with Amine

by Knoll A.-G.

700 ccs. of alcohol, 82 grams. (1/2 mol.) of *p*-methoxybenzyl-methyl-ketone, 75 ccs. of 40% methylamine solution, 50 ccs. of water and 50 grams of activated aluminum turnings are refluxed with thorough stirring for 6 to 8 hours. On completion of the reaction the solid matters are separated by suctional filtration, repeatedly washed with alcohol and the alcoholic solution evaporated to dryness. The residue (87.5 grams) is dissolved in 260 ccs. of alcohol, the solution is rendered acid to Congo with alcoholic hydrochloric acid and 1300 ccs. of alcoholic hydrochloric acid and 1300 ccs. of alcohol are added, thereto. After standing for one hour in ice the solution is suctionally filtered and impurities are removed by washing with ether.

Yield: 98.5 grams of hydrochloride of melting point 174° C. A further 1.5 grams of hydrochloride of melting point 155 to 160° C. can be recovered from the mother liquors. The total yield accordingly amounts to 93% theory. Source: Knoll A.G.1937a Ref.: Laboratories Amido 1964; Hildebrandt 1944; Knoll A.G.1937b

Reduction; Aluminum Amalgam & Nitromethane

A mixture of substituted phenyl-2-propanone (0.25 moles), nitromethane (25 grams, 0.40 mole) and 150 mL ethanol are added dropwise while stirring to a mixture of 40 grams of aluminum amalgam in 650 mL ethanol. This mixture is refluxed for three hours. The solution is then decanted from the aluminum and concentrated. The residue is dissolved in a minimum quantity of ether or acetone, acidified with hydrochloric acid and cooled to crystallize the substituted N-alkylamphetamine. The amphetamine salt is collected by suction filtration. The product is washed with ether or acetone. Approximate yield is 0.21 moles of substituted N-alkylamphetamine. By replacing the nitromethane with equal molar quantities of nitroethane (30 grams, 0.40 mole) should produce the N-ethyl-amphetamine.

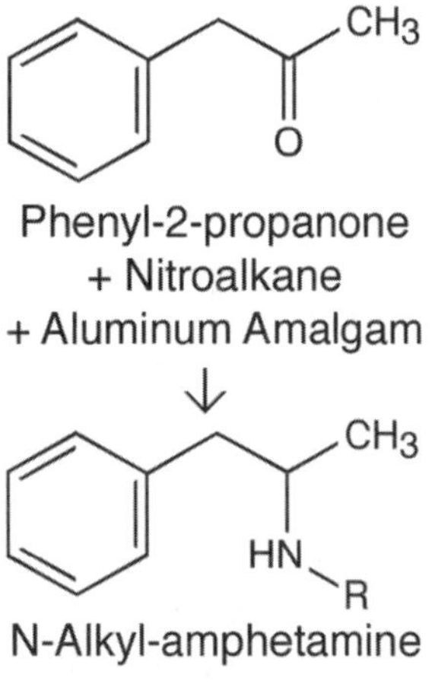

Phenyl-2-propanone
+ Nitroalkane
+ Aluminum Amalgam
↓

N-Alkyl-amphetamine

Starting M.: 2-Methoxyphenyl-2-propanone & nitromethane
Pdct.: 2-Methoxy-N-methylamphetamine   Ref.: (Tanaka 1957)

"When reduction is carried out with nascent hydrogen it is preferred to use activated aluminum in an alcoholic medium. Alternatively, an alkaline or acidic medium may be used, in dissolving-metal reductions or when reductions or with alloys soluble in bases, e.g. with activated aluminum, zinc, Degvarda's alloy or amalgams," Chinoin Gyogyszer.

Phenylethylamines from ß-Nitrostyrene: Zinc and Mercuric Bichloride

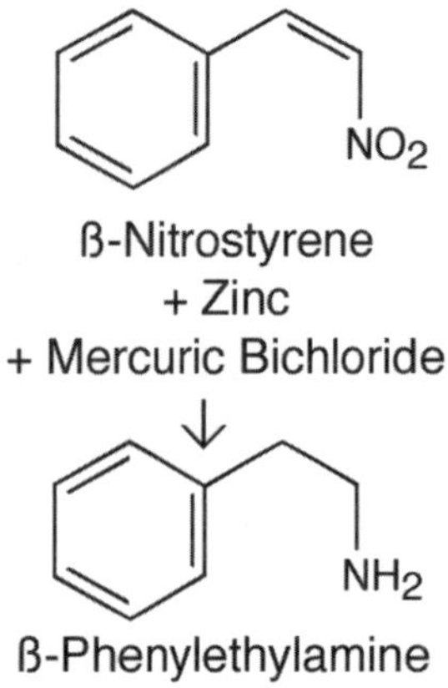

ß-Nitrostyrene
+ Zinc
+ Mercuric Bichloride
↓
ß-Phenylethylamine

0.1 Mole of ß-nitrostyrene is mixed in a solution of 500 mL of ethanol containing 100 grams of powdered zinc and 10 grams of mercuric bichloride. The mixture is stirred rapidly as concentrated hydrochloric acid is added until the yellow tinge disappears from the solution. The reaction mixture is rapidly stirred for one half hour following the color disappearance. The solution is filtered to remove excess zinc amalgam. The ethanol is then evaporated to leave a residue of the phenylalkylamine hydrochloride and impurities. The residue is made alkaline with ammonium hydroxide and extracted with ether or appropriate water insoluble solvent. The extract is cooled and cold hydrochloric acid is added to precipitate the phenylethylamine hydrochloride.

Starting Molecule: 3-Bromo-4,5-methylenedioxy-ß-nitrostyrene
Product: 3-Bromo-4,5-methylenedioxy-ß-phenylethylamine
Reference: (Tomita 1968)

Reduction of Phenylnitroalcohols with Zinc Phenylpropanolamine Preparation
by William F. Bruce

6 grams of phenyl-2-nitropropane compound are dissolved in 50 mL. of 95% ethanol, and 20 grams of zinc pellets (20 mesh) are added, together with a few drops of ferric chloride. Then while stirring and with temperature maintained at 40° C., 35 mL. of 12 N sulfuric acid are added, dropwise, during the course of 1 hour. Stirring is continued at 40° C. for six hours, then for an additional 18 hours at 20-25° C. The solution is then decanted from the zinc, made very alkaline, and extracted with ether. Concentration of the latter yielded crystals of phenylpropanolamine. Source: Bruce 1952

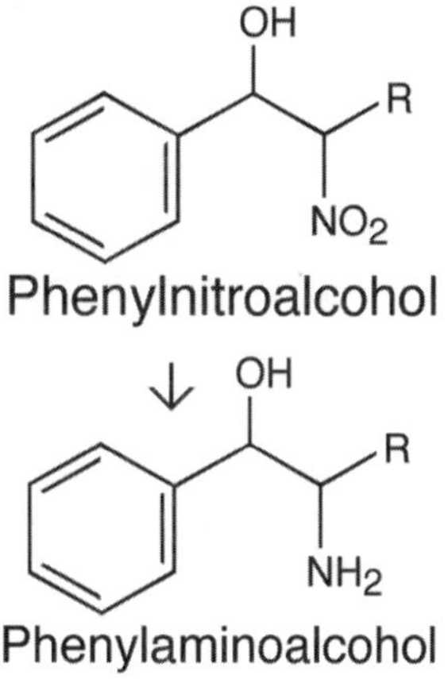

Immediate Precursor	R	Product
Phenyl-2-nitroethanol	H	Phenylethanolamine
Phenyl-2-nitropropanol	CH3	Phenylpropanolamine

Phenylnitroalcohol

For use of formaldehyde to N-methylate the amine see (Kanao 1929).

St. Mol.: 2-Methyl-2-nitro-1-phenyl-1-propanol
Product: 2-Amino-2-methyl-1-phenyl-1-propanol
(ephedrine) Refs.: Bruce 1952; Nagai 1929

Phenylaminoalcohol

St.g Mol.: 2-Nitro-1-phenyl-1-propanol Prdct: *dl*-Norephedrine & *dl*-norpseudo-ephedrine
Refs.: (Hoover 1947) (Kanao 1928) (Nagai 1929; Fe + H2SO4)

Starting Molecule: 3,4-Diacetoxyphenylnitroethanol
Product: 1-(3,4-Diacetoxyphenyl)-2-aminoethanol Reference: (Kanao 1929)

Starting Molecule: 1-(3,4-Diacetoxyphenyl)-2-nitropropanol
Product: 1-(3,4-Diacetoxyphenyl)-2-aminopropanol Reference:(Kanao 1929)

Reductions Using Iron Filings
Phenylnitroalcohols to Phenylaminoalcohols
Preparation of Phenylethanolamine (1-Phenyl-2-amino-ethan-1-ol)

by Alexander Nagai

An alcoholic solution of 167 grams of phenylnitroethanol... , dissolved in 800 c.c. of alcohol, is reduced by adding 1600 grams of 25% sulphuric acid and 240 grams of iron filings alternately, and the iron sulfate thus formed is then precipitated by means of alcohol. The alcoholic solution is made alkaline by adding potassium carbonate to it, then the upper layer is separated from the lower layer, and is neutralized by adding sulphuric acid, thus precipitating potassium sulfate which is filtered off. When the alcohol in the filtrate is distilled away, and the residue is crystallized from alcohol by recrystallization, a sulfate of rhombic tabular form is obtained. When to this aqueous solution, caustic soda is added and is shaken with ether, and the ether is then distilled away from this ethereal solution, a base shown in the title of this example having a melting point of about 40° C. remains.
Source: Nagai (1934).

Ephedrine from 1-Phenyl-1,2-propanedione

by Wilfrid Klavehn

15 grams of phenylpropanedione are dissolved in 250 cc. of an ethereal solution of methylamine containing 3.4 grams of the latter. While cooling, 32 grams of activated aluminium are introduced. In the course of 3-5 hours, 30 grams of water are allowed to drop in, whereby the ether is kept gently boiling. When the evolution of hydrogen has ceased, the whole is filtered from the aluminium hydroxide which has been formed and the colourless ethereal solution, after repeated extraction of the residue, is shaken with diluted hydrochloric acid, extract the base, or the later may be precipitated in the form of the hydrochloride by introducing gaseous hydrochloric acid. By crystallization from alcohol, the hydrochloride of phenylmethylamino propanol (*l*-ephedrine) of melting point 185-186° C. is obtained in very good yield. Source: Kalvekhn (1929) Ephedrine can be obtained by reducing phenylpropanedione with iron filings (Sugino 1953).

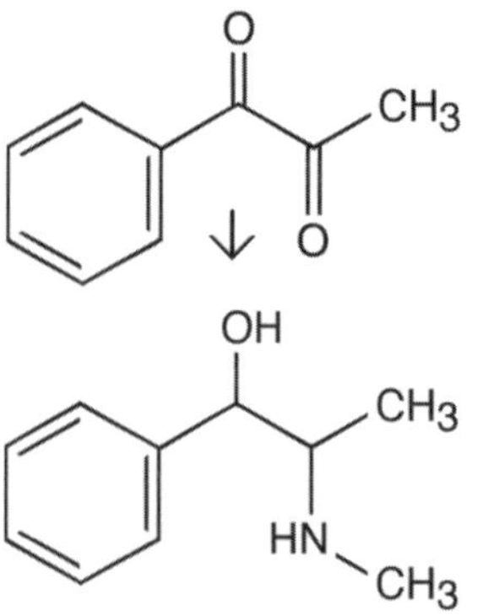

Ephedrine from 1-Phenylpropan-1-ol-2-one

(1-Phenylpropanol-1-one-2); (Phenylpropanolone)
(Phenylacetylcarbinol), (L-PAC)
by Gustav Hildebrandt and Wilfrid Klavdhn

120 grams of the fermentation product containing phenylpropanolone obtained by extraction with ether (see page 150) are allowed to run, without further purification, in the course of about two hours into a solution of 10 grams of methylamine in 500 cc. of ether in presence of 20 grams of activated aluminium whilst stirring. Simultaneously 20-30 grams of water are added, drop by drop. The vigorous reaction which at once sets in is moderated by periodical cooling. When the reaction is complete the ethereal solution is filtered and the optically active base which has been formed is extracted from the filtrate by means of dilute hydrochloric acid. The product is worked up in the usual manner.

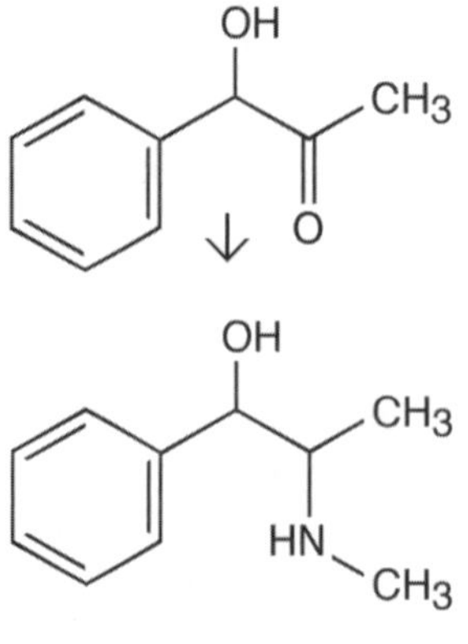

There is obtained the hydrochloride of levo-1-phenyl-2-methyl-amino-propanol-1 (ephedrine) having a melting point of 214° C. and having the optical rotation given in the literature. The yield amounts to 25-45 grams of the hydrochloride depending upon the nature of the parent material. Source: Hildebrandt 1931, 1934 Ref.: Neuberg 1922

Preparation of Mercuric Bichloride
Caution: mercury containing chemicals are poisonous!

Mercury bichloride can be prepared by several different reactions.

A mixture of 12 grams of mercury are boiled with 18 grams of sulfuric acid on a sand bath until a dry white residue remains. This white residue is mercury sulfate. The residue of mercury sulfate is ground with 9 grams of sodium chloride (salt) in an earthenware mortar. The powder is then placed in a sublimation apparatus. A vacuum is drawn on the apparatus and the stopcock is closed to keep the vacuum. The sublimation apparatus is gradually heated to sublime the mixture which condenses mercury bichloride on the walls of the apparatus.

Mercury bichloride can also be produced by dissolving mercuric oxide (red) in hydrochloric acid and evaporating the solution to leave a residue of mercury bichloride.

Mercury bichloride can also be produced by the direct reaction of chloride gas with mercury vapor.

Methylamine Hydrochloride Preparation

$$2HCHO + NH_4Cl \rightarrow CH_3NH_2\ HCl + HCO_2H$$

Prepared by C. S. Marvel and R. L. Jenkins.
Checked by J. B. Conant and F. C. Whidden.

1. Procedure

IN a 5-L. round-bottom flask fitted with a stopper holding a condenser set for downward distillation and a thermometer which will extend well into the liquid, are placed 4000 g. of technical formaldehyde (35-40 per cent; sp. gr. 1.078 at 20°) and 2000 g. of technical ammonium chloride. The mixture is heated on the steam bath until no more distillate comes over and then over a flame until the temperature of the solution reaches 104°. The temperature is held at this point until no more distillate comes over (four to six hours). The distillate, which consists of methylal, methyl formate and water, may be treated as described in Note 3.

The contents of the reaction flask are cooled to room temperature (Note 1), and the ammonium chloride which separates is filtered off and centrifuged (Note 2). The mother liquor is concentrated on the steam bath under reduced pressure to 2500 cc., and again cooled to room temperature, whereupon a second crop of ammonium chloride is obtained. The total recovery of ammonium chloride up to this point amounts to 780-815 g.

The mother liquor is again concentrated under reduced pressure until crystals begin to form on the surface of the solution (1400-1500 cc.). It is then cooled to room temperature and a first crop of methylamine hydrochloride, containing some ammonium chloride, is obtained by filtering the cold solution and centrifuging the crystals (Note 2). At this point 625-660 g. of crude product is obtained. The mother liquor is now concentrated under reduced pressure to about 1000 cc. and cooled, a second crop of methylamine hydrochloride (170-190 g.) is then filtered off and centrifuged. This crop of crystals is washed with 250 cc. of cold chloroform, filtered and centrifuged, in order to remove most of the dimethylamine hydrochloride which is present; after the washing with chloroform the product weighs 140-150 g. The original mother liquor is then evaporated under reduced pressure, as far as possible, by heating on a steam bath, and the thick syrupy solution (about 350 cc.) which remains is poured into a beaker and allowed to cool, with occasional stirring, in order to prevent the formation of a solid cake (Note 1). The thick paste so obtained is centrifuged, and the crystals (170-190 g.) are washed with 250 cc. of cold chloroform; the solution is filtered and the crystals are centrifuged, thus yielding 55-65 g. of product. There is no advantage in further concentrating the mother liquor.

The total yield of crude centrifuged methylamine hydrochloride is 830-850 g. This product contains, as impurities, water, ammonium chloride, and some dimethylamine hydrochloride. In order to obtain a pure product, the crude methylamine hydrochloride is recrystallized from absolute alcohol (Note 4). The crude salt is placed in a 5-L. round-bottom flask fitted with a reflux condenser protected at the top with a calcium chloride tube; 2 L. of absolute alcohol is added and the mixture heated to boiling. After about half an hour the undissolved material is allowed to settle and the clear solution is poured off. When the alcoholic solution is cooled, methylamine hydrochloride crystallizes out. It is filtered off and centrifuged, and the alcohol used for another extraction.

The process is repeated until the alcohol dissolves no more of the product (about five extractions are necessary). In the flask 100-150 g. of ammonium chloride remains, making the total recovery of ammonium chloride 850-950 g. The yield of recrystallized methylamine hydrochloride is 600-750 g. (45-51 per cent of the theoretical amount, based on the ammonium chloride used up in the process).

Notes

1. The methylamine hydrochloride solutions should be cooled rapidly in order to bring the salt down in small crystals which may be easily purified.

2. Centrifuging the precipitates is the only satisfactory method of drying, as all of the products tend to take up water when allowed to stand in the air.

3. Methylal and sodium formate may be obtained from the first distillate of the main reaction mixture. The crude distillate is placed in a flask fitted with a reflux condenser and to it is added a solution of 200 g. of sodium hydroxide in 300 cc. of water. The methyl formate is hydrolyzed to sodium formate. The methylal layer is separated, dried over calcium chloride and distilled. In this way 240-260 g. of methylal, boiling at 37-42°, is obtained. By evaporating the watery portion to dryness there is obtained a residue of about 280 g. of crude sodium formate.

4. Since ammonium chloride is not absolutely insoluble in 100 per cent ethyl alcohol (100 g. dissolve 0.6 g at 15°) the methylamine hydrochloride purified in the manner described contains appreciable traces of it. A purer product can be prepared by recrystallizing from n-butyl alcohol, in which the solubility of ammonium chloride even at the boiling temperature is negligibly small. Methylamine hydrochloride is somewhat less soluble in this solvent than in ethyl alcohol, but as a rule three extractions carried out at 90-100° with 4-6 parts of fresh butyl alcohol for each extraction result in a substantially complete separation. Since the last traces of the solvent are not readily removed by exposure to air, a solution of the recrystallized material in a small quantity of water should be distilled until free of alcohol, and allowed to crystallize.

5. The literature (ref. 1) claims a yield of methylamine hydrochloride amounting to 79 per cent of the weight of ammonium chloride used up in the reaction. This figure is probably based on the weight of crude methylamine hydrochloride and not of the recrystallized material.

Other Methods of Preparation

Methylamine occurs in herring brine (ref. 2) in crude methyl alcohol from wood distillation (ref. 3) and in the products obtained by the dry distillation of beet molasses residues (ref. 4). It has been prepared synthetically by the action of alkali on methyl cyanate or isocyanurate (ref. 5); by the action of ammonia on methyl iodide (ref. 6), methyl chloride (ref. 7), methyl nitrate (ref. 8), or dimethyl sulfate (ref. 9); by the action of methyl alcohol on ammonium chloride (ref. 10), on the addition compound between zinc chloride and ammonia (ref. 11), or on phospham (ref. 12), by the action of bromine and alkali on acetamide (ref. 13); by the action of sodamide on methyl iodide (ref. 14) by the reduction of chloropicrin (ref. 15), of hydrocyanic or of ferrocyanic acid (ref. 16), of hexamethylenetetramine (ref. 17), of nitromethane (ref. 18), or of methyl nitrite (ref. 19); by the action of formaldehyde on ammonium chloride (ref. 20).

1. *J. Chem. Soc.* 111, 850 (1917).
2. *Ber.* 18, 1922 (1885).
3. *Jahresb.* 1873, 686; *Ann. chim. phys.* (5) 1, 444 (1874).
4. *Ann. chim. phys.* (5) 23, 316 (1881).
5. *Ann.* 71, 332 (1849).
6. *Ann.* 79, 16 (1851).
7. *Bull. soc. chim.* 45, 499 (1886).
8. *Compt. rend.* 48, 344 (1859); *Ann.* 110, 255 (1859); *Jahresb.* 1862, 327; *Ann. chim. phys.* (5) 23, 321 (1881).
9. *Ber.* 43, 139 (1910); *J. Chem. Soc.* 117, 236 (1920).
10. *Ber.* 8, 458 (1875)
11. *Ber.* 17, 639 (1884)
12. *D. R. P.* 64,346, *Frdl.* 3, 13 (1890-94).
13. *Ber.* 15, 765 (1882); *Compt. rend.* 147, 430, 680,983 (1908).
14. *Compt. rend.* 156, 328 (1913).
15. *Ann.* 109, 282 (1859); 184, 51 (1877); *J. Chem. Soc.* 115, 159 (1919).
16. *Ann.* 121, 139 (1862); 128, 201 (1863); Z. physik. Chem. 72, 674 (1910); *D. R. P. 264,528, Frdl.* 11, 110 (1912—14).
17. *D. R. P.* 73,812, *Frdl.* 3, 15 (1890 94); *Bull. soc. chim.* (3) 11, 23 (1894); *D. R. P.* 143,197, *Frdl.* 7, 24 (1902-04); *D. R. P. 148,054, Frdl.* 7, 26 (1902-04); *C. A.* 9, 2232 (1915).
18. *Bull. soc. chim.* (3) 21, 783 (1899); (4) 7, 954 (1910); *Ber.* 44, 2403 (1911).
19. *Bull. soc. chim.* (4) 7, 824 (1910); *Ann. chim. phys.* (8) 25, 136 (1912).
20. *Bull. soc. chim.* (3)13, 534 (1895); *Compt. rend.* 147, 429 (1908); *J. Chem. Soc.* 111,848 (1917); *J. Am. Chem. Soc.* 40, 1411 (1918).

References: Jones 1918; Werner 1917.

N-Methylation of Amphetamines

Preparation of N-Methyl-PMA from PMA and Benzaldehyde
by Gordon Alles

One mole of 1-(*para*-methoxyphenyl)-2-aminopropane base and one mole of benzaldehyde are mixed and after the initial reaction is completed, water is distilled from the mixture by heating above 100° C. under atmospheric pressure. The resultant Schiff base may be used without further treatment...

One mole of anhydrous 1-(*para*-methoxyphenyl)-2-benzalamino-propane and one mole of methyl iodide are mixed and placed in a sealed container. After heating a few hours in a boiling water bath there is formed a glassy mass of the quaternary ammonium salt product above mentioned.

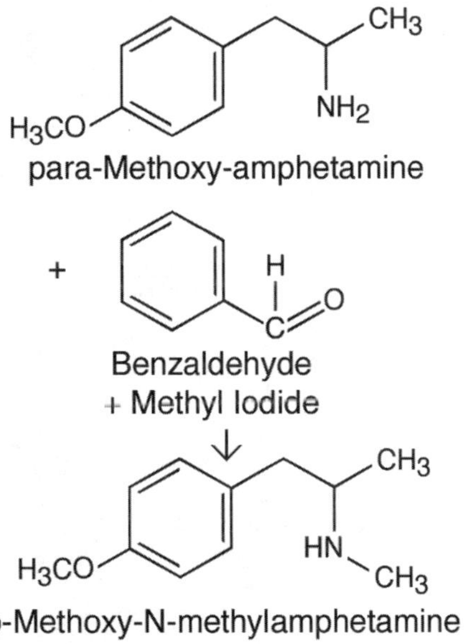

Solution of this product in 200 cc. methanol followed by addition of 100 cc. concentrated hydrochloric acid and 300 cc. water, followed by warming for a short time in a hot water bath hydrolyses benzaldehyde off from the quaternary ammonium salt, and extraction with ether removes the benzaldehyde from the aqueous mixture. Sodium hydroxide is then added to liberate the base present which is then removed by extraction with benzene. This benzene extract contains the desired 1-(*para*-methoxyphenyl)-2-methyl-amino-propane, which may be obtained as the free base by distilling off the benzene... Source: Alles 1935

para-Methoxy-amphetamine

+

Benzaldehyde
+ Methyl Iodide

p-Methoxy-N-methylamphetamine

CHAPTER 10 ELECTROLYTIC REDUCTIONS

Electrolytic reductions elevate the need to use hazardous reducing agents, metals etc. Electricity is used instead. The following small apparatus suits the needs of most amateur as well as professional chemists. It does not require much space and can be disassembled and stored when not in use. Electrolytic reductions are used to produce amines, alcohols, aldehydes etc.

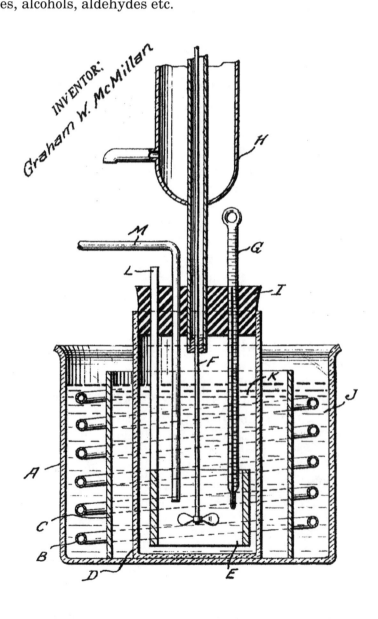

ELECTROYLIC PRODUCTION
by Graham W. McMillan

Electrolytic reduction processes are based on the fact that the cathode, or negative pole of an electrolytic cell establishes a reducing atmosphere in which reactants involving a transfer of electrons from electrode to components of the solution are promoted. Thus, under such conditions, a nitro group will tend to be reduced to an amino group with the gain of electrons from the cathode pole...

In the acid reduction of the nitro... compound to the amino compound the mechanism of reduction proceeds first to the nitroso compound, next to a hydoxylamino compound and only then to the amino compound as represented below:

$$RNO2 \xrightarrow{2H} RNO \xrightarrow{2H} RNHOH \xrightarrow{2H} RNH2$$

Thus, the reaction is a step wise one and the reaction therefor, can be no faster than the slowest or most limiting step, nor can it be complete unless the intermediate products are preserved from the side reactions until they can be made to undergo the desired reduction reactions. I have found that the limiting step in the preparation... is usually the last one in which reduction of the hydroxyamino compound to the amine takes place. Under a wide variety of conditions the nitro and nitroso compounds react swiftly and completely to form the hydroxylamino compound, but on the other hand, very little amine compound forms until after nearly all the nitro compound has been transformed to the hydroxyamine compound and then only under carefully controlled conditions which not only tend to prevent side reactions of the auxiliary materials present, but also which protect the aminohydroxyl compound from undesired reactions with the other materials present in the cell, including dehydration, deammonation, reactions of the nitro compound with the hydroxylamine compound and the like...

...high yields of the order of 80-95% or higher of amino... compounds can be obtained with purities of 90% or more, usually between about 95-99%...

I first prepare an electrolytic cell consisting of anode and cathode compartments filled with anolyte and catholyte solutions, respectively, as described, the anolyte consisting preferably of about a 10-20% solution of sulfuric acid, the catholyte solution preferably of a solution of hydrochloric acid of less than about 10%, or sulfuric acid of about 25% or somewhat less. Anode and cathode poles or suitable conducting material are placed in their respective chamber filled with anolyte and catholyte respectively. The nitro... compound to be reduced is placed in the cathode compartment of the cell in the concentrations described, and an electric current is passed through the cell at a current density at least as high as about 0.1 to 0.2 ampere per square centimeter, probably in most cases at the higher figure. The temperature of the cell is maintained between about 50°-100° C., depending somewhat on the compound being reduced, throughout the electrolysis (see Alles in this chapter). After about six faradays of current per mole of nitro compound have been passed, the amount of current theoretically required to completely reduce the nitro compounds of my invention to the corresponding amino compound, the electrolysis is continued but the current density may be lowered, for example, to about 0.10-0.13 ampere per square centimeter and continued at this intensity until samples of catholyte solution are negative to Fehling's solution test or other tests indication absence of oxidizing agents, that is, completion of the reduction of nitro compound to amino compound. Or, successive reduction in current density may be made as the reaction bears completion.

The recovery of the (amine) can be effected either as an acid salt or as the free amine. The salt is readily obtained simply by evaporating the catholyte solution to dryness. The amine may then be obtained from the acid salt by any desired known method, for recovering amines from aqueous solutions of their salts, for example, any distillation or neutralization and filtration depending on the nature of the amine and of the particular acid salt involved...

One type of electrolytic cell which is suitable for use in my invention, and the one used in specific examples described below, is illustrated in the figure of the drawing, and comprises a glass vessel A containing a cylindrical lead anode C, and a cylindrical unglazed porcelain diaphragm D. The annular space between the diaphragm cup and the glass vessel holds, in addition to the anode C, a glass cooling-coil B through which hot or cold water can be passed as required to control the temperature. the diaphragm cup serves as a container for the catholyte solution and depolarizer K and for a cylindrical lead cathode E whose active area is 150 square centimeters. The diaphragm cup is closed off by a rubber stopper I though which are passed a reflux condenser H, stirrer F, thermometer G, cathode connector L and a glass sampling tube M into which samples of the catholyte can be drawn periodically for analysis. Direct current is used. Best results are obtained when the lead cathode is highly polished. Source: McMillan 1949

Preparation of Amphetamine
from Phenyl-2-nitropropene
by Gordon Alles

The preferred method of synthesizing the 1-phenyl-2-aminopropane, is by the reduction of the phenyl-2-nitropropene. This reduction may be carried out by sodium-mercury amalgam in an ethanol-acetic acid solution or by electrolytic reduction at a metal cathode in a suitable solution. This cathodic reduction can be carried out with good yield in the following manner:

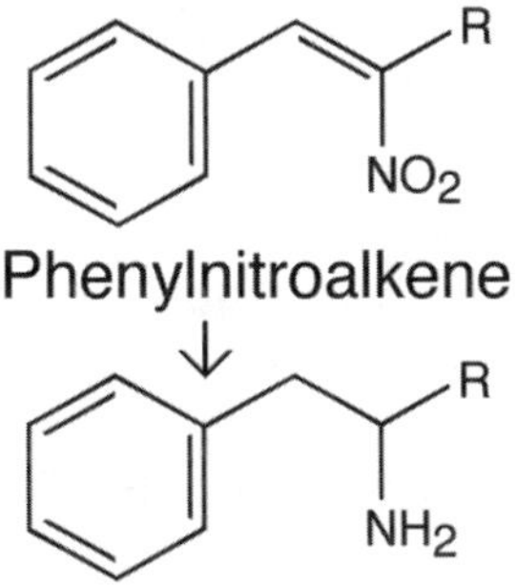

Phenylnitroalkene

Phenylalkylamine

One mole of the phenyl-2-nitropropene is dissolved with a solvent prepared by mixing one liter of ethanol with one-half liter of acetic acid and one-half liter of twelve normal sulphuric acid. The resultant solution is placed in the cathode compartment of a divided cell containing a metallic cathode of mercury, copper, or other metal of similar nature. Current is passed, using a current density of about two-tenths ampere per square centimeter of cathode surface. The temperature is kept about 40° C. during the electrolysis which is continued until at least eight Faradays of electricity have been passed.

When the reduction is completed, the 1-phenyl-2-aminopropane may be separated from the solution. A convenient way of doing this is by removing the ethanol and ethyl acetate present by evaporation and then making the residual solution strongly alkaline by addition of caustic alkali. The basic layer thus formed is separated from the aqueous solution and contains the desired 1-phenyl-2-aminopropane.
Source: Alles 1932

Preparation of Methoxy-amphetamine
by Gordon Alles

One-fifth gram-mol methoxyphenyl-2-nitropropene, in a mixture of two-fifths liter, ethanol, one-fifth liter acetic acid, and one-fifth liter twelve normal sulfuric acid, is placed in the cathode compartment of an electrolytic cell with a mercury cathode. For the anode division of the cell a porous cup containing a lead anode and a six normal sulfuric acid anolyte is used. Electric current is passed through the cell at such voltage that the amperage passing gives a cathode current density of about one-tenth ampere per square centimeter, and the temperature of the catholyte is maintained preferably between 25° and 35° C. by cooling. An excess of electric energy over the theoretically required eight farradays per mole of methoxyphenyl-2-nitropropene used completes the reaction. Addition of water to the catholyte product and removal of the ethanol and acetic acid present, by distillation, and then making strongly alkaline with caustic soda, causes a basic layer to separate... and is purified by distillation under reduced pressure. Source: Alles 1944

APPARATUS COMPONENTS

The electrolytic reduction apparatus has several components. All of these components can be purchased readily or made with locally obtained materials. I will list the various components:

1) The porous porcelain cylindrical cell. It is composed of unglazed cylindrical porous porcelain cup with the approximate external dimensions of 3 x 6.6 inches. It can be purchased from a laboratory supply company or made at a local ceramics shop. A filtros plate or thin corkpine wood sealed by the use of paraffin may also be used. Porous porcelain cells are commonly used in chemistry class battery experiments.

"*An inexpensive substitute for these cups may be made as follows: Wet a sheet of paper, wrap it several times about a large test-tube, folding in to close the bottom. Mold the paper into shape, then coat it, inside and out, with a hot solution made by dissolving 75 grams of gelatin and 100 g. K4Fe(CN)6 in one liter of water. When the cup has drained and cooled, it may be removed, and inverted until dry.*" From: *Exercises in General Chemistry* (1924)

2) The glass coil. The reason for the glass coil is to lower the heat from the reduction mixture. It can be made. I would suggest learning how to work with glass as in the chemistry laboratory it saves a lot of money (repairing breaks). The coils are available from laboratory supply companies or can be manufactured to specifications at glass work shops. The glass coils surround the anode and fit with in the porous porcelain cell (the anode chamber).

3) The anode (+). It is usually composed of lead, carbon, or platinum. Carbon rods can be purchased in art supply stores.

4) The cathode (-). It is usually composed of lead, mercury or platinum. In this apparatus, the cathode is a piece of lead flashing which is bent to surround the porous porcelain cup and fit within a 500 mL beaker. The lead cathode should have the approximate dimensions of 8.5 x 3.5 x 3/32 inches. A strip of lead is extended upward from the lead

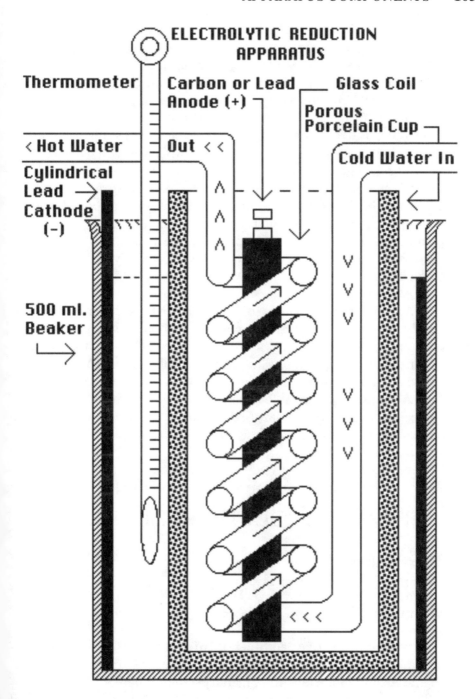

ELECTROLYTIC REDUCTION APPARATUS

Thermometer

Carbon or Lead Anode (+)

Glass Coil

Porous Porcelain Cup

< Hot Water

Out <<

Cold Water In

Cylindrical Lead → Cathode (−)

500 ml. Beaker →

sheet for attachment to the negative pole of the power source. The lead cathode should be 'shined' before each reaction to increase conductivity.

This can be done by use of circular fine wire brush attached to a drill. The surface of the cathode is 'polished' (slightly scratched) from (dull gray) till the surface is shiny, like freshly cut lead.

5) A 500 mL beaker is used to hold the apparatus.

6) The DC power supply. The power supply must produce 12 volts DC at 6 amps. Variations of these currents will produce variable yields. Battery chargers should not be used as a power source. There is no resistance in the reduction apparatus and will over load the battery charger. The current of electricity must be constant. A battery charger will not do this. Battery chargers usually produce a large current in the beginning of charging a battery and tapper off as the battery stores charge and builds resistance. The power supply for the apparatus is available from electronics supply houses. Alligator clips are wired to the output wires so that they can be easily attached to the anode and cathode.

7) A thermometer.

8) A small water circulator. This is used to circulate the water through the glass coils. A circulator will not waste tap water and run up the water bill. These circulators are used to circulate water in small water fountains and can be purchased in any place that supplies lawn ornaments such as garden centers etc.

9) A large container for the reduction apparatus. The reduction apparatus is placed in a large glass bowl which holds ice and the water circulator. The cold water is circulated through the glass coils and back into the bowl of ice.

References: (Ingersoll; *Organic Syntheses Col* 1: *Organic Syntheses* 9) (McMillan 1949) (Norris 1925) (Slotta 1933)

THE ELECTROLYTIC REDUCTION

Immediate Precursor	R	Product
ß-Nitrostyrene	H	Phenylethylamine
Phenyl-2-nitropropene	CH3	Amphetamine

Low temperature reduction of 1-(phenyl)-1-acetoxy-2-nitropropane will produce *d,l*-norephedrine (racemic phenylpropanolamine) and also racemic kathine (*d,l*-norpseudo-ephedrine).

This apparatus will work equally well with trimethoxy, ethoxy and various other substitutes. Hydroxy groups should be protected (OH groups should be methylated or acetylated) as they may also be reduced.

For use of methylamine hydrochloride to N-methylate the amine see (Sugino 1951). For use of formaldehyde to N-methylate the amine see (Kanao 1929).

The cathode compartment contains a solution of 30 grams of substituted phenylnitroalkene in 100 mL of glacial acetic acid and 100 mL of absolute alcohol which contains 50 mL of concentrated hydrochloric acid.

The anode compartment is filled to the same level as the cathode liquor with a solution of 14% hydrochloric acid.

The alligator clips from the power source are connected to the appropriate electrodes, the water is circulated through the coils and the power is turned on. The catholyte is held at 20 degrees for the first six hours and then allowed to rise to 40 degrees for the last six hours. The reduction takes approximately 12 hours.

The catholyte liquor is filtered and poured into 300 mL of water. The unreduced nitroalkene is extracted with ethyl acetate or any other appropriate solvent that the amine hydrochloride is not soluble in (e.g. acetone, ether).

The crude amine hydrochloride, remains in the water solution. The water can be distilled off to leave a mush of the crude amine salt, traces of hydrochloric acid, water and impurities. This mush must be dried of water by use of anhydrous Epson salt (magnesium sulfate) or calcium chloride.

Drying agent: Epson salt or calcium chloride is placed in a Pyrex dish and heated in the oven at 120 degrees C. The Epsom salt will become anhydrous (loose the extra H_2O that is attached to the molecule). It takes on a white very hard constancy. Take the dish of drying agent out of the oven with oven gloves (so as not to get burned). Break up the anhydrous Epsom salt and store in a air tight bottle so as not to absorb atmospheric moisture.

Starting Molecule: *dl-threo*-1-(Acetoxy-phenyl)-2-nitropropane
Product: *dl*-Norpseudoephedrine Reference: (Drefahl 1958)

Starting Molecule: 2,5-Dimethoxy-ß-nitrostyrene
Product: 2,5-Dimethoxyphenylethylamine
Reference: (Leaf 1948)

Catholyte: 150 mL. MeOH, 40 mL. concd. HCl
Starting Molecule: 3,4-Dimethoxy-ß-nitrostyrene (10 grams)
Anolyte: 20%, H2SO4, c.d. 0.07 amp./ cm2, 20-22°, 6 hours
Product: 3,4-Dimethoxyphenylethylamine Reference: (Ban 1954)

Cathodic Fluid: 200 cc. 5% HCl plus pinch of EtOH
Starting Molecule: 3-Methoxy-4-ethoxy-ß-nitrostyrene (5 gr.)
Anodic Fluid: 20% H2SO4 Temp. 65° , 12 v., 5 amps, 3 hours.
Product: 3-Methoxy-4-ethoxy-phenylethylamine
Reference: (Kondo 1928)

S.M.:2-(*alpha*-Methoxy-4-nitropropyl)-4,5-methylenedioxytoluene (15 gr.)
Reduction: 6-7 amp./100 cm2 cathode, 25°
Product:ß-Methoxy-ß-(3,4-methylenedioxy-6-methyl)-amphetamine
Reference: (Sugasawa 1954)

Starting Molecule: 6-Methyl-ß-nitroisosafrole
Product: 6-Methyl-3,4-methylenedioxy-amphetamine
Reference: (Sugasawa 1954)

Starting Molecule: ß-Nitro-asarone
Product: 2,4,5-Trimethoxyamphetamine Reference: (Bruckner 1933)

Starting Molecule: ß-Nitroisosafrole
1-(3,4-Methylenedioxyphenyl)-2-nitropropene-1
Product: 3,4-Methylenedioxy-amphetamine
Reference: Dal Cason 1990

Catholyte: MeNH2 HCl (15 gr.), 50 gr. 68% EtOH
Starting Molecule: PhCOCOMe (7.7gr.)
Anolyte: 15 gr. H2SO4, c.d. 46 amp./ dm2, 12-15°
Product: Ephedrine Reference: (Sugino 1951)

Starting Molecule: 3,4,5-Timethoxy-ß-nitrostyrene
Product: Mescaline (3,4,5-Trimethoxyphenylethylamine)
Reference: (Slotta 1933)

Drying of The
Phenylalkylamine Hydrochloride (a salt)

Sprinkle the anhydrous drying agent on the bottom of a large Pyrex dish. Place the 'wet' phenylalkylamine hydrochloride in a smaller dish, set it in the large dish on the anhydrous Epsom salt and place a cover on the large dish. The moisture from the phenylalkylamine salt will be absorbed by the anhydrous drying agent much like an open box of bicarbonate of soda absorbs the odors in the refrigerator. Allow to stand till the weight of the dish containing the phenylalkylamine hydrochloride remains constant.

Purification And Precipitation of The Substituted Phenylalkylamine Salt

The amine salt is placed in a beaker. A minimal quantity of hot acetone or ether are added. Just enough to dissolve the amine salt. Ether or acetone (or appropriate solvent which the amine salt is insoluble) is used. Cover the solution so as not to absorb moisture and cool in a refrigerator. The amine salt precipitates from the solution and is then filtered from the solvent by vacuum filtration using a water aspirator. The amine salt is again dried with anhydrous drying material and stored in an air tight container.

Purification of The Crude Phenylalkylamine Hydrochloride Salt From The Catholyte Liquor

Another purification can be done. To the crude amine salt solution (catholyte liquor), that has been purified of the phenylnitroalkene with solvent washing, 100 grams of concentrated sodium hydroxide solution is added to basify the amine salt and make it soluble in acetone, ether etc. The base amine is then extracted from the sodium hydroxide solution with ether or acetone, concentrate the solution and cool. Hydrochloric acid is added to the cooled solution to precipitate the purified amine hydrochloride salt. Vacuum filter and dry.

This reduction produces 75% theoretical yields or better of purified amine salt.

Amphetamine from Electrolytic Reduction of P-2-P/P-2-P Oxime
by Fred P. Nabenhauer

This invention relates to a method for the production of substituted benzyl carbinamine having the formula C_6H_5-CH_2-CHx-NH_2, in which X is an alkyl or alphyl group group and to the products produced in accordance with the method. More particularly, this invention relates to a method for producing benzyl methyl carbinamine and to the product produced in accordance with the method.

Heretofore various methods have been know for the production of substituted benzyl carbinamines, but variously they have been open to objections from the standpoint of economy, facility in practice, low yield and from the standpoint of lack of purity of product.

The method in accordance with this invention will be found to be economic, readily carried out in practice on a commercial scale, productive of a high yield and directly of products of a high degree of purity.

The method in accordance with this invention involves in essence the production of a substituted benzyl carbinamine by electrolytic reduction of a benzyl ketone oxime to a corresponding benzyl carbinamine. Thus, more specifically, the method in accordance with this invention involves the electrolytic reduction of benzyl methyl ketone oxime to benzyl methyl carbinamine (amphetamine)...

Having indicated in a general way the procedure in accordance with this invention, it will now be exemplified in detail with reference to practical procedure for the preparation of benzyl methyl carbinamine (amphetamine), all with reference to the accompanying drawing by which is diagrammatically illustrated a suitable form of apparatus for carrying out the essential procedure embodying this invention.

With reference to the drawing. A indicates a bath containing brine b. Within the bath A is positioned a glass jar C containing a layer of mercury h and a supply of electrolyte, as, for example, battery acid d comprising, for example, sulphuric acid solution having a specific gravity of 1.4 In the jar C enough mercury is added to cover the bottom completely. This is connected by wire E and a suitable lead wire f to a source of direct current G, which may, for example, be a motor generator. Within the jar C and submerged in the battery acid is a stirring device, as, for example, a paddle i adapted to be operated in any suitable manner to effect agitation of the electrolyte.

Within the jar C and submerged in the electrolyte contained therein is positioned a porous porcelain cup J, in which is contained a supply of electrolyte K, as, for example, battery acid comprising sulphuric acid having a specific gravity of 1.4 Within the cup J and immersed in the electrolyte is suspended a lead anode L connected with the source of current by a suitable lead wire f'.

In carrying out the method in accordance with this invention, for example, 1500 cc. of sulphuric acid, specific gravity of 1.4, are placed in the cup J, sufficient mercury, and sulphuric acid, specific gravity 1.4, are placed in jar C, and brine is placed in brine bath A. The brine is suitably cooled to maintain a temperature in jar C of about 25° C. or lower. To the sulphuric acid in the jar C there will then be added 150 grams of benzyl methyl ketone oxime obtained from any suitable source or produced as indicated above. A current of about 6 to 10 volts and about 36 ampere corresponding to a current density of about 11 to 14 amperes per square decimeter with then be maintained as the reaction proceeds. At the end of four hours a further addition of 150 grams of benzyl methyl ketone oxime will be made to the jar C.

The benzyl methyl ketone oxime with be dissolved in the sulphuric acid solution in the jar C and as a result of the electrolytic action hydrogen will be discharged from the solution at mercury cathode h. The hydrogen will combine with the oxime to form amine in the form of acid amine sulphate in solution in the sulphuric acid.

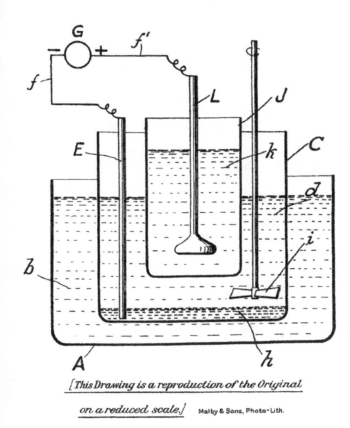

[This Drawing is a reproduction of the Original on a reduced scale.] Malby & Sons, Photo-Lith.

When the reduction of the total of 1500 grams of benzyl methyl ketone oxime to the jar C is complete, the jar C will contain acid benzyl methyl amine sulphate in concentrated solution.

On completion of the reduction, the concentrated solution of acid benzyl methyl amine sulphate will be diluted with water and oily impurities permitted to separate. The oily impurities having been removed, an alkali, as caustic soda, will be added to the solution to neutralize the acid and free the amine, which may be separated from the aqueous solution by decantation or other means. The oily layer or free amine, which is strongly basic, is then neutralized by dissolving it in hydrochloric acid, which converts the amine into a neutral hydrochloride. Oily impurities are then removed from the resultant solution of neutral amine hy-drochloride by extraction of the solution with an organic solvent, as, for example, isopropyl ether.

The amine hydrochloride in solution is then converted to free amine by the addition of alkali. The free amine, which is the benzyl methyl carbinamine (amphetamine) product, will settle from the solution as an oily layer, which may be readily separated. The separated benzyl methyl carbinamine is then desirably distilled in vacuo for recover of the pure product. The distillation in vacuo may be carried out within a wide range of temperatures and under varying pressures. By way of example, the distillation will desirably be carried out at a temperature of about 80°-90° C. and under a pressure of about one mm. mercury.

It will now be noted the method in accordance with this invention involves, from the broad standpoint, electrolytic reduction of abenzyl ketone oxime, more particularly benzyl methyl ketone oxime, to the corresponding amine sulphate and freeing the amine. More specifically, the purity of the final product is assured by the separation of by-products from the original solution of amine sulphate obtained, freeing the amine, as by the addition of alkali, the formation of amine hydrochloride by dissolving the amine in hydrochloric acid, extracting the amine hydrochloride solution with an organic solvent, converting the amine hydrochloride to free the amine and finally distilling in vacuo.

As will be appreciated, the unit of apparatus described above with reference to the accompanying drawing may be duplicated and the units arranged in batteries. As will be obvious, the precise arraignment and capacity of the unit as described for illustrative purposes may be widely varied.

The method is accordance with this invention will be found to be really carried out on a commercial scale and will be found to be highly efficient and economic, it having been found that the yield obtained from the oxime runs in the neighborhood of 60% of theoretical. Economy in commercial practice will further be obtained from the fact that the oily impurities removed in connection with recovery of the substituted benzyl carbinamine (amphetamine) may readily be reoxidized to the ketone, which in turn may be readily converted to oxime for use in carrying out the method of this invention. Thus, for example, in carrying out the method in accordance with this invention for the production of benzyl methyl carbinamine one may readily recover benzyl methyl carbinol from the oily impurities and such may be readily oxidized to benzyl methyl ketone, which in turn may be readily converted into benzyl methyl ketone oxime.

The method is accordance with this invention will further be found to be distinctly advantageous over methods heretofore known for the production of substituted benzyl carbinamine in that, for example, it will display increased safety in that no sodium is used. The method affords easy control and will give uniform yields. Objectionable impurities are not formed and side products may be readily recovered and reused. Production of hydroxylamine and phenyl-2-propanone oxime see Semon 1923. Source: (Nabenhauer 1936)

For prepartion of substituted phenyl-2-propanone oxime from substituted phenyl-2-nitropropene see (Dessi 1952). For replacement of hydroxylamine with methylamine hydrochloride to N-methylate the amine see (Sugino 1951). For use of formaldehyde to N-methylate the amine see (Kanao 1929). Preparation of hydroxylamine see Adams 1918, Raschig 1888.

Electrolytic Preparation of Methamphetamine from 1-Phenyl-1-chloro-2-methylaminopropane

The cathode solution is composed of 5 grams of phenyl-1-chloro-2-methylaminopropane which is dissolved in 200 mL. 20% H_2SO_4. The cathode is a sheet of lead 60 square cm. 2000 mL. of 50% H_2SO_4 which surrounds the lead anode. The two solutions and electrodes are separated by an unglazed porous porcelain cylinder (as illustrated earlier in this book). The temperature of the alcoholysis is kept a 10° C, 15 amps at 3.5 v. for a period of 4 hours.

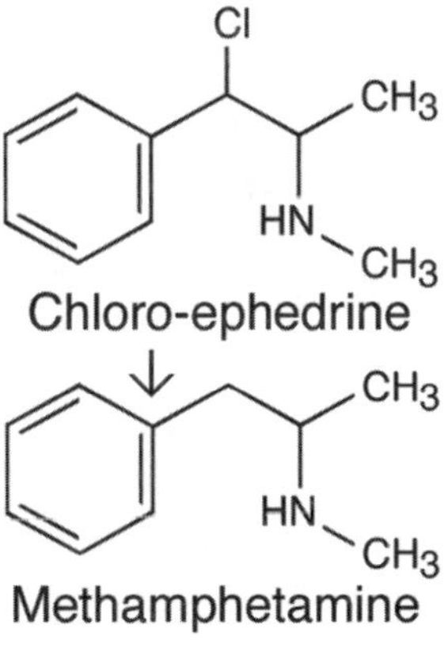

The cathode solution is neutralized with NaOH and extracted with ether or appropriate solvent. The solvent is evaporated to reduce volume and worked up in usual manner to yield 3.8 grams of methylamphetamine. Reference: Fujisawa 1946

Chloro-ephedrine

Methamphetamine

CHAPTER 11:
PHENYL-2-NITROALKENE PREPARATION
Phenylnitroalkenes From
Benzaldehydes & Nitroalkanes

50 Grams of the substituted benzaldehyde is mixed with 50 mL of nitroalkane, 20 grams of ammonium acetate and 200 mL of glacial acetic acid. A Dean & Stark moisture receiver is attached to the reflux apparatus. The solution is heated on a boiling water bath for three hours and then poured into ice-water. The product will precipitate as an oil or as a solid. Solid precipitates may be collected by vacuum filtration. The oils may be extracted by washing the solution with ether (or any water insoluble solvent). The oils are then obtained by distillation or evaporation of the solvent-phenylnitroalkene solution.

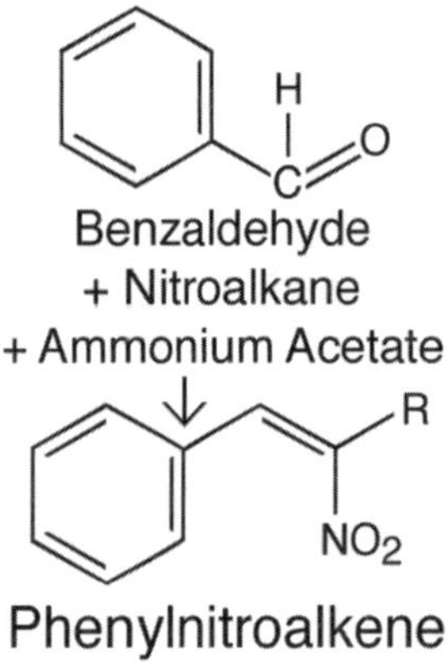

Benzaldehyde
+ Nitroalkane
+ Ammonium Acetate

Phenylnitroalkene

The phenylnitroalkene is purified by recrystallization. Phenylnitroalkene is dissolved in a minimum quantity of ethanol, methanol or acetic acid and then cooled to crystallize the product (this may take several hours in the refrigerator or freezer). Some products may not crystallize and will remain as oils. Yields are approximately 75% plus.

Nitroalkane	Product
Nitromethane	ß-Nitrostyrene (R = H)
Nitroethane	Phenyl-2-nitropropene (R = CH3)
1-Nitropropane	Phenyl-2-nitro-1-butene (R = CH2CH3)

Starting Molecules: Benzaldehyde & nitroethane
Pdct.: 1-Phenyl-2-nitropropene References: Hass 1950; Gairaud 1952.

Starting Molecules: Benzaldehyde & nitropropane
Product: 1-Phenyl-2-nitro-1-butene Reference: Hass 1950

Starting Molecules: 4-Bromo-2,5-dimethoxybenzaldehyde & nitroethane
Prdct: 1-(4-Bromo-2,5-dimethoxyphenyl)-2-nitropropene-1
References: (Barfknecht, 1970; 1971) (Nichols 1970)

Starting Molecules: 2-Bromo-4,5-dimethoxybenzaldehyde & nitroethane
Product: 1-(2-Bromo-4,5-dimethoxyphenyl)-2-nitropropene-1
References: (Barfknecht 1970) (Sepulveda 1972)

Starting Molecules: 4-Bromo-3,5-dimethoxybenzaldehyde & nitroethane
Product: 1-(4-Bromo-3,5-dimethoxyphenyl)-2-nitropropene-1
References: (Barfknecht 1971) (Sepulveda 1972)

Starting Molecules: 5-Bromo-2,4-dimethoxybenzaldehyde & nitroethane
Product: 1-(5-Bromo-2,4-dimethoxyphenyl)-2-nitropropene-1 Reference: (Sepulveda 1972)

Starting Molecules: 2-Bromo-5-methoxybenzaldehyde & nitroethane
Product: 1-(2-Bromo-5-methoxyphenyl)-2-nitropropene-1 Reference: (Barfknecht 1970)

Starting Mols.: 3-Bromo-5-methoxybenzaldehyde & nitroethane
Product: 1-(3-Bromo-5-methoxyphenyl)-2-nitropropene-1 Reference: (Barfknecht 1970)

Starting Mols.: 4-Bromo-3-methoxybenzaldehyde & nitroethane
Product: 1-(4-Bromo-3-methoxyphenyl)-2-nitropropene-1 Reference: (Barfknecht 1970)

Starting Molecules: 2-Bromo-4,5-methylenedioxybenzaldehyde & nitroethane
Product:1-(2-Bromo-4,5-methylenedioxyphenyl)-2-nitropropene-1 Ref.: (Sepulveda 1972)

Starting Molecules: 2,5-Dimethoxybenzaldehyde & nitroethane
Product: 1-(2,5-Dimethoxyphenyl)-2-nitropropene-1
References: (Coutts 1973) (Bollinger 1962) (Merck & Co. 1962)

Starting Molecules: 2,4-Dimethoxybenzaldehyde & nitromethane
Product: 2,4-Dimethoxy-ß-nitrostyrene References:(Kondo 1928) (Gairaud 1952)

Starting Molecules: 3,4-Dimethoxybenzaldehyde & nitroethane
Product: 1-(3,4-Dimethoxyphenyl)-2-nitropropene-1 Reference: (Gairaud 1952)

Starting Molecules: 3,4-Dimethoxybenzaldehyde & nitromethane
Product: 3,4-Dimethoxy-ß-nitrostyrene   Reference: (Gairaud 1952)

Starting Molecules: 2,5-Dimethoxy-4-ethylbenzaldehyde & nitroethane
Product: 1-(2,5-Dimethoxy-4-ethylphenyl)-2-nitropropene-1 Reference: (Nichols 1973)

Starting Mols.: 2,5-Dimethoxy-4-methylbenzaldehyde & 1-nitropropane
Product: 1-(2,5-Dimethoxy-4-methyl-phenyl)-2-nitro-1-butene Reference: (Standridge 1976)

Starting Molecules: 2,5-Dimethoxy-p-tolualdehyde & nitromethane
Product: 2,5-Dimethoxy-4-methyl-ß-nitrostyrene Reference: (Ho 1970)

Starting Molecules: 4-Methoxybenzaldehyde & nitromethane
Product: 4-Methoxy-ß-nitrostyrene
References.: (Kondo 1928) (Gairaud 1952)

Starting Molecules: 3-Methoxy-4-ethoxybenzaldehyde & nitromethane
Product: 3-Methoxy-4-ethoxy-ß-nitrostyrene
Reference: (Kondo 1928)

Starting Molecules: 2,3,4,5-Tetramethoxybenzaldehyde & nitromethane
Product: 2,3,4,5-Tetramethoxy-ß-nitrostyrene
Reference: (Benington 1955)

Starting Molecules: 2,3,4,6-Tetramethoxybenzaldehyde & nitromethane
Product: 2,3,4,6-Tetramethoxy-ß-nitrostyrene
Reference: (Benington 1955)

Starting Molecules: 2,4,6-Trimethoxy-benzaldehyde & nitromethane
Product: 2,4,6-Trimethoxy-ß-nitrostyrene
Reference: (Benington 1953)

Phenyl-2-nitropropenes from Propenylbenzenes

A solution is made with a mixture of 14 grams (192 mmoles) of sodium nitrite mixed with 9 grams (144 mmoles) of either ethylene glycol or propylene glycol in 20 mL. of water. 48 mmoles of propenyl-benzene are mixed with 150 ethyl acetate and added to the solution. 18 grams (72 mmoles) of iodine are added at 0° C. The mixture is then stirred for 2 days under nitrogen. The solution is extracted (separated) using ethyl acetate. The ethyl acetate solution is repeatedly washed with water and then aqueous 10% thiosulfate and aqueous saturated sodium chloride solution. The washed ethyl acetate solution is dried with magnesium sulfate and evaporated to leave the crude phenyl-2-nitropropene which can be purified by chromatography or fractional crystallization. Yields are approximately 80% theoretical. References: Jew 1986, Sy 1985

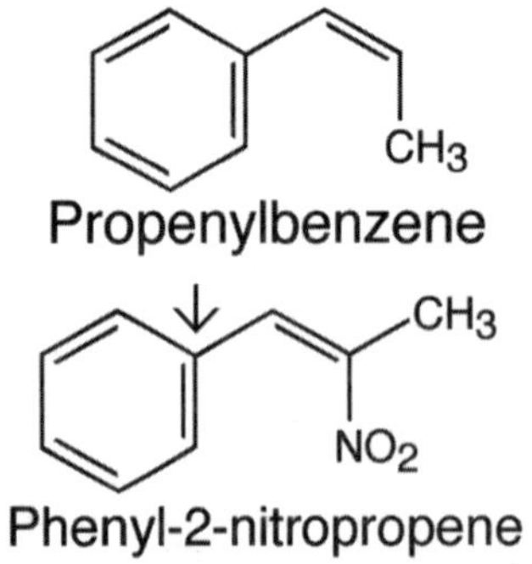

Propenylbenzene

Phenyl-2-nitropropene

Phenyl-2-nitropropenes from Pseudonitrosites

Method A: Propenylbenzene pseudonitrosite (0.25 mole) is dissolved in 430 mL of 8% alcoholic potassium hydroxide by gentle heating (maximum of 25 degrees) and shaking. 1.1 Kilograms of ice is added, acidified with 720 mL of dilute hydrochloric acid and placed in an ice bath for one-half hour. The precipitate is filtered by suction, washed with water, dried in a vacuum desiccator over calcium chloride, giving 0.2 mole of substituted phenyl-2-nitropropene.

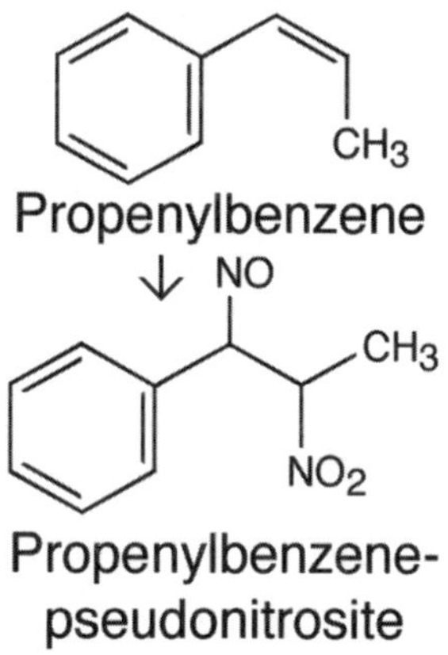

The mixture should not be heated at a high temperature because substantial amounts of substituted benzaldehyde will be obtained as a by product. The longer the time of reaction, or at a high temperature will result in more by product being obtained.

Example: One mole of pseudonitrosite, at boiling temperature, will produce 0.4 moles of substituted phenyl-2-nitropropene and 0.48 moles of substituted benzaldehyde. This is a very poor yield.

Caution! Reactions give off toxic fumes!

Starting Mol.: 2,4,5-Trimethoxypropenylbenzene pseudonitrosite
Product: 2,4,5-Trimethoxyphenyl-2-nitropropene Reference: (Bruckner 1933)

Method B: Substituted propenylbenzene pseudonitrosite (0.25 mole), 430 mL ether and 2.2 liters of 30% aqueous potassium hydroxide are warmed at 20 degrees for three hours. The ether layer is then concentrated, and the residue recrystallized from alcohol to give 0.20 moles of the substituted phenyl-2-nitropropene.

Starting Molecule: 2-Methoxypropenylbenzene pseudonitrosite
Product: 2-Methoxyphenyl-2-nitropropene   Reference: (Horii 1957)

Method C: Substituted propenylbenzene pseudonitrosite (0.25 mole) is slowly added to a refluxing mixture of 1.5 liters anhydrous ethanol and 150 mL of ammonia saturated ethanol. The mixture is cooled to 0 degrees, and poured into 5.5 liters cold water which precipitates the substituted phenyl-2-nitropropene. The nitropropene is collected by suction filtration, washed with water and dried in a vacuum desiccator over calcium chloride.

Starting Molecule: Anethole pseudonitrosite
Prduct: ß-Nitro-anethole; 1-(4-Methoxyphenyl)-2-nitropropene-1
Reference: (Dessi 1952)

Pseudonitrosites
From Substituted Propenylbenzenes

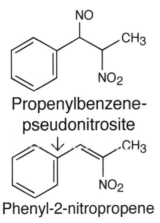

Propenylbenzene-pseudonitrosite

Phenyl-2-nitropropene

Substituted propenylbenzene (0.25 moles) in 280 mL ether is combined with 75 grams of sodium nitrite in 150 mL of water. The mixture is stirred at approximately 0 degrees while 270 mL 20% sulfuric acid is added dropwise and stirred for one more hour at no higher than 5 degrees. The solution is kept cold to precipitate the pseudonitrosite which is collected by suction filtration. The pseudonitrosite is washed with ether, water and ethanol to give 0.20 to 0.23 moles of propenyl-benzene pseudonitrosite.

Starting Molecule: Anethole; 4-Methoxypropenylbenzene
Product:Anethole pseudonitrosite
References: (Dessi 1952) (Krámli 1937)

Starting Molecule (Common Name) ß-Asarone
(Chemical Name) 2,4,5-Trimethoxypropenylbenzene
Product: Asarone pseudonitrosite   Reference: (Rao 1937)

Starting Molecule: 2,5-Dimethoxypropenylbenzene
Product: 2,5-Dimethoxypropenylbenzene pseudonitrosite
Reference: (Govindachari 1953)

Starting Molecule (Common Name): Isoelemicin
(Chemical Name): 3,4,5-Trimethoxypropenylbenzene
Product: Isoelemicin pseudonitrosite   Ref.: (Sugasawa 1937)

Starting Molecule: 2-Methoxypropenylbenzene
Product: 2-Methoxypropenylbenzene pseudonitrosite
Reference: (Horii 1957)

Starting Molecule: 6-Methyl-isosafrole
Product: 6-Methyl-isosafrole pseudonitrosite
Reference: (Sugasawa 1954)

Preparation of Phenylnitropropanols
by Nagayoshi Nagai

In a closed vessel, a mixture of benzaldehyde and nitroethane in equi-molecular proportions is agitated for several hours at room temperature in the presence of a small quantity of a solution of inorganic or organic weak alkaline substances, such as alkali metal-carbonates, bicarbonates, phosphates, or pyridine etc. To separate the condensation product form the two unaffected substances, benzaldehyde and nitroethane, the whole body of material is extracted with ether, and the ether solution separated from the aqueous layer is washed with water and being mixed with a concentrated solution of sodium bisulphite is vigorously shaken. In this way the unchanged benzaldehyde combines with sodium bisulphite and the compound formed dissolving in the aqueous solution present, the ether solution is separated from the bisulphite solution by means of a separating funnel. The ether solution is then washed with water and the ether is distilled off. This distillation is continued in a vacuum to remove the remainder of nitroethane thus leaving the condensation product in the form of an oily mass. The mass, phenylnitropropanol, is then dissolved in a sufficient quantity of dilute alcohol and reduced in the presence of formic aldehyde (formaldehyde) solution in the molecular quantity proportion at as low a temperature as possible by adding the necessary quantity of dilute acetic acid and zinc dust thereto. The acid liquid is filtered from the remaining zinc and... (is processed as known in the art). Source: Nagai 1918

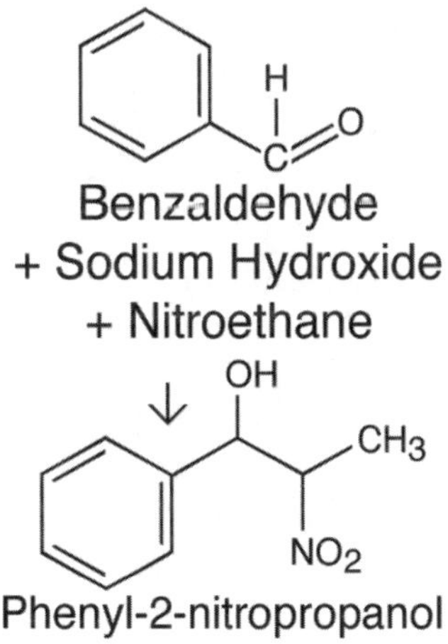

Benzaldehyde
+ Sodium Hydroxide
+ Nitroethane

Phenyl-2-nitropropanol

Manufacture of Phenyl-2-nitropropanol
by Jonas Kamlet

10.7 kilograms of technical benzaldehyde is vigorously agitated with a solution of 11.0 kilograms of sodium bisulphite in 50.0 liters of water until the formation of the addition-product is complete. Simultaneously, 8.25 kilograms of nitroethane is dissolved in a solution of 4.5 kilograms of caustic soda in 20.0 liters of water and the resultant warm solution is added, with vigorous stirring to the magma of benzaldehyde sodium bisulphite. the mixtures is agitated for thirty minutes and then allowed to stand overnight.

The aqueous portion of the mixture is now siphoned off from the supernatant layer of oily phenylnitropropanol, and replaced with a fresh solution of 11.0 kilograms of sodium bisulphite in 50.0 liters of water. The mixture of phenylnitropropanol and bisulphite solution is now vigorously agitated for fifteen minutes in order to remove and recover small amounts of unreacted benzaldehyde, and is then again allowed to stratify. This time, the phenylnitropropanol is siphoned off and filtered to remove a small amount of resinous material. The aqueous solution of sodium bisulphite remaining behind is reacted with benzaldehyde, as described above, thus making the process continuous.

The 1-phenyl-2-nitropropanol thus obtains is a colorless oil, specific gravity 1.14 at 20° C., odorless with pure, volatile with steam and boiling at 150°-165° C. under a pressure of 5 mm. of mercury. It is soluble in alcohol, ether, acetone, chloroform, carbon tetrachloride, benzene and glacial acetic acid.

The yield of 1-phenyl-2-nitropropanol obtained by this procedure is 17.1 to 17.7 kilograms. On reduction in the presence of formaldehyde, it forms *dl*-ephedrine. Source: Kamlet 1939

Starting Molecules: Anisaldehyde & nitromethane
Product: 1-(p-Methoxyphenyl)-2-nitroethanol Reference: (Jacob 1951)

Starting Molecules: Benzaldehyde & nitroethane Product: 2-Nitro-1-phenyl-1-propanol
Refs.: (Hoover 1947) (Kamlet 1939) (Kanao 1927; 1929) (Nagai 1929) (Vanderbilt 1940)

Starting Molecules: Benzaldehyde & nitroethane & formaldehyde
Product: 2-Methyl-2-nitro-1-phenyl-1-propanol Reference: (Nagai 1929)

Starting Molecules: p-Ethoxybenzaldehyde & nitromethane
Product: 1-(p-Ethoxyphenyl)-2-nitroethanol
Reference: (Jacob 1951)

Starting Mols.: 3,4,5-Trimethoxybenzaldehyde & nitromethane
Product: 1-(3,4,5-Trimethoxyphenyl)-2-nitroethanol
Reference: (Heacock 1961)

----

d,l-threo-1-(Acetoxy-phenyl)-2-nitropropane From Propenylbenzene

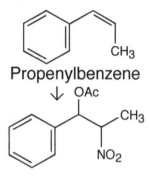

Propenylbenzene

0.5 Mole of substituted propenylbenzene is mixed with 120 mL of acetic anhydride. The solution is stirred at 0 degrees for over 3 hours into 45 mL of 70% nitric acid containing 180 mL of acetic anhydride. The entire mixture is poured on ice, extracted with ether and distilled to give *d,l-threo*-1-(acetoxy-phenyl)-2-nitropropane.

Starting Molecule: Anethole
Product: alpha-(4-Methoxyphenyl)-ß-nitropropanol acetate
Reference: (Kramli 1937)

Starting Molecule: 2-Methoxypropenylbenzene
Product: *alpha*-(2-Methoxyphenyl)-ß-nitropropanol acetate
Reference: (Horii 1957)

Starting Molecule: Propenylbenzene
Product: *dl-threo*-1-(Acetoxy-phenyl)-2-nitropropane Refs.: (Drefahl 1958) (Fodor 1948)

ß-Nitropropenylbenzenes from phenyl-ß-nitropropanol acetate:
(Drefahl 1958; Horii 1957; Kramli 1937; Sugasawa 1937; 1957).

Preparation of Sodium Nitrite

Pb (lead) + $NaNO_3$ (sodium nitrite) forms
PbO (lead oxide) + $NaNO_2$ (sodium nitrite)

One part of sodium nitrate is fused with approximately 2.5 parts of lead. The sodium nitrite that is formed is composed of approximately 3 times its weight in litharge.

Sodium nitrate mp 308° C, sodium nitrite mp 271° C, decomposes above 320° C., lead mp 327.4° C, and the litharge which forms, melts at approximately at 880° C.

The reaction apparatus has been described as a long handled lead melting ladle, 6 in. in diameter.   This can be held with a clamp. The bowl is held on a strong retort ring. (Do not use porcelain). The ladle is heated with a Bunsen burner, and stirred with spatula with a long blade. The reaction product is obtained in two layers, one a mixture of lead and sodium nitrate and the other a thick pasty composition of largely litharge and sodium nitrite.

180 grams of sodium nitrite are heated to reaction temperature, 400°-450° C. The temperature is continuously checked with a thermocouple protected by a sheath of Pyrex tubing. Small amounts of lead are added to a total of at least 450 grams. The reaction occurs quickly on the surface and mixture must be completely and continuously mixed as it takes place. The lead forms globules and must be mixed to make sure that the bottom layers of reaction do not over heat. This heating and stirring are continued for at least 60 minutes.

The mixture is then cooled a little. Water is added and stirred into the mixture to dissolve all clumps of chemicals that are formed and allowed to settle.

The strongly caustic liquid is decanted from the mixture. CO_2 is bubbled through the liquid to free the lead from the solution. The solution is slowly neutralized by adding a dilute solution of nitric acid which decomposes some of the sodium nitrite (red fumes).

(Caution! Fumes are toxic! Nitric acid can cause serious burns!)

A more productive way of doing this is to add low nitrite containing liquors or crystals. Then the dilute nitric acid is slowly added to neutralize the solution. Nitric acid fumes are formed, but are released through the alkaline solution. The solution is evaporated in several porcelain evaporating dishes.

The reaction forms a mixture composed of sodium nitrate and sodium nitrite. The first crystals formed during the evaporation are more concentrated with sodium nitrite, as the evaporation is continued, the sodium nitrite concentration decreases with an increase in sodium nitrate being crystallized. Smaller crops of crystals produce higher concentrations of sodium nitrite.

It is more economical to make sure that the reaction (fusion) is allowed to be as complete as possible instead of depending on fractional crystallization.

The evaporating dishes are heated to boiling temperature (up to approximately 120° C) and a crust will form. On cooling, crystals are formed which appear as fine needles, leaflets and prisms. As nitrite is not oxidized in the solution, mixed crystals are not formed. A magnifying glass is used to see if there is an increased concentration of cubical sodium nitrate crystals.

Determination of sodium nitrite concentration can be done by permanganate titration.

First crops of crystals are usually 85 to 95% sodium nitrite. Following crops decrease in sodium nitrite concentration and can be recycled to increase nitrite concentration.

Low grade crystals are fused again with appropriate proportion of lead to increase first crop yields of sodium nitrite. In fact, it is much easier to do this as less lead oxide is formed during the fusion, the mixture is more fluid which allows the fusion reaction mixture to be stirred easier.

The following are examples on recycling low grade sodium nitrite residues:

300 grams of residues, 62% nitrite, 290 grams lead.
1st crop, 40 grams of 95%
2nd crop, 60 grams of 96%
3rd crop, 90 grams of 86%

100 grams of residues, 54% nitrite, 175 grams lead.
1st crop, 30 grams of 93%
2nd crop, 19 grams of 85%
3rd crop, 28 grams of 82%

Recrystallization.

200 grams of (about) 88% nitrite content.
1st crop, 80 grams of 96%
Residue: 120 grams of 85%

405 grams of about 81% nitrite content.
1st crop, 160 grams of 93%
2nd crop, 110 grams of 79%
3rd crop, 55 grams of 74%

References: Cooke 1944; Mellor 1928; Oswald 1914; Pelet, Shields 1949, Turner 1915; Vanion 1925; Wachter 1943.

Manufacture of Sodium Nitrite

by Gilbert T. Morgan

J. Soc. Chem. Ind., 27, 483-5 (May 30) - The author reviews various methods for the production of nitrite from nitrate by reduction with metals (see C.A. 1908, 1330). The non-metal, sulphur, has been used with success by Messers, Read, Holiday & Sons. The mixture of nitrate, sulphur and caustic alkali is fused in open pans, fitted with stirring gear. The following reaction takes place: $3NaNO_3 + S + 2NaOH = Na_2SO_4 + 3NaNO_2 + H_2O$. The hot, fused product is added to sufficient warm water to dissolve the whole of the nitrite, leaving most of the sulphate behind in a granular condition. The nitrite is filtered through vacuum filter and crystallized in fractions from the small amount of dissolved sulphate. Product is good nitrite, and troublesome by-products are eliminated. Source: Morgan 1909

Preparation of Ether from Ethanol
by James F. Norris

Caution-Ether is very inflammable and very volatile; as its vapor readily ignites, vessels containing ether should not be brought near a flame or allowed to stay in a warm place. Place 50 cc. of ethyl alcohol in a 500 cc. distilling flask and add slowly, with constant shaking, 50 cc. of concentrated sulphuric acid. Close the neck of the flask with a two-holed stopper bearing a thermometer and a dropping funnel, both of which reach to the bottom of the flask. Place the flask on a sand-bath and connect it by means of a tightly fitting stopper with a long condenser, through which a rapid stream of cold water is passing. Use as a receiver a filter-bottle which is connected with a long condenser, through which a rapid stream of cold water is passing. Use as a receiver a filter-bottle which is connected with the condenser by a tightly fitting stopper. Attach to the side-arm of the filter-bottle a long rubber tube, which extends almost to the floor. This tube serves to conduct the vapor of the ether, which is very heavy, away from any flames present on the desk. Heat the contents of the flask slowly. When the temperature reaches 140° C. and the ether distills over, add through the funnel 100 cc. of alcohol, allowing the latter to drop at about the same rate as that at which the ether distills over, add through the funnel 100 cc. of alcohol, allowing the latter to drop at about the same rate as that at which the ether distills over, add at about the same rate as that at which the ether distills (about 2 drops per second). During the entire time the temperature of the mixture in the flask should be maintained at 140° - 145° C.

Take the receiver from the immediate vicinity of any flames, and transfer the contents to a separatory funnel. Shake the ether with about one-fourth its volume of a solution of sodium hydroxide. Draw off the lower aqueous layer, which should still be alkaline, add to the ether about one-fifth its volume of a cold mixture of equal volumes of concentrated sulphuric acid and water. Shake thoroughly, let the mixture stand until the two layers become clear. Draw off the acid layer and run the ether into a distilling flask. Distill from a water-bath, and collect the distillate in a receiver in the way described above. Record the boiling point and the weight of the product obtained.

Ether boils at 35° C. Source: Norris 1924

Preparation of Ether
by W.R. Orndorff

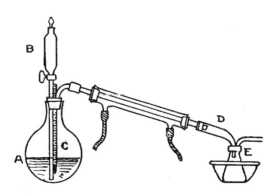

A is a round-bottomed, wide-necked flask of 2 liters' capacity.

B is a cylindrical separating-funnel reaching to the bottom of A.

C, a short thermometer, the bulb of which must dip below the surface of the liquid.

D, an adapter which is connected with the receiver by a doubly bored stopper.

E, a receiver, which must be surrounded with a freezing mixture (ice and salt).

Into the flask A put a cooled mixture of 325 grams of concentrated sulphuric acid and 170 grams of alcohol (95%). Heat the mixture in the flask A until the temperature reaches 140° C. Then cautiously open the stopcock of the separating-funnel and let a slow stream of alcohol in the form of vapor bubble through the liquid, regulating the flow of the alcohol so that the temperature of the mixture is kept as nearly 140° C. as possible (not below 140° and not above 145°). When 250 grams of alcohol have been run in, the operation is stopped. The distillate consists of two layers, and contains, besides ether, water, alcohol, and sulphurous acid. The watery layer is removed by means of a liter separating-funnel, and the ether is washed first with dilute caustic soda solution, then two or three times with small quantities of distilled water.

(Drying the ether). The washed ether is now treated with one-half its weight of fused calcium chloride, and distilled on a water-bath through a Hempel or Vigreux distilling-tube, taking care that the temperature does not rise above 50° C. The distillate must be kept cold by ice-water.   Source: Orndorff 1913

CHAPTER 12: PREPARATION OF KETONES

Phenyl-2-Propanone From Phenylacetic Acid

This is the most popular synthesis of phenyl-2-propanone. The reaction can be used to produce other ketones other than P-2-P, e.g. acetophenone can be produced in similar yields from benzoic acid. The phenyl-2-propanone or other ketones are obtained from the reaction mixture by fractional distillation to remove diketone impurities.

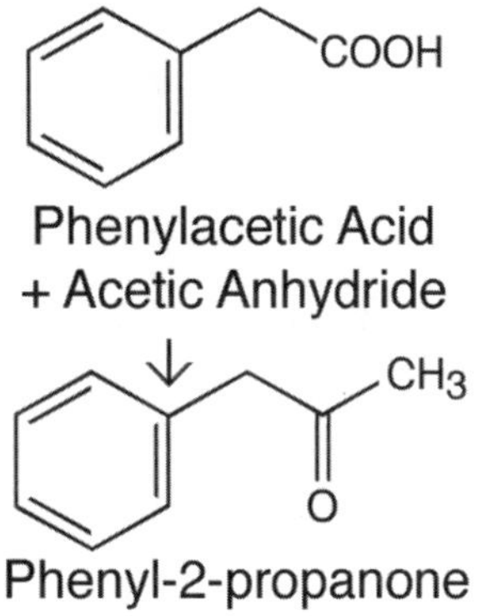

0.5 Mole of phenyl acetic acid is refluxed at 140 to 150 degrees for 18 hours with 115 grams of acetic anhydride and 35 grams of sodium acetate. Approximately 0.4 mole of phenyl-2-propanone can be obtained by fractional distillation. Phenyl-2-propanone distills between 210-215 degrees at atmospheric pressure.

COOH

Phenylacetic Acid + Acetic Anhydride

CH3

O

Phenyl-2-propanone

Starting Molecule: Benzoic Acid and Acetic Anhydride
Product: Acetophenone Reference: Adams 1924

Starting Molecule: Phenyl Acetic Acid and Acetic Anhydride
Product: Phenyl-2-propanone Reference: Magidson 1941

----

p-Methoxyphenyl-2-propanone Reference: (Fusco 1948)
See Bodranskii; Percy; Zaputryaev; for P-2-P from acetoacetonitrile.
See Allen 1992 for extensive review of phenyl-2-propanone syntheses.

Phenyl-2-propanone Using Pyridine

2 Moles of phenyl acetic acid are mixed and refluxed for 6 hours with 100 mL. of acetic anhydride and 100 mL. of pyridine. Carbon dioxide is rapidly formed during the first of the reaction.

The solvent is removed, the residue dissolved in benzene and 10% sodium hydroxide is added. The benzene layer is separated and distilled. The benzene is distilled off and then the phenyl-2-propanone (56% yield) is distilled followed by phenylhydrazone and then diphenylacetone (24% yield). Reference: King 1951

Dehydrocarboxylation of Carboxylic Acids to Form Phenyl-2-propanone

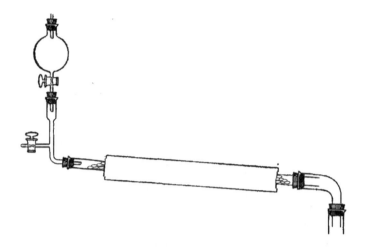

The dehydrocarboxylation of two carboxylic acids to produce ketones has been used for almost a century. It is used both for industrial production and laboratory scale synthesis. The basic reaction involves the vaporization of a mixture of carboxylic acids over a catalyst to form the ketone. The apparatus is composed of a thermocouple or pyrometer, wrapped with asbestos or heat resistant cloth, heated by a heating coil (eg. nichrome wire no. 30, heating tape) and insulated with more heat resistant cloth. Pyrex, iron and steel have been used for reaction tubes.

A gentle stream of an inert gas such as nitrogen or argon is run through the apparatus. The end products are condensed and then the catalyst is washed with acetic acid. The end products and acetic acid wash are mixed; water and ice are added and made slightly alkaline with 50% sodium hydroxide. The oily layer is separated and the aqueous layer is extracted with benzene. The benzene extract and the oil are combined, the benzene is distilled off and then the ketone is fractionally distilled. The yields are from 60 to 70%. Many different ketones can be produced using this apparatus. Phenyl-2-propanone is produced when phenylacetic acid and acetic acid are used.

References: Herbst 1943; Cowan 1940

Phenyl-2-propanone can also be obtained by the dehydration of ethylene alcohols, see Grignard 1926.

Gas Phase Production of Phenyl-2-propanone from Phenyl Acetic Acid and Acetic Acid

by Noboru Saito

... in a gas phase in the presence of a catalyst containing at least either of MgO and CaO. The process allows for production of an intended ketone at a high yield at high productivity...

As an example of the process for synthesis of ketone from carboxylic acid by gas-phase catalytic reaction, there is reported, in *Organic Synthesis*, Vol. II, p. 389 (1943), a process for synthesis of phenylacetone from phenylacetic acid and acetic acid using ThO_2 (catalyst). The process, however, is difficult to carry out in industry because the thorium compound used as a catalyst is radioactive and its handling is restricted...

The gas-phase catalytic reaction aimed at by the present invention is a decarboxylation reaction. It is generally thought that since an alkaline earth metal oxide generally becomes an alkaline earth metal carbonate in a decarboxylation reaction, MgO or CaO is unusable as a catalyst in the reaction. In the present process, however, MgO and CaO can both act as a catalyst by setting the reaction temperature at 250° C. or above (when a MgO-containing catalyst is used) and at 450° C or above (when a CaO-containing catalyst is used). For example, when a reaction is conducted at a temperature of 450° C. or above using CaO as a catalyst, at the initial stage of the reaction, a ketone is formed but no CO_2 is formed because part of CaO is converted to $CaCO_3$. However, after this reaction has been continued for 1 hour or more and a CaO-$CaCO_3$ decomposition equilibrium has been reached, a ketone is formed by the catalysis of the CaO moiety and CO_2 is formed simultaneously. Interestingly, BaO, although being an alkaline earth metal oxide, shows no catalysis in the present process. The reason is that since $BaCO_3$ has a high decomposition equilibrium temperature of 1,450° C. at 1 atm., BaO is completely converted to $BaCO_3$ at a reaction temperature of, for example, 500° C. or below.

The catalyst used in the present process is not restricted to a catalyst containing at least either of MgO and CaO, and may be one obtained by adding, to the catalyst, P_2O_5, Sb_2O_3, ZnO, Fe_2O_3, SnO_2, CuO, an alkali metal oxide or the like in order to adjust the acidity or basicity of the catalyst. The catalyst of the present invention is used by loading the catalyst on a powdery carrier (e.g. SiC, alumina or diatomaceous earth) or on a cylindrical, spherical, ring-shaped or crushed carrier, or by molding the catalyst itself into pellets or other form.

The catalysts used in Examples and Comparative Examples were obtained by molding MgO or CaO (each of special grade quality) or its mixture with the above-mentioned additive (this was as necessary added for acidity or basicity adjustment) and grinding the resulting molding into 10-24 mesh. 8 cc of each ground catalyst was filled in a stainless steel tube having an inside diameter of 10 mm. The stainless steel tube was then immersed in a molten salt to set the tube at an intended reaction temperature. From the inlet of the tube and through the tube was passed a vapor of a raw material carboxylic acid(s) together with nitrogen as a carrier gas (flow rate=480 ml/min) at 1 atm. to give rise to a gas-phase catalytic reaction. The reaction mixture gas containing a reaction product and an unreacted carboxylic acid(s) was analyzed by gas chromatography using FID as a detector.

MgO was used as a catalyst. A material gas consisting of 5-22% by volume of phenyl acetic acid (2 parts) and glacial acetic acid (20 parts) and 95-78% by volume of nitrogen as a carrier gas was passed at a gas hourly space velocity (GHSV) of 3,700 hr.-1 or more (e.g. 4615 hr.-1 GHSV) and subjected to a reaction at 440° C. The conversion of carboxylic acid was 80.1%; the yield of ketones formed was 68.2%; and the selectivity of intended ketone, i.e. phenyl-2-propanone was 85.1%.
Source: Saito 1998

Preparation of P-2-P Using Magnesia
By Albert C. Zettlemoyer et al.

A mixture of phenyl acetic acid and acetic acid in a mol. ratio of 1 to 5 was vaporized, preheated and passed through a reaction zone containing an active magnesium oxide supported on pumice, The said magnesia having an iodine number of 130 and an ignition loss of 7 at a velocity of 0.36 liter/liter of catalyst hour. The product then obtained was then treated to recover the phenyl acetone by neutralizing any unreacted acid with a solution of sodium bicarbonate and then separating the oil and water layers. The oil layer was then fractionated and the fraction collected between 210° and 230° C., This product being the phenyl acetone. The amount collected represented 70% conversion of the phenyl acetic acid.

The supported catalyst may be satisfactorily obtained by soaking a volume of the pumice or other carrier in an equal volume of magnesium nitrate for a period of 30 minutes with constant agitation. At the end of this period the liquid is decanted and the magnesium hydroxide is precipitated on the surface of the carrier by the addition of ammonium hydroxide. The resulting mass is dried at 110° C and then activated by heating the same in a reactor over night at an elevated temperature of 300°-400° C in the presence of a slow stream of nitrogen passed over the same. Source: Zettlemoyer (1952 Ref.: Potapov 1958.

Preparation of Manganous Oxide Catalyst

Manganous carbonate is precipitated from manganous chloride and sodium carbonate.   Small pieces of pumice (3-8 mesh) are mixed with a water slurry of manganous carbonate. Only enough water is used to absorb onto the pumice, too much and the carbonate will not be absorbed. The mix is heated and stirred till lumps do not stick to each other. Overheating can be a problem.

The manganous carbonate pumice is activated by packing in the tube furnace, running a slow stream of nitrogen through the apparatus and heating to 400-450° C. for 8 hours. The carbonate is transformed into the oxide catalyst and allowed to cool. Reference: Cowan 1940

Benzyl-Methyl-Ketone Preparation Using Manganese Dioxide

by Les Usines De Melle

Into a vigorously stirred bath maintained at a temperature of 335° C. and compound of 550 cc's of a Pennsylvania paraffin oil having a distillation range of from 220° to 400° C. at a pressure of 5 mm. Hg. and which 20% distills between 260° and 320° C. in which is suspended 25 grams of manganese dioxide there is slowly fed a liquid mixture of 65 grams of acetic acid and 50 grams of phenylacetic acid. The distillate which is obtained is condensed and fractionally distilled, there being obtained 50% of the theoretical yield of acetone and 47% of the theoretical yield of benzyl-methyl-ketone.

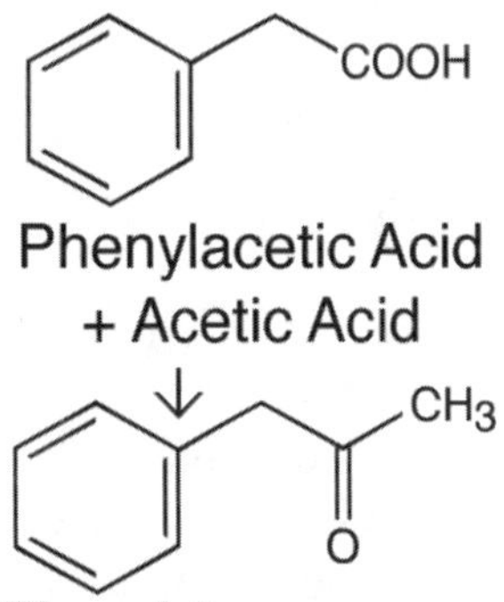

COOH

Phenylacetic Acid
+ Acetic Acid

CH₃

O

Phenyl-2-propanone

Source: Les Usines De Melle1946

Preparation of Propiophenone
from Benzoic Acid and Propionic Acid

by Charles A. Smith et al.

The reactor used for the preparation of propiophenone in accordance with this invention consisted of a reactor fabricated from 1-inch by 48-inch stainless steel pipe, insulated and electrically heated. Temperatures were determined at four points by thermocouples positioned in a 1/4" thermowell which extended through the entire length of the reactor.

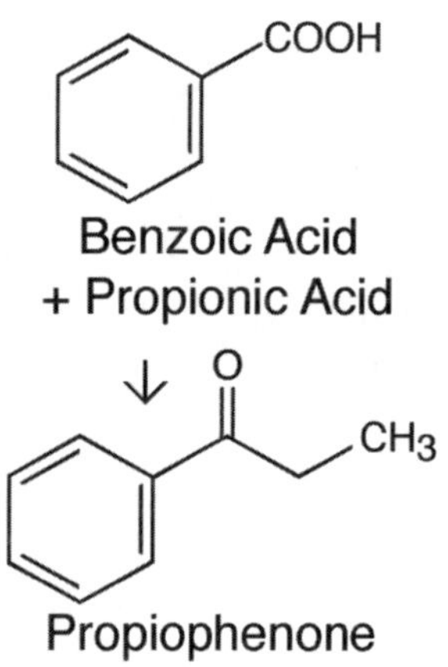

Benzoic Acid
+ Propionic Acid

Propiophenone

Reactants were fed, via a small diaphram pump from a calibrated feed tank through a steam-jacketed line to the top of the reactor. The feed tank and pump were warmed by infrared heat lamps to prevent crystallization of benzoic acid.

The catalyst bed consisted of two layers. A 13" bed of inert material in the top end of the vertically oriented reactor served as a preheat section. The bottom 31" consisted of calcium acetate on alumina.

Activated alumina (Alcoa F-1 grade, 4-8 mesh) is immersed in a 25 percent aqueous solution of calcium acetate for 2 to 24 hours. The calcium acetate solution is drained off, and most of the excess water adhering to the alumina is removed by vacuum evaporation. The impregnated catalyst is then heated overnight at 500° C. to remove the last traces of water. The amount of calcium impregnated on the catalyst depends on how long the alumina is dipped in the calcium acetate solution and on how many times the procedure is repeated. The catalyst used in these examples contained 2.95 percent calcium by weight (3.87 percent by weight when calculated as calcium oxide).

Using the reactor described above, together with ancillary equipment, a mixture containing 2 moles of propionic acid per mole of benzoic acid was fed to the reactor together with 4 moles of water per mole of benzoic acid at a rate of 249 ml/hr. for 4.5 hours. The reaction temperature was maintained between 445° C. and 450° C. Analysis of the condensed organic layer by gas chromatography indicated that 4.68 pounds of isobutyrophenone were produced per 100 pounds of propiophenone... The instrument used was a Bendix Model 2300 dual column programmed temperature gas chromatograph having a thermal conductivity detector. The bridge current was 200 ma. with a 0-1 mv. recorder. The column consisted of two, 10 feet by 1/8 inch stainless steel tubing packed with silicone on an inert support. The column temperature was 190° C. The carrier gas was helium at 30 cc/minute.

Large Scale Production of Propiophenone

In a plant scale run, a charge consisting of propionic acid, benzoic acid and steam was charged to a vaporizer at a rate of 625 lbs/hr., 375 lbs/hr., and 175 lbs/hr., respectively. This mixture exited from the vaporizer at a temperature of 135° C. The vaporized charge was heated in a preheater to 325° C. and thence to the first of three catalyst bed zones maintained at a temperature of 470° C. The catalyst was calcium acetate on alumina. The stream of reactants and products was led from the first to the second catalyst bed zone maintained at a temperature of 490° C., together with steam at 0 to 25 lbs/hr. The second catalyst zone effluent was passed to the third catalyst bed zone maintained at a temperature of 510° C., together with steam at a rate of 25-50 lbs/hr. Analysis of the organic layer of the product mixture by gas chromatography indicated the following:

> Diethyl ketone -- 43-44%
> Propiophenone -- 54-56%
> Acetophenone -- 0.5-1.0%
> Isobutyrophcnone -- 0-0.15%
> Butyrophenone -- 0
> Source: Smith 1979

Phenyl Acetic Acid Preparation
$$C_6H_5CH_2CN + 2 H_2O + H_2SO_4 \rightarrow C_6H_5CH_2CO_2H + NH_4HSO_4$$

Prepared by Roger Adams and A. F. That:.
Checked by O. Kamm and A. O. Matthews.

1. Procedure
IN a 5-L. round-bottom flask, fitted with a mechanical stirrer and reflux condenser, are mixed 1150 cc. of water, 840 cc. of commercial sulfuric acid and 700 g. of benzyl cyanide. The mixture is heated under a reflux condenser and stirred for three hours, cooled slightly and then poured into 2 L. of cold water. The mixture should be stirred so that a solid cake is not formed; the phenylacetic acid is then filtered off. This crude material should be melted under water and washed by de-

cantation several times with hot water. These washings, on cooling, deposit a small amount of phenylacetic acid which is filtered off and added to the main portion of material. The last of the hot water is poured off from the material while it is still molten and it is then transferred to a 2-L. Claisen distilling flask and distilled in vacuo. A small amount of water comes over first and is rejected; about 20 cc., containing an appreciable amount of benzyl cyanide, then distills. This fraction is used in the next run. The distillate boiling 176-180°/50 mm. is collected separately and solidifies on standing. It is practically pure phenylacetic acid, m. p. 76-76.5°; it amounts to 630 g. (77.5 per cent of the theoretical amount). As the fraction which is returned to the second run of material contains a considerable portion of phenylacetic acid, the yield actually amounts to at least 80 per cent.

For the preparation of small quantities of phenylacetic acid, it is convenient to use the modified method given in the Notes.

2. Notes

The standard directions for the preparation of phenylacetic acid specify that the benzyl cyanide is to be treated with dilute sulfuric acid prepared by adding three volumes of sulfuric acid to two volumes of water. There action, however, goes so vigorously that it is always necessary to have a trap for collecting the benzyl cyanide which is blown out of the apparatus. The use of the more dilute acid, as described in the above directions, is more satisfactory.

The phenylacetic acid may also be made by boiling under a reflux condenser for eight to fifteen hours, without a stirrer, but this method is not nearly so satisfactory as that described in the procedure.

When only small quantities of the acid are required, the following modified procedure is of value. One hundred grams of benzyl cyanide are added to a mixture containing 100 cc. of water, 100 cc. of concentrated sulfuric acid, and 100 cc. of glacial acetic acid. After this has been heated for forty-five minutes under a reflux condenser, the hydrolysis is practically complete. The reaction mixture is then poured into water, and the phenylacetic acid isolated in the usual manner.

The odor of phenylacetic acid is disagreeable and persistent.

3. Other Methods of Preparation

The standard method of preparation of phenylacetic acid is by the hydrolysis of benzyl cyanide with either alkali (1) or acid (2). The acid hydrolysis runs by far the more smoothly and so was the only one studied. There are numerous other ways in which phenylacetic acid has been formed, but none of them is of practical importance for its preparation. These methods include the following: the action of water on phenyl ketene (3); the hydrolysis and subsequent oxidation of the product between benzaldehyde and hippuric acid (4); the reduction of mandelic acid (5); the reduction of benzoylformic acid with hydriodic acid and phosphorus (6); the hydrolysis of benzyl glyoxalidone (7); the fusion of atropic acid with potassium hydroxide (8); the action of alcoholic potash upon chlorophenylacetylene (9); the action of benzoyl peroxide upon phenylacetylene (10); the alkaline hydrolysis of triphenylphloroglucinol (11); the action of ammonium sulfide upon acetophenone (12); the heating of phenylmalonic acid (13); the hydrolysis of phenylacetoacetic ester (14); the action of hydriodic acid upon mandelonitrile (15). Source: Adams 1922

References:
1) *Ann.* 96, 247 (1855); *Ber.* 14, 1645 (1881); *Compt. rend.* 151, 236 (1910).
2) *Ber.* 19, 1950 (1886).
3) *Ber.* 44, 537 (1911).
4) *Ann.* 370, 371 (1909).
5) *Z. Chem.* (2) 1, 443 (1865); *Ber.* 14, 239 (1881).
6) *Ber.* 10, 847 (1877).
7) *J. prakt. Chem.* (2) 82, 52, 58 (1910).
8) *Ann.* 148, 242 (1868).
9) Ann. 308, 318 (1899).
10) *J. Russ. Phys. Chem. Soc.* 42, 1387 (1910); *Chem. Zentr.* 1911 (1) 1279.
11) *Ann.* 378, 263 (1911).
12) *Ber.* 21, 534 (1888); *J. prakt. Chem.* (2) 81, 384 (1910).
13) *Ber.* 27, 1094 (1894).
14) *Ber.* 31, 3163 (1898).
15) Inaugural Dissertation of A. Kohler (1909), Univ. of Bern.

Benzyl Cyanide
$$C6H5CH2Cl+NaCN \rightarrow C6H5CH2CN+NaCl$$

Prepared by Roger Adams and A. F. That:.
Checked by 0. Kamm and A. O. Matthews.

1. Procedure

IN a 5-L. round-bottom flask, fitted with a stopper holding a reflux condenser and separatory funnel, are placed 500 g. of powdered sodium cyanide (96-98 per cent pure) and 450 cc. of water. The mixture is warmed on a water bath in order to dissolve most of the sodium cyanide, and then 1 kg. of benzyl chloride (b.p. 170-180°) mixed with 1 kg. of alcohol is run in through the separatory funnel in the course of one-half to three-quarters of an hour. The mixture is then heated with a reflux condenser on the steam bath for four hours, cooled and filtered with suction to remove most of the sodium chloride. It is well to wash the filtered salt with a small portion of alcohol in order to remove any benzyl cyanide which may have been mechanically held. The flask is now fitted with a condenser, and as much alcohol as possible is distilled off on the steam bath. The residual liquid is cooled, filtered if necessary, and the layer of benzyl cyanide separated. This crude benzyl cyanide is now placed in a Claisen distilling flask and distilled in vacuo, the water and alcohol coming over first, and finally the cyanide. It is advantageous to use a fractionating column or, better still, a Claisen flask with a modified side-arm (1) (Vol. 1, p. 40, Fig. 3) which gives the same effect as a fractionating column. The material is collected from 135-140°/38 mm. (115-120°/10 mm.). The yield is 740-830 g. (80-90 per cent of the theoretical amount).

2. Notes

The quality of the benzyl chloride markedly affects the yield of pure benzyl cyanide. If a poor technical grade is used, the yields will not be more than 60-75 per cent of the theoretical, whereas consistent results of about 85 per cent or more were always obtained when a product was used that boiled over 10°. The technical benzyl chloride at hand yielded on distillation about 8 per cent of high-boiling material; a technical grade from another source was of unusual purity and boiled over a 2° range for the most part.

It is advisable to distill off the last portion of alcohol and water in vacuo and also to distill the benzyl cyanide in vacuo, since under ordinary pressures a white solid invariably separates during the distillation.

One method of purifying the benzyl cyanide is to steam distill it after the alcohol has been first distilled from the reaction mixture. At ordinary pressures, this steam distillation is very slow and, with an ordinary condenser, requires eighteen to twenty hours in order to remove all of the volatile product from a run of 500 g. of benzyl chloride. The distillate separates into two layers; the benzyl cyanide layer is removed and distilled. The product obtained in this way is very pure and contains no tarry material, and, after the excess of benzyl chloride has been removed, boils practically constant. This steam distillation is hardly advisable in the laboratory.

The benzyl cyanide, prepared according to the procedure as outlined, is collected over a 5° range. It varies in appearance from a colorless to a straw-colored liquid and often develops appreciable color upon standing. For a product of special purity, it should be redistilled under diminished pressure and collected over a 1-2° range. For most purposes, such as the preparation of phenylacetic acid or ester, the fraction boiling 135-140°/38 mm. is perfectly satisfactory.

3. Other Methods of Preparation

Benzyl cyanide occurs naturally in certain oils (2). The only feasible method of preparing it that has been described in the literature is the one in which alcoholic potassium cyanide and benzyl chloride (3) are employed. The cheaper sodium cyanide is just as satisfactory as the potassium cyanide and therefore is the best material to use. Gomberg has recently prepared benzyl cyanide from benzyl chloride and an aqueous solution of sodium cyanide (4). Source: Adams 1922

1) *J. Am. Chem. Soc.* 39, 2718 (1917).
2) *Ber.* 7, 519, 1293 (1874); 32, 2337 (1899).
3) *Ann.* 96, 247 (1855); *Ber.* 3, 198 (1870); 14, 1645 (1881); 19, 1950 (1886).
4) *J. Am. Chem. Soc.* 42, 2059 (1920).
References: *Chemical Abstracts* (1947) 41: 6252 c-d;
Chem Abstracts (1948) 42: 2606 b

More Preparations of Phenyl Acetic Acid

Method 1: One mole of benzylmagnesium chloride is added to a dry ice/ether slush. The mixture is shaken frequently to break up any formation of lumps and allowed to warm to 15°. The mixture is decomposed with a dilute solution of sulfuric acid. The crude product is obtained in 40% yields after purification by crystallization from water. Phenylacetic acid mp. 76-77°. Reference: Austin 1932

Method 2: (Modified Willgerodt Reaction)

0.5 mole of acetophenone is mixed with 0.8 mole of sulfur and 60 ml. of morpholine and refluxed for 5-8 hours. The product is slowly poured onto water. The crude phenylacetic acid begins to crystallize and the rest of the mixture is poured onto the water. The crystallized mixture is filtered to leave crude product. The crude phenylacetic acid is ground and mixed with water, filtered again and air dried. Yields range from 45% to 98%. Refs.: Schwenk 1942; Schwenk 1946

0.25 Mole of substituted propiophenone is mixed with 0.4 mole of sulfur, 30 mL of morpholine, refluxed for 8 hours to produce an oily substituted phenylacetothiomorpholide. The phenylacetothiomorpholide is mixed with 250 mL of 10% alcoholic sodium hydroxide and then refluxed for a total of 6 hours. An equal volume of water is added, the alcohol is evaporated. The solution is then acidified to Congo Red paper with hydrochloric acid and extracted with ether. The ether is evaporated to leave a residue of substituted hydrocinnamic acid. Yields 60 to 98%

Starting Molecules: *p*-Bromoacetophenone
Reagents: Sulfur, Morpholine, Sodium Hydroxide, Ether
Product: *p*-Bromo-phenylacetic Acid Reference: (Schwenk 1942)

Starting Molecules: 2,5-Dimethoxyacetophenone
Reagents: Sulfur, Morpholine, Sodium Hydroxide, Ether
Product: 2,5-Dimethoxy-phenylacetic Acid Reference: (Schwenk 1942)

Starting Molecules: *p*-Methoxyacetophenone
Reagents: Sulfur, Morpholine, Water
Product: *p*-Methoxyphenyl Acetic Acid Reference: (Schwenk; 1942; 1946)

Method 3: One mole of ethylbenzene is mixed with one mole of sodium chromate dihydrate and 200 mL. of water. The mixture is rapidly heated to 275° in a rocking autoclave for 60 minutes and then cooled, filtered to remove green inorganic precipitate.   The filtrate is extracted with ether to remove ethylbenzene. The aqueous layer is acidified with 6N sulfuric acid and filtered to remove dibasic acids. The monobasic acid extracted by extracting the acid solution with ether. Yields of phenylacetic acid are 96%. Reference: Reitsema 1962

Benzyl Chloride from Toluene

by Chauncey C. Loomis

...dry bleaching powder (calcium hypochlorite, or other equivalent hypochlorite) and toluene are mixed in proportions varying according to the extent of chlorination desired. For example, 200 kilograms of toluene are heated, as in a steam jacketed iron mixing kettle to a high temperature, say 90° C. Dry bleaching powder is then slowly added to this, the temperature being gradually raised until it approximates the boiling point of toluene, which, of course, cannot be exceeded. When 200 kilograms of bleaching powder have been added the mixture is held at the high temperature attained, (i. e., to secure the best results, from 100° C. to 105° C.) for about one hour, or, until the reaction is effected, with continuous thorough mixing. The escape of toluene vapor during the operation may be prevented by means of a reflux condenser fitted to the mixing vessel.

The resulting mixture is then cooled down and allowed to settle and as much oil as possible is siphoned off from the top. The oil left adhering to the line residue is then removed by steam distillation and added to that siphoned off. In this way 200 to 210 kilos of oil are obtained, having a specific gravity of .940 to .960 at 20° C. and containing from 30 to 35 per cent. of benzyl chloride and from 70 to 65 per cent. of toluene. These can then be separated by fractional distillation. A higher percentage of chlorinated product can be obtained by using a greater proportion of the bleaching powder. Source: Loomis 1918

Benzyl Chloride from Benzyl Alcohol

A 2 liter flask equipped with a stirrer (paddle) is poured 1 mole of benzyl alcohol (substituted benzyl alcohols will work eg. methoxy). 500 mL. of concentrated hydrochloric acid are added and then stirred vigorously for approximately a quarter of an hour. The mixture is then separated using a separatory funnel. The lower layer of benzyl chloride is separated. The benzyl chloride is dried for half an hour with 45 grams of granular calcium chloride. The calcium chloride is then filtered from the solution. Crude benzyl chloride is unstable and is prepared for use the same day. Reference: Rorig

Substituted Phenyl-2-Propanones From Substituted Phenyl-2-Nitropropenes

0.35 Moles of substituted phenyl-2-nitropropene is mixed with 100 mL of toluene. The mixture is stirred and heated to dissolve the phenyl-2-nitropropene. The solution is then vigorously refluxed and stirred while 100 grams of iron powder and 5 grams of ferric chloride (hydrated ferric chloride maybe used) are added. The mixture is refluxed with stirring at 75 degrees. 180 mL of concentrated hydrochloric acid is added over the next two to three hours and heated for another 45 minutes.

The solution is steam distilled until 4 to 5 liters are collected. The steam distillate forms two layers; one aqueous and one non-aqueous (containing: toluene, substituted phenyl-2-propanone and substituted benzaldehyde). The toluene layer is decanted and the aqueous layer is washed with fresh toluene. The toluene layers are combined. The toluene mixture is agitated with 14 grams of sodium bisulfite and filtered to remove aldehydes. The toluene solution is then washed with water to remove sodium bisulfite traces.

The toluene is distilled from the substituted phenyl-2-propanone under reduced pressure (water aspirator) while heating on a steam bath. A yellow liquid of substituted phenyl-2-propanone is left after the distillation of the toluene. Yields are approximately 75% theoretical.

Starting Molecule: 1-(2,5-Dimethoxy-4-ethylphenyl)-2-nitropropene
Product: 1-(2,5-Dimethoxy-4-ethylphenyl)-2-propanone Reference: (Nichols 1973)

Starting Molecule: 1-(2,5-Dimethoxy-4-methyl-phenyl)-2-nitro-1-butene
Product: 1-(2,5-Dimethoxy-4-phenyl)-2-butanone Reference: (Standridge 1976)

Starting Molecule: 1-(2,5-Dimethoxyphenyl)-2-nitropropene-1
Product: 1-(2,5-Dimethoxyphenyl)-2-propanone References: Bollinger 196; Merck 1962

Starting Molecule: 1-(2-Methoxyphenyl)-2-nitropropene-1
Product: 1-(2-Methoxyphenyl)-2-propanone Reference: (Heizelman, 1953)

Starting Molecule: 1-(3-Methoxyphenyl)-2-nitropropene-1
Product: 1-(3-Methoxyphenyl)-2-propanone Reference: (Heizelman, Organic Syntheses)

Starting Molecule: 1-(3-Methoxy-4-hydroxyphenyl)-2-nitropropene-1
Product: 1-(3-Methoxy-4-hydroxyphenyl)-2-propanone Ref.: (Bollinger 1962) (Pearl 1950)

Starting Molecule: 1-Phenyl-2-nitro-1-butene
Product: 1-Phenyl-2-butanone Reference: (Hass 1950)

Starting Molecule: 1-Phenyl-2-nitropropene
Product: 1-Phenyl-2-propanone Reference: (Hass 1950)

Phenyl-2-Propanone From Monochloroacetone

Equipment:

1) A three necked boiling flask.

2) A condenser for reflux. The top of the condenser is attached to an acid trap then vented through a gas absorption bottle and out a window.

3) A separatory funnel for the addition of chloro-acetone to the boiling flask.

4) A stirrer with a vapor seal.

The fumes are highly irritating.

The system must be sealed tight and then vented.

165 Grams of anhydrous aluminum chloride is mixed with 420 mL anhydrous benzene. Water is run through the condenser. The stirrer is turned on and the boiling flask is refluxed on an oil bath. 55 Grams (0.6 mole) of chloroacetone is dripped slowly into the reaction flask over a period of two hours. The solution is refluxed for a total of five hours. The solution becomes blackened. The reaction is cooled to room temperature. Water is added through the separatory funnel into the boiling flask, while stirring, until the evolution of hydrogen chloride gas ceases. When the evolution of gas has stopped 90 mL of water and 85 mL of concentrated hydrochloric acid is added. Two layers will form. The benzene layer is decanted from the solution and the aqueous layer is extracted with 500 mL of benzene or toluene. The benzene (or

toluene) solutions are combined. The benzene (or toluene) is distilled to leave an oily residue of phenyl-2-propanone and contaminants. The phenyl-2-propanone is fractionally distilled from the residue. The B.P. of phenyl-2-propanone is 216.5 degrees. Yields are 30% theoretical.

Starting Molecule: Methoxybenzene
Product: *p*-Methoxy-phenyl-2-propanone Reference: (Fusco 1948) (Mason 1940)

Preparation of Monochloroacetone
ClCH2COCH3
by Michael Heidelberger

If acetone be treated with a chlorinating agent such as phosphorus pentachloride, the keto group is attacked and 2,2-dichloro-propane, CH3CCl2CH3, results. If, however, elementary chlorine is used, the hydrogen atoms of the methyl groups are successively replaced. Not only is a mixture of mono- and poly-chlorinated acetones formed, but the hydrochloric acid liberated condenses the acetone to products of higher molecular weight, of which mesityl oxide may be taken as an example:

Thus, unless some substance is at hand to bind the hydrochloric acid as fast as formed, exceedingly complex mixtures are obtained from which it is virtually impossible to isolate pure products, mesityl oxide, for instance, boiling at practically the same point as monochloroacetone. Fritsch (1894) found that small pieces of marble were very satisfactory, as these reacted at once with the hydrochloric acid liberated, and his method is accordingly the basis of that given below.

Chlorination of Acetone

21 g. of marble, broken into small pieces, and 84 g. of acetone are placed in a flask provided with an inlet tube, dropping funnel, and reflux condenser, and warmed to 40° in a water bath. A slow stream of chlorine is then passed in and enough water (a total of 50 to 60 cc. slowly dripped in to keep in solution the calcium chloride formed by interaction of the marble and hydrochloric acid. This is also aided by frequent agitation of the flask. The reaction must be very carefully watched, for if a yellow color develops (and according to Kling (1905) this usually happens at the lower reaction temperature originally given by Fritsch (1894) it indicates the formation of hypochlorous acid, and this, if it accumulates, may react explosively with the acetone. In the event, then, that the solution turns yellow the stream of chlorine is at once interrupted until the coloration disappears. When only a little marble is left, the reaction is discontinued, for although a large excess of acetone is

present the main product would be the symmetrical dichloro derivative, ClCH2COCH2Cl, if this excess were not maintained. The mixture is allowed to stand at 40° until the evolution of carbon dioxide ceases, making sure that an excess of marble is present, and is then poured off from the marble into a separatory funnel. The two layers formed are separated and the lower, consisting of a strong aqueous solution of calcium chloride, is discarded.

Fractionation

The upper layer of acetone and its chlorination products is fractionated with the aid of a good distilling column, the mono-chloroacetone boiling at 118-20°.

The yield is 16.8 g., plus an additional 5 g. on refractionation of the lower and upper fractions.

The chloro-acetones are extremely irritating, both in vapor form and if dropped on the skin. Gloves should be worn and all operations conducted under the hood. This applies to the next experiment as well.
Source: Heidelberger 1923 References: Fritsch; *Ann.* 279, 313 (1894); Kling; *Bull. soc. chim.* [3] 33, 322 (1905).

Starting Molecule: Acetone Product: mono-Chloroacetone
References: Okeda 1956 see also: Rahrs 1941

Stablization of Chloroacetone

by Emil J. Rahrs

Relatively small amounts of the calcium carbonate, as for example 1 to 6 grams of calcium carbonate added to 100 grams of chloracetone would be sufficient. However, a surplus causes no injury and may be added if desired. Chloracetone treated accordance with my invention, even after several months' storage was satisfactory for use without redistillation. If desired, the chloracetone in accordance with my invention, may be stored in colored containers as, for example, amber colored glassware, but this is not necessary. Source: Rahrs 1941

Phenyl-2-propanones From Propenylbenzenes

0.7 Mole of substituted propenylbenzene is mixed with 800 mL of glacial acetic acid. To this solution is added, in proportions, 400 grams of lead tetroxide. This is stirred for one hour at 40 degrees. A small quantity of water is added and the solution is distilled under reduced pressure to leave a residue. The residue is extracted with ether or appropriate solvent and evaporated or distilled under reduced pressure to leave the substituted phenyl-1,2-propanediol diacetate.

Substituted Phenyl-2-Propanones From Substituted Phenyl-1,2-Propanediol Diacetates

The previous solution containing the substituted phenyl-1,2-propanediol diacetate is mixed with 600 mL of 20% sulfuric acid and refluxed for 3 hours. This solution is then extracted with ether or appropriate solvent. The solvent is distilled under reduced pressure to leave 0.3 moles of the substituted phenyl-2-propanone.

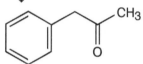

Phenyl-1,2-propanediol Diacetate

Phenyl-2-propanone

Starting Mol.: 2-Methoxypropenylbenzene
Product: 2-Methoxyphenyl-1,2-propanediol
References: (Tanaka 1957). See (Dal Cason 1984).

Starti. Mol.: 2-Methoxy-phenyl-1,2-propanediol diacetate
Product: 2-Methoxyphenyl-2-propanone
Refs.: (Tanaka 1957); Also check (Sunagawa 1952)

Starting Molecule: Phenyl-1,2-propanediol
Product: Phenyl-2-propanone
References:: (Hamada 1950) (Murahashi 1950)

Preparation of Propiophenone
Preparation of Phenylethylcarbinol

A Grignard solution of 12 grams of magnesium and 60 grams of ethyl bromide in 250 cc. of dry ether is gradually introduced drop by drop into a solution of (0.47 moles) of benzaldehyde in 400 cc. of dry ether. The whole is poured on ice and well acidified, with concentrated hydrochloric acid. The ether solution is separated and shaken at first with a bisulphite solution, and finally with water. After drying by means of sodium sulphate, the ether is evaporated and the residue is distilled in a vacuum. (The phenylethylcarbinol is distilled under reduced pressure).

Phenylpropiophenone is formed from the carbinol by oxidation with chromic acid. For this purpose the phenylethylcarbinol is slowly introduced drop by drop into a solution of 150 grams of potassium dichromate and 125 grams of sulphuric acid in 750 cc. of water. After several hours the oxidation is complete. The ketone is extracted by means of ether and distilled, after washing the ethereal solution and evaporating the ether, in a vacuum. (The propiophenone is distilled under reduced pressure). The propiophenone obtained with a yield of (0.24 to 0.26 moles). Source: I.G. Farbenindustrie 1932

FRIEDEL-CRAFTS REACTION; KETONES FROM PHENOLS

---

tarting Molecule: Pyrogallol; (2,3-Dihydoxy-phenol)
Reagents: Zinc Chloride, Caproic Acid
Product: 2,3,4-Trihydoxyphenyl-n-Amyl Ketone Reference: (Hart 1936)

Starting Molecule: Resorcinol; (2-Hydroxy-phenol)
Reagents: Zinc Chloride, Glacial Acetic Acid
Product: 2,4-Dihydroxyacetophenone Ref.: (Cooper 1941)   See also: (Noller 1924)

Methylation of Dihydroxy Ketones:
2,6-Dimethoxyacetophenone from 2,6-dihydroxyacetophenone
(Borche 1907); 4-O-Benzoyl-2,6-dimethoxyacetophenone from
4-O-Benzoylphloracetophenone (Sugasawa 1934).

Preparation of P-2-P and *alpha*-Phenylpropionaldehyde; 2-Phenylpropanal from Allybenzene

One hundred and thirty grams of bromine and 98 grams of allybenzene are added to 1 L. of 15% H2SO4 and heated at 80° with stirring for 8 hours. The reaction was cooled and an oily layer separates.   It is diluted with benzene and dried with sodium sulfate. The mixture is distilled to give an oil, bp 75-85°/8 mm. The oil was further purified as addition compound of sodium bisulfite. The mixture was was then fractionally distilled to obtain *alpha*-phenyl-propionaldehyde and P-2-P (yields 48% and 51%). Reference: Inoi 1969

Preparation of P-2-P from 2-Phenylpropanal and Phosphoric Acid

by Canter et al. (exemplified for P-2-P)

Water and (2-phenylpropanal) were fed through separate pumps and were vaporized in a coiled stainless steel vaporizer. The vapors were passed downwardly through the tubular reactor... the catalyst being in the form of 4 mm. x 4 mm. pellets. The catalyst bed was maintained at the desired reaction temperature. A condenser, water-scrubber and distillation column were used to collect the product, the distillation column being operated at 80° C. overhead temperature.

In preparing the catalyst, 1/4" ceramic Berl saddles are soaked in 85% phosphoric acid and drained. The catalyst is placed in a reactor tube heated at 300-350° C., and (2-phenylpropanal) is passed through with an equimolar amount of steam. Sufficient phosphoric acid is added to replace any which is lost into the product vapors. At a contact time of 10 seconds, 8.2% of the (2-phenylpropanal) fed is converted per pass into (phenyl-2-propanone). Satisfactory results have also been obtained with phosphoric acid on diatomaceous earth (Celatom) at various temperatures, contact times, pressures and water to (2-phenylpropanal) rations. Source: Cantor 1968

References: Hargis 1969; Hoelderich 1987; Linstid 1985; Tohzuka 1980; Young 1969; Velenyi 1982;

For use of lithium oxide catalyst see Fleischer 1968.

2-Phenylpropanal from 2-Phenyl-1-propanol
by Wolfgang Sauer

Aromatic and araliphatic aldehydes are prepared by oxidizing corresponding alcohols with oxygen in the presence of a silver catalyst of a defined particle size, and under defined temperature conditions. The products are starting materials for the preparation of dyes, pesticides, plastics and scents...

For large-scale industrial operation, the catalyst bed diameter is preferably at least 0.05 meter, advantageously from 0.1 to 3 meters. The reaction is advantageously carried out continuously at from 450° to 700° C., preferably from 475° to 650° C., especially from 500° to 625° C., under atmospheric or superatmospheric pressure...

An installation comprising a vaporizer and a vertical tubular reactor is used. At its top, the reactor comprises the inlet for the vapor starting mixture, and the reactor cover. The catalyst bed is located below the reactor top, and a cooling zone is provided below the catalyst bed. The reactor is connected to 4 absorption columns.

A catalyst comprising 84 parts of silver crystals of the following composition is introduced into the reactor:

	Proportion of the catalyst (% by weight)	Particle size mm
Layer 1	20	0.1-0.4
Layer 2	50	0.4-0.75
Layer 3	30	0.75-1

The height of the catalyst bed is 30 mm. Per hour, a mixture of 150 parts of 2-phenyl-1-propanol, 60 parts of nitrogen and 185 parts of air is fed to the vaporizer and the 2-phenyl-1-propanol is vaporized. The vapor starting material is passed through the catalyst and reacted at 550° C. and 1.1 bar. The residence time is 0.08 second and the through-

put is 0.2 tonne/m2.h. 108 parts of 2-phenylpropanal (in the form of an 78 percent strength by weight solution) are obtained per hour, corresponding to a yield of 73% of theory, based on 2-phenyl-1-propanol employed. The conversion is 92 percent and the space-time yield is 5 grams of 2-phenylpropanal per cm3 of catalyst volume per hour.
Source: Sauer 1980; Refs: Chalk 1978; Ogata 1980

1-Phenylpropan-1-ol-2-one (L-PAC)
Preparation from Benzaldehyde

by Andrew Smallridge, Maurice Trewhella and Margaret Del Guidice, Robert Coughlin, Wafaa Mahmoud; A. Halim El-Sayed and John W. Rothrock

Ephedrine (*alpha*-[1-(methylamino)ethyl]benzene-methanol), originally isolated from plants of the genus *Ephedra*, occurs as the naturally-occurring isomers *l*-ephedrine and *d*-pseudoephedrine, and other pharmacologically active isomers include *d*-ephedrine and *l*-pseudoephedrine. These compounds are adrenergic sympathomimetic agents and have antihistamine activity; *l*-ephedrine is widely used as a bronchodilator, while *d*-pseudoephedrine is widely used as a decongestant. Compounds of these groups are present in a very wide range of prescription and over-the-counter pharmaceutical formulations.

The production of l-phenylacetylcarbinol, a precursor of *l*-ephedrine, by catalysis using whole baker's yeast cells in aqueous medium was one of the first microbial biotransformation processes to be used commercially Neuberg (1921); see also Hildebrandt (1934). This reaction involves the yeast-induced condensation of benzaldehyde with acetyl-coenzyme A. The reaction has been widely investigated, and has been shown to be mediated by the enzyme pyruvate decarboxylase Groger (1966). It has also been shown that the reaction has a relatively broad specificity for the substrate, enabling a variety of substituted aromatic aldehydes to be converted to the corresponding substituted optically-active phenylacetylcarbinols Long (1989)...

We have now surprisingly found that yeast-mediated acyloin condensation of benzaldehyde can be achieved in an organic solvent using non-fermenting yeast, and that addition of a small proportion of ethanol to the reaction mixture suppresses formation of undesired side-products. Even more surprisingly, by performing the reaction at reduced temperature, an even greater reduction of side-reactions can be achieved, without loss of catalytic activity. The effect of reduction in temperature appears to be generally applicable to both aqueous and non-aqueous systems utilizing a non-fermenting yeast...

Any yeast capable of effecting reduction may be used. It is economically advantageous to use the cheapest yeast available, and ordinary baker's yeast, *Saccharomryces cerevisiae*, is preferred. Strains of yeast adapted to other purposes, including brewing yeast and wine or sherry yeasts could also be employed. Strains specifically adapted to an organic solvent environment or for enhanced reduction efficiency may be used; such strains include conventionally-selected and genetically modified strains. For maximum efficiency of reaction, it is advisable to present the maximum surface area of yeast for contact with the reactants. This can be effected by using "active" dried yeast, which is readily commercially available as "instant dry yeast", and may be stored at room temperature. Alternatively, well-pulverised dry baker's yeast may be used. Other yeasts, such as those described in Leuenberger (1988), or fungi such as those disclosed in Chenevert (1992) may also be used. The person skilled in the art will readily be able to test whether any specific organism will function for the purposes of the invention, using the methods described herein.

Preferably the aliphatic alcohol or aliphatic aldehyde is ethanol or acetaldehyde, suitably 0.1 mL per gram yeast. This results in a significant increase in the yield of carbinol, and reduces the amount of aromatic alcohols produced as a side-reaction. Ethanol is preferred, since this results in superior conversion of the aromatic aldehydes to the desired carbinol, and lower yield of undesired reduction product. Without wishing to be bound by any particular theory, it is believed that the ethanol or acetaldehyde provides an alternative substrate for the reductase enzymes thus inhibiting the formation of side products such as benzyl alcohol. Therefore, it is predicted that other aliphatic alcohols or aliphatic aldehydes could perform the same function.

Although the reaction can be performed at ambient temperature, suitably 16-24° C., preferably 20° C., we have surprisingly found that significantly better results are obtained at lower temperatures, in the range 0-5° C. The reason for the improved performance and further reduction of side-reactions which is observed is not presently understood; however, we have observed that the activity of the yeast at these reduced temperatures is comparable to that at ambient temperature. This result is particularly surprising, because it would normally be expected that a yeast-mediated reaction would demonstrate a temperature optimum at ambient or slightly elevated temperature, although Shiu (1996), have shown that isolated pyruvate decarboxylase, the enzyme involved in the acyloin condensation reaction, exhibits increased activity at 4° C.

It is known that in order to preserve functioning of an enzyme in an organic solvent environment it is necessary for the enzyme to be fully hydrated by being surrounded by a few layers of water molecules. This requirement is satisfied by providing a ratio of 0.6 to 1.2 mL water/g of yeast, preferably 1.0 mL water/g of yeast. This results in a single phase organic system as all of the water is absorbed into the yeast. A two-phase system reduces the yield of the product and makes isolation of the product considerably more difficult.

Once the yeast-mediated reaction has been completed, the yeast can readily be separated from the reaction mixture by filtration and washing. The reaction mixture, comprising product, unreacted starting material, solvent and minor impurities, is subjected to conventional purification, for example by flash distillation, to yield the purified product. Optionally the yeast can be extracted with an organic solvent such as ethyl acetate to yield a marginal amount of further product.

While the ratio of yeast to substrate will vary depending on the individual system, and is readily determined experimentally using routine trial and error methods, we have found that for the conversion of benzaldehyde to phenylacetylcarbinol the optimum ratio is 5 grams yeast/mmol benzaldehyde; increasing the amount of yeast results in only a small increase in conversion, and lower amounts of yeast provide lower conversion.

Similarly, the optimum reaction time may readily be determined, and for the benzaldehyde-phenylacetyl-carbinol system we have investigated reaction times from 12 to 72 hours, and have found that when the reaction is continued for longer than 24 hours there is very little improvement in conversion, and that there is an increase in production of by-products.

In a particularly preferred embodiment, production of undesired side-products is reduced by performing the catalysis reaction at below ambient temperature. Preferably the temperature is 0-5° C.
Source: Smallridge (2001)

Saccharomyces cerevisiae accession number ATCC 834 of the American Type Culture Collection, 12301 Parkland Drive, Rockville, Md., 20852 USA. was maintained on a medium that contained (per liter): 10 g of yeast extract, 10 grams of malt extract, 4 grams of dextrose, 20 grams of agar. The liquid medium used for growing the yeast cells and for production of L-PAC contained (per liter): 6 grams of yeast extract, 4 grams of NH4SO4, 0.6 grams of MgSO4, 1 g of KH2PO4, 100 grams of dextrose, with the balance water. For sterilization, a solution of dextrose and a solution containing the other ingredients were autoclaved separately, then mixed and the pH adjusted to 6.2. The yeast was grown for 24 hrs on the liquid medium at 28°-30° C., centrifuged, re-suspended in sterile water then re-centrifuged.

The washed and centrifuged cells were re-suspended in a solution containing 3% (w/v) of sodium alginate (Aldrich Chemical Company). The latter cell suspension was extruded as drops into a 2% calcium chloride solution thereby forming beads which were kept in the CaCl2 solution for 1 hour before filtering and washing them on a Buchner funnel. These beads of immobilized yeast were then used to inoculate the medium in the shake flasks so that the cell dose was 2.8 grams (cell wet weight) per 100 mL of medium in 250 mL Erlenmeyer flasks. After shaking under aerobic conditions for 1 hour, shaking was continued under anaerobic conditions. Pre-purified (by distillation) benzaldehyde was added in four equal aliquots at 1 hour intervals during the anaerobic shaking. The total amount of benzaldehyde added was 6 g per liter of medium. Thereafter, with continued shaking under anaerobic conditions, small samples were withdrawn over the ensuing 24-hour period and assayed for L-PAC by the method of Groger (1966). The maximum liter of L-PAC was 5.5 g/L. Source: Coughlin (1992)

A 3,4-substituted benzaldehyde compound, wherein the 3 and 4 substitutes are hydroxy, alkoxy, or when taken together an alkylenedioxy (e.g. methylenedioxy) substitute, is contacted with a growing culture of an acyloin-producing microoranism at a temperature of abut 25-30° C. and the L-acyloin produced is isolated from the fermentation broth by extraction, chromatography and crystallization.

The acyloin-producing microorganisms utilized is the process of my invention are preferably commercially available yeast strains ordinarily employed as "wet compressed yeast" is the baking and brewing industries, in particular selected strains of *Saccharomyces* cerevisiae. In addition, selected strains of microorganisms belonging to the *Schizomysetes*, *Myxomycetes*, and *Eumycetes* are effective in carry-ing out the desired stereospecific conversion to the L-acyloin.

For any given species of microorganisms it is necessary to select acyloin-producing strains of microorganisms, by a simple test. This test includes growing the selected microorganism in contact with a 3,4-disubstituted-benzaldehyde, and filtering and extracting the fermen-tation broth with ethyl acetate. A portion of the extract is then spotted on filter paper and chromatographed using n-butanol saturated with 3% aqueous ammonium hydroxide solution. A positive blue tetrazolium spot test indicates the presence of the desired acyloin and the strains showing a positive tetrazolium test are then utilized in the fermenta-tion process...

A suitable sterile nutrient medium containing assimilable sources of carbon and nitrogen are inoculated with a selected strain of microorganism and aerated and agitated until substantial growth of the microorganism has occurred. Generally, a period of 1-7 days is required. Typical media utilized in the process of my invention are indicated in the following tables.

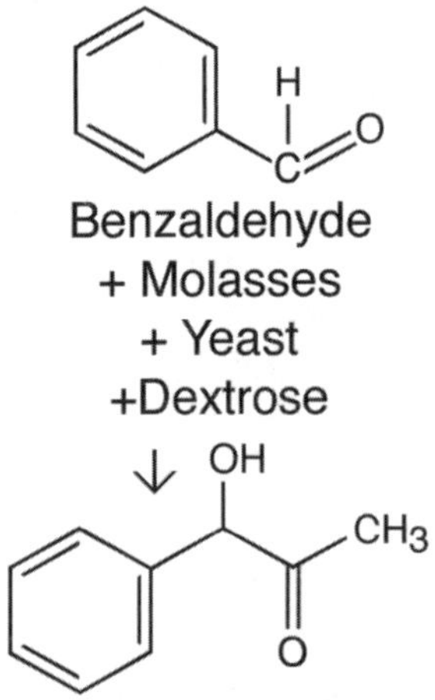

Medium I

Molasses .... 6 grams
Water: sufficient to make 100 mL.
pH adjusted to 5.5 with phosphoric acid.

Medium II

	Grams
Commercial yeast extract ...	20
Dextrose	20
MgSO4-7H2O	0.5
KH2PO4	0.2
NaHPO4	0.2
Water .... (sufficient to make 1.0 liter).	

pH adjusted to 7.

Benzaldehyde
+ Molasses
+ Yeast
+Dextrose

1-Phenylpropan-1-ol-2-one

Following the growth period, the selected 3,4-disubstituted-benzaldehyde is added to the medium in a concentration of approximately 1-10 grams of the compound per liter of medium, and the medium containing the test compound incubated with agitation at about 28° C. for a period of from 1-10 hours.

Following the incubation period, the fermented broth containing the desired compound along with other products of metabolism is extracted with a water-immiscible solvent for the acyloin such as an ester of a lower aliphatic acid, preferably ethyl acetate.

The solvent extract contains, in addition to the desired acyloin, unreacted aldehyde as well as the corresponding substituted benzyl alcohol and the substituted benzoic acid. The desired acyloin compound is separated from the related compounds by processes including partition chromatography, by fractional crystallization and by extraction with aqueous sodium bisulfate solution.

Piperonal Acyloin
L-3,4-Methylenedioxyphenylacetyl Carbinol

A fermentation medium having the composition of Medium II is inoculated with a strain of *Saccharomryces cerevisiae* selected from a commercial wet compressed yeast available from the Atlantic Yeast Company. The medium is then aerated and agitated at 28° C. for approximately 48 hours to achieve optimal growth of the *Saccharomryces cerevisiae* organisms. Aeration and agitation, and to the medium is added piperanal in a concentration of 10 grams per liter of medium. Following introduction of the piperonal, the medium is again aerated and agitated at 28° C. for a period of about 7 hours to produce the desired L-3,4-methylenedioxyphenyl-acetyl carbinol.

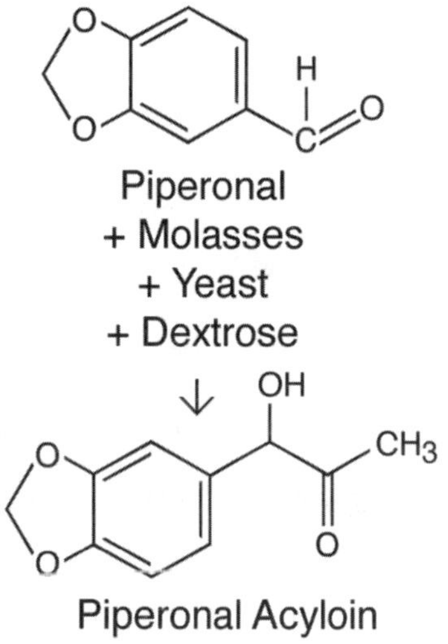

The resulting fermentation broth containing the desired product is sterilized by autoclaving and then filtered to remove the yeast cells. The filtrate containing the product is then saturated with sodium chloride and extracted four times with 1/3 volume ethyl acetate. The crude product is obtained by evaporation of the ethyl acetate leaving a brown oil containing the product in crude form admixed with by-products.

Piperonal
+ Molasses
+ Yeast
+ Dextrose

Piperonal Acyloin

The desired product is purified by extraction with ethyl acetate, and aqueous bisulfite followed by partition column chromatography and fractional crystallization from ethyl acetate solution to give substantially pure L-3,4-methylenedioxyphenylacetyl carbinol. M.P. 44-46° C. [∂] D25=228°; c.=1.2 ethyl acetate. Source: Rothrock (1967)

Refs: Chenevert 1992; Coughlin 1992; Groger 1966 ; Hildebrandt 1934; Leuenberger 1988; Long 1989; Nagai 1934; Neuberg 1921; Rothrock 1967; Shiu 1996; Smallridge 2001

CHAPTER 13:
METHAMPHETAMINE PRODUCTION: MORE METHODS
Preparation of Methamphetamine from Chloro-ephedrin

Chloro-ephedrine

Methamphetamine

150 mL. of water is mixed with 8.5 grams of anhydrous sodium acetate. 20 grams of chloroephedrine are added. 8.5 grams of copper are added. The mixture is stirred for 12 or more hours. Excess alkali is added and the solution is steam distilled to hydrolyze chloroephedrine and to distill ephedrine and pseudoephedrine by-products. Ether is used to extract the residue. Evaporation of the ether leaves an oil containing both desoxyephedrine (methamphetamine) and also didesoxyephedrine. Yields are approximately 30% The reaction has been reported to be incomplete as the copper had not completely dissolved and the yield was too low. Reference: Gero 1951

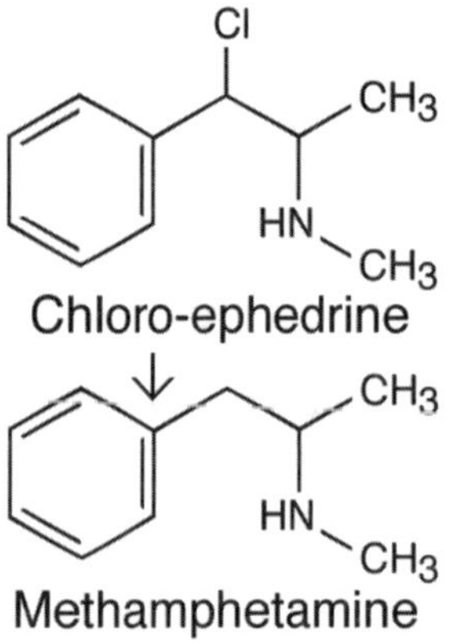

Preparation of Chloroephedrine

50 Grams of phenylpropanolamine is mixed with 800 mL of concentrated hydrochloric acid in a bomb tube. The tube is heated at 110-115 degrees for four hours. The solution is then cooled to precipitate the phenyl-1-chloro-2-aminopropane which is then collected by suction filtration. Yields are approximately 50% theoretical.

References: (Allen 1987) (Cantrell 1988)

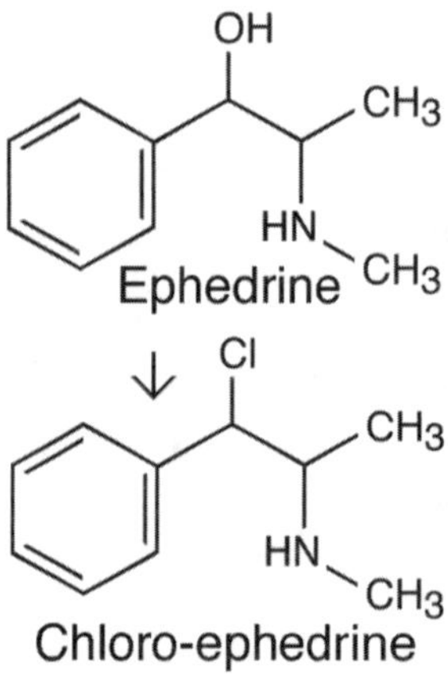

Ephedrine

Chloro-ephedrine

Methamphetamine from Ephedrine Using Phosphorus and Hydriodic Acid

0.2 moles of ephedrine are mixed with 10 grams of red phosphorus and 85 mL. of 57% hydriodic acid. The mixture is refluxed for 24 hours and let stand for 12 hours. 350 cc. of water are added and the phosphorus is filtered (asbestos filter) from the the mixture. A few crystals of sodium thiosulfate are added (to remove iodine) and then basified with 40% sodium hydroxide.

The methamphetamine is extracted with ether; the ether washed with water and dried with anhydrous sodium carbonate. The ether is reduced and cooled. Cold hydrochloric acid is added to precipitate the methamphetamine hydrochloride. The methamphetamine hydrochloride is dried over anhydrous sodium carbonate. Yields are 80 to 88%. References: Ho 1975; Shaw 1956: Zenitz 1948

Catalytic Hydrogenation Preparation of Methamphetamine

by John Tindall

Preparation of Catalyst

Method 1.

To a suspension of 80 grams of lime, technical, in 500 mL. water was added with agitation during a period of 50 minutes at room temperature one liter of a solution containing 250 grams of technical hydrated cupric sulfate in water. The mixture was then held at 90° C. for 3 hours and continuously agitated. The precipitate which formed was then recovered by filtration, dried at 70° C., and ground to pass a 120 mesh screen. The yield of catalyst was 225 grams.

Method 2.

A solution of 29.8 pounds of technical hydrated cupric sulfate in 119 pounds of water was added in a steady stream over a period of 25 minutes to 9.6 pounds of calcium hydroxide in 60 pounds of water. The resulting mixture was then heated in a water bath to 90° C. and agitated at this temperature for 3 hours. The mixture was next cooled, filtered and the precipitate dried by heating with hot air for 19 hours at 70° C. The dried precipitate was ground and screened, yielding 30.1 pounds of finished catalyst.

Preparation of Desoxyephedrine (meth)

(Thirty grams) of the catalyst prepared above were added to a mixture of 200 grams of phenylacetone and 500 mL. of methanol, and the mixture placed in a rocking bomb of 1840 mL. capacity. After cooling the bomb with solid carbon dioxide to avoid loss of methylamine, 85 mL. of anhydrous methylamine was added and the resulting mixture subject to hydrogenation for a period of 5 hours at a pressure ranging from 1000 to 1500 p.s.i. and a temperature of 160° C.

The contents of the bomb were then filtered to remove the catalyst, and treated with a solution of 130 mL. of 12 N hydrochloric acid to 500 mL. of water. The filtered mixture was subjected distillation to remove methanol and non-basic products. The distillation residue was next diluted with 250 mL. of water and extracted once with 100 mL and three times with 50 mL. portion of benzene. This benzene containing any remaining non-basic products was discarded. The extracted residue was then treated with 70 grams of sodium hydroxide n 200 mL. of water and the resulting oily layer separated. The lower or aqueous layer was next extracted twice with 100 mL. and twice with 50 mL. portions of benzene. Finally, the separated oil layer and the benzene extract from the water layer were mixed an subjected to distillation through a packed column at atmospheric pressure until the oil was free of water and benzene, and then distillation continued at 10 mm. pressure...

A yield of 203 grams of product was obtained containing 99.6% desoxyephedrine boiling with the range of 84°-90° C. at 10 mm. pressure. This represented a yield of 92% based on the phenylacetone used. Source: Tindall 1958 Reference: Metzger 1960

Methamphetamine from Ephedrine
Birch Reaction

The reaction is carried out using a large three necked boiling flask equipped with a magnetic stirrer. A condenser, a glass tube to introduce ammonia gas into the bottom of the flask and separatory funnel are attached to the three necks. The reaction flask is cooled in a dry ice/acetone bath. l-Ephedrine is mixed with appropriate solvent (eg. tetrahydrofuran) and poured into the separatory funnel. Ammonia gas is introduced into the reaction flask and condensed as a result of the dry ice/acetone bath. Pieces of lithium are washed with naphtha, dried and introduced into the liquid ammonia; the solution will turn deep royal blue.

The *l*-ephedrine solution is added dropwise over a period of 10 to 15 minutes with simultaneous stirring. The solution is quenched by the slow addition of ammonium chloride with stirring.

A side arm is attached to a trap cooled by a dry ice/acetone bath to condense ammonia. The dry ice/actone bath is removed from the reaction flask containing the methamphetamine, and ammonia. The flask is allowed to warm to room temperature. The ammonia is then condensed in the dry ice/acetone trap for containment.

The solution is then placed in a separatory funnel and the aqueous layer is discarded. The tetrahydrofuran/methamphetamine solution is dried with magnesium sulfate (Epson salts) and filtered. The solution is then cooled and hydrogen chloride gas is bubbled through the solution to precipitate the *d*-methamphetamine hydrochloride.

Methamphetamine hydrochloride can also be precipitated from the THF/methamphetamine solution by cooling the solution and adding hydrochloric acid. The precipitated methamphetamine hydrochloride is dried over magnesium sulfate.

Refs: Allen 1989; Augustine in *Techniques and Applications in Organic Synthesis* 1968; Birch 1945; Ely 1990, Hall 1971; Small 1975.

Substituted N-Alkyl-Amphetamine From Substituted Phenylisopropyl-N-Alkylformamides Amines From Formamides

by Harry E. Albert and Richard W. Kibler

It is known to produce amines by hydrolyzing a formamide in the presence of an aqueous alkali metal hydroxide. However, this method of producing amines is not particularly satisfactory because an aqueous mixture of the amine results. Separation of the pure anhydrous amine form such mixtures by distillation is very difficult because of the tendency of these amines to form azeotropes containing large percentages of water. An additional disadvantage of the use of aqueous alkali for the hydrolysis is that water is present with the sodium formate by-product after removal of the amine. This interferes with the recovery of concentrated formic acid from the sodium formate because the formic acid-water azeotrope (B.P. 107° C., 77.5% formic acid) boils so close to water (B.P. 100° C.). Further, the yield of amine resulting from the use of previously known methods has been low and consequently, these methods have not been commercially feasible...

Carrying out the reaction in the absence of water greatly enhances the smoothness of the reaction. The formamides used in the practice of the invention can be obtained by any suitable means and are rendered anhydrous in any suitable manner. One convenient method for rending a formamide anhydrous is to dry it over a suitable drying agent such as anhydrous sodium carbonate. Another suitable manner of rendering the formamide anhydrous is to dissolve the formamide in benzene or toluene and distill off the benzene or toluene; any water present is removed along with the benzene or toluene as azeotrope...
Source: Albert 1956

Method 1: 0.5 Mole of the substituted phenyl-2-(formyl-N-alkyl-amino)propane is refluxed for 5 hours with 600 mL of 25% sodium hydroxide. The mixture is steam distilled. The steam distillate containing the N-alkyl amphetamine is extracted with ether or appropriate water insoluble solvent and   concentrated. Hydrochloric acid is added to the solvent and chilled to precipitate the   substituted phenyisopropyl-N-alkyl-amine hydrochloride salt which can be suction filtered. Approximately 90% theoretical yields can be obtained.

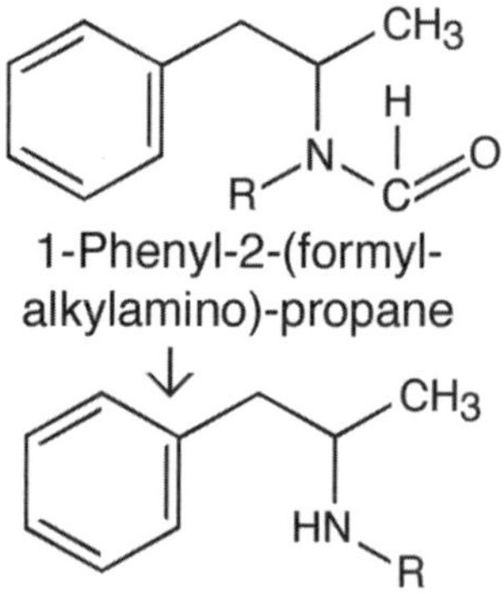

1-Phenyl-2-(formyl-alkylamino)-propane

N-Alkyl-amphetamine

Start. Molecule: 1-(2-Chloro-phenyl)-2-(formylamino)propane
Product: 2-Chloro-amphetamine
Reference: (Johns 1938)

Starting Molecule: N-(Dimethylbenzylcarbinol)-formamide
Product: Dimethylbenzylcarbinamine (Phentermine) Ref.: (Ritter 1948)

Start. Molecule: 1-(4-Fluoro-phenyl)-2-(formylamino)propane
Pduct: 4-Fluoro-phenylisopropylamine (4-Fluoro-amphetamine)
Reference: (Suter 1941)

Starting Molecule: N-Methyl-N-formyl-MDA
Prduct: 3,4,-Methylenedioxy-N-methamphetamine Ref.: (Dal Cason 1990)

Starting Molecule: Phenyl-2-(formylamino)propane
Product: Phenylisopropylamine (Amphetamine)
Reference: (Magidson 1941)

Method 2:

0.5 Mole of phenyl-2-(formyl-N-alkylamino)-propane is refluxed with 150 mL of concentrated hydrochloric acid for one hour. Water may be added to keep the 1-phenyl-2-(formyl-N-alkyl-amino)propane in solution. The reaction solution is then basified with sodium hydroxide and extracted with benzene or appropriate water insoluble solvent. The solvent is concentrated by distillation, hydrochloric acid is added and the solution is refrigerated to precipitate the amphetamine hydrochloride salt. The product is collected by suction filtration.

Starting Molecule: N-(Benzylmethylcarbinyl)-acetamide
Product: Methylbenzylcarbinamine (amphetamine) Reference: (Ritter 1948)

Starting Molecule: N-Methyl-N-formyl-MDA
Product: 3,4,-Methylenedioxy-N-methamphetamine Reference: (Dal Cason 1990)

Starting Molecule: 1-(3,4-Methylenedioxyphenyl-2-formylamino)propane
Product: 3,4,-Methylenedioxyamphetamine Reference: (Fujisawa 1956)

Starting Molecule: 1-(2-Methoxyphenyl-2-formylamino)-propane
Product: 2-Methoxyamphetamine Reference: (Heizelman, 1953)

Starting Molecule: 1-Phenyl-2-(formylamino)-propane
Product: Amphetamine Reference: (Bobranski 1941)

Leuckart-Wallach Reaction:
1-Phenyl-2-(formylamino)propane From Phenyl-2-propanone And Ammonium Formate

The reaction is done in a distillation apparatus. As the boiling flask is heated, a mixture of water and ketone is distilled into the receiving flask. When the water is not simultaneously distilled, the reaction will not occur. During the course of this reaction the original mixture, which is composed of two layers, becomes homogeneous. The ketone is transferred back into the boiling flask.

100 Grams of ammonium formate and 0.5 moles of substituted P-2-P are placed in a boiling flask along with boiling stones

Phenyl-2-propanone
+ Ammonium Formate

1-Phenyl-2-(formyl-
amino)propane

(several pieces of porcelain) to prevent bumping. The mixture is heated on a small flame. The contents will melt and form two layers. The mixture begins to distill at 140 degrees. The mixture becomes homogeneous between 150 to 160 degrees. The heating is stopped when the temperature reaches 185 degrees.

The distillate forms two layers. The water insoluble layer is the top layer and contains the substituted phenyl-2-propanone. The upper layer of the distillate is separated from the bottom aqueous layer and is poured back into the boiling flask.

The solution is refluxed for two more hours until the temperature reaches 185 degrees. The solution is then extracted with an appropriate solvent and evaporated to leave the 1-phenyl-2-(formylamino)propane.

Formamide can be recycled from the aqueous layer of the distillate by distilling to 165 degrees. The formamide can be purified by crystallization or fractional distillation. This is unnecessary as long as the recovered formamide is going to be used with the same ketone in future reactions.   Reference: (Ingersoll 1936)

Starting Molecule: 1-(2-Methoxyphenyl)-2-propanone
Product: 1-(2-Methoxyphenyl)-2-(formylamino)propane
Reference: (Heizelman 1953)

Starting Molecule: 1-(4-Methoxyphenyl)-2-propanone
Product: 1-4-Methoxyphenyl)-2-(formylamino)propane
Reference: (Alles 1935)

Starting Molecule: 3,4-Methylenedioxyphenyl-2-propanone
Product: 1-(3,4-Methyledioxyphenyl)-2-(formylamino)propane
References: (Dal Cason 1990), (Elks 1943)

Starting Molecule: Phenyl-2-propanone
Product: Phenyl-2-(formylamino)propane. References:(Bobranskii 1941)

1-Phenyl-2-(formylalkylamino)propane
From Substituted P-2-P and N-Alkylformamide

0.5 Mole of substituted 1-phenyl-2-propanone is refluxed at 180 to 195 degrees for five to nine hours with 2 moles of formamide or N-alkylformamide.

Amide Used	Product
Formamide	1-Phenyl-2-(formylamino)propane
N-Methylformamide	N-methyl homolog
N-Ethylformamide	N-ethyl homolog

The mixture is extracted with chloroform or appropriate solvent. The solvent is distilled to leave the 1-phenyl-2-(formylamino)propane or 1-phenyl-2-(formylalkylamino)-propane.

Starting Molecule: 1-(2-Chloro-phenyl)-2-propanone
Product: 1-(2-Chloro-phenyl)-2-(formylamino)propane Ref.: (Johns 1938)

Starting Molecule: 1-(4-Fluoro-phenyl)-2-propanone
Product: 1-(4-Fluoro-phenyl)-2-(formylamino)propane Ref.: (Suter 1941)

Starting Molecule: 1-(3,4-Methylenedioxyphenyl)-2-propanone
Product.: 1-(3,4-Methylenedioxyphenyl-2-(formylamino)propane
References: (Dal Cason 1990) (Elks 1943) (Fujisawa 1956)

Starting Molecule: Phenyl-2-propanone
Product: 1-Phenyl-2-(formylamino)propane Ref.: (Magidson 1941)

Preparation of
4-Methoxy-phenyl-2-methylaminopropane
Using Methylamine Hydrochloride
By Gordon Alles

One mole of *para*-methoxybenzyl methyl ketone, one mole of methylamine hydrochloride, one mole of sodium formate and over a mole of ninety per cent formic acid are mixed and heated together, preferably in a flask fitted with a reflux condenser for a suitable period, such as six hours, maintaining the temperature between 120 and 130° C. The product is mixed with water and the insoluble layer that separates is taken up with ether. The ether extract may be freed of ether by distillation and the residue distilled under reduced pressure, yielding a fraction boiling between 210 and 220° C. under 8 mm. mercury pressure and consisting substantially of 1-(*para*-methoxyphenyl)-2-formylmethyl-aminopropane. Source: Alles 1935

Preparation of Phenyl-2-ethylaminopropane
By Don P.R.L. Giudicelli

13 mL. (0.2 mol.) of ethylamine are introduced into a 250 mL. two-necked flask equipped with an air condenser and a dropping funnel and cooled on an alcohol-carbon dioxide ice bath. 9.65 (0.25 mol.) of formic acid are added dropwise. The reaction mixture is allowed to return to ambient temperature and 65 mmols of phenyl-2-propanone are added. the contents of the flask are heated for 20 hours at 150° C. After cooling 20 mL. of concentrated hydrochloric acid and 20 mL. of water are added., and the mixture is heated for 5 hours at the reflux temperature. A large amount of water is added and the product is extracted with 100 mL. of diethyl ether. The aqueous layer is rendered alkaline with sodium hydroxide solution and extracted three times in succession with 100 mL. of diethyl ether each time. The combined ether extracts are washed several times with water, dried over sodium sulphate, and filtered. The ether is evaporated from the filtrate in vacuo on a water bath.

The residue is rectified. 70% yield of phenyl-2-ethylaminopropane are thus obtained as a liquid...

To prepare the hydrochloride, the above base is dissolved in anhydrous diethyl ether and a solution of hydrogen chloride in diethyl ether is added until precipitation has ended, so as to obtain phenyl-2-ethylaminopropane hydrochloride... Source: Gludicili 1979
References: Alles 1935; Giudicelli 1976; Giudicelli 1978

Amphetamine From *alpha*-Bromophenylpropane

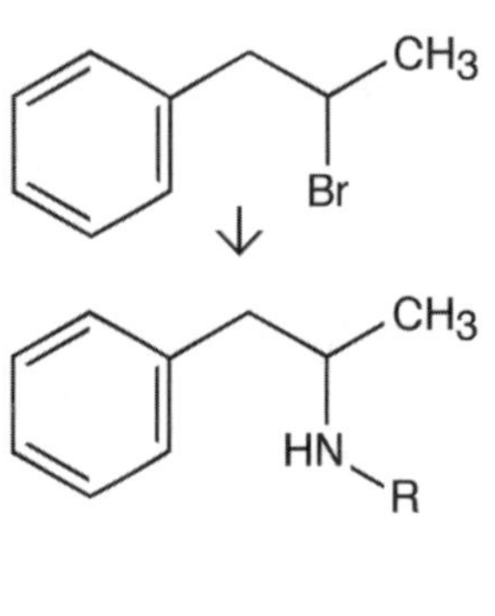

A mixture of 0.02 mole of phenyl-2-bromopropane is heated at 130 degrees with a solution of approximately 18% methylamine solution. The solution is evaporated to leave a residue of methamphetamine. The methamphetamine is then dissolved in a minimal solution of ether or appropriate solvent and cooled to precipitate the crystals of methamphetamine hydrochloride.

St.Mol.: 3,4-Dimethoxyphenyl-2-bromopropane
Prduct: 3,4-Dimethoxy-N-methylamphetamine
Reference: (Biniecki 1960)

Starting Molecule: *p*-Fluorophenethyl Bromide   Reagents: Ammonia
Product: *p*-Fluorophenylethylamine   Reference.: (Suter 1941)

Starting Molecule: *p*-Fluorophenethyl Bromide
Reagents: Methylamine
Product: N-Methyl-*p*-fluorophenylethylamine Reference: (Suter 1941)

Starting Molecule: Methoxyphenyl-2-bromopropane
Reagents: Ammonia
Product: Methoxyamphetamine   Reference: (Horii 1957)

Starting Molecule: 3,4-Methylenedioxyphenyl-2-bromopropane
Reagent: Methylamine
Product: 3,4-Methylenedioxy-N-methylamphetamine
Common Name: (MDMA)   Reference: (Biniecki 1960) (Merck 1912)

Starting Molecule: 2-Chloro-1-phenylpropane
Reagents: Ammonia
Product: Amphetamine   Reference: (Patrick 1946)

Starting Molecule: 2-Chloro-1-phenylpropane
Reagents: Methylamine
Product: N-Methylamphetamine   Reference: (Patrick 1946)

2-Bromo-1-phenylpropane from Allybenzene

At 0 degrees, a 0.06 mole of allybenzene is dropwise added to a solution of 40 grams of a 70% hydrogen bromide solution. The mixture is continued to be cooled at 0 degrees for a period of approximately 15 hours. The mixture is poured on ice at 0 degrees and then extracted with ether or appropriate solvent. The distillation of the mixture is done under reduced pressure to obtain the 2-bromo-1-phenyl-propane.

Starting Molecule: Allybenzene
Product: ß-Bromopropylbenzene
Reference: (Carter 1935) (Riegel 1946)

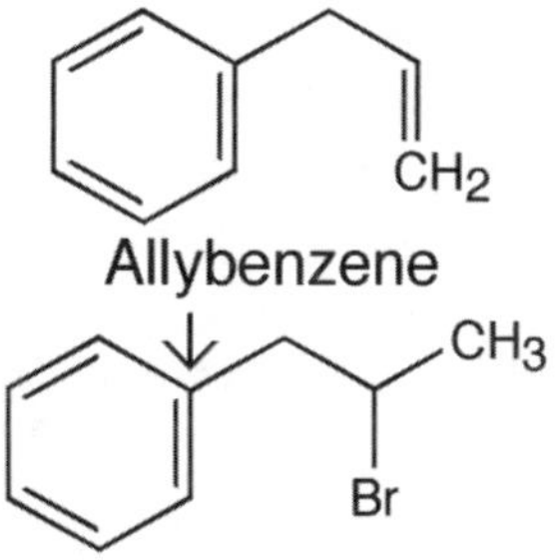

Starting Molecule: 3,4-Dimethoxy-allybenzene
Prduct: 3,4-Dimethoxyphenyl-2-bromopropane
Reference: (Biniecki 1960)
2,5-Dimethoxyphenyl-2-bromopropane (Shishido 1951)

Star. Mol.: 3,4-Methylenedioxyallybenzene (safrole)
References.: Biniecki 1960, Merck 1912
Product: 3,4-Methylenedioxyphenyl-2-bromopropane

Allybenzene

Starting Molecule: Methoxyallybenzene
Product: Methoxyphenyl-2-bromopropane Reference: (Horii 1957)

Ritter Reaction
Preparation of Phentermine
by Dom Vincent Fioncchio

To a Grignard reagent (prepared from (0.31 moles) 39.55 grams of benzyl chloride and 7.45 grams of magnesium in diethyl ether) is added 18.0 grams of acetone at such a rate that constant reflux is maintained. The reaction mixture is allowed to stand overnight at room temperature, and is then poured onto a mixture of 20 percent sulfuric acid and ice. The organic layer is separated, washed with water, an aqueous solution of sodium hydrogen carbonate and again with water, dried over magnesium sulfate and evaporated to dryness. The residue is distilled under reduced pressure to an approximate yield of (0.23 moles) 39.56 grams of 1-(phenyl)-2-methyl-2-propanol.

To 29.0 mL. of glacial acetic acid, cooled to 15° C. is added 11.5 grams of sodium cyanide (98 percent) while stirring, and then dropwise 32.4 mL. of concentrated sulfuric acid, dissolved in 29 ml. of glacial acetic acid, while maintaining a temperature of 20° C. The 1-(phenyl)-2-methyl-2-propanol is added moderately fast, allowing the temperature to rise spontaneously. After completing the addition, the reaction mixture is heated to 70° C. and stirred, and is then poured onto a mixture of water and ice. The aqueous mixture is neutralized with sodium carbonate and extracted with diethyl ether. The organic solution is washed with water, dried over magnesium sulfate and evaporated to dryness.

The oily residue is taken up in 100 mL. of 6 N aqueous hydrochloric acid and refluxed until a clear solution is obtained. The later is made basic with aqueous ammonia and extracted with diethyl ether; the organic solution is separated, washed, dried and evaporated to yield of approximately (0.16 moles) 20.96 grams of 1-(phenyl)-2-methyl-2-propylamine.

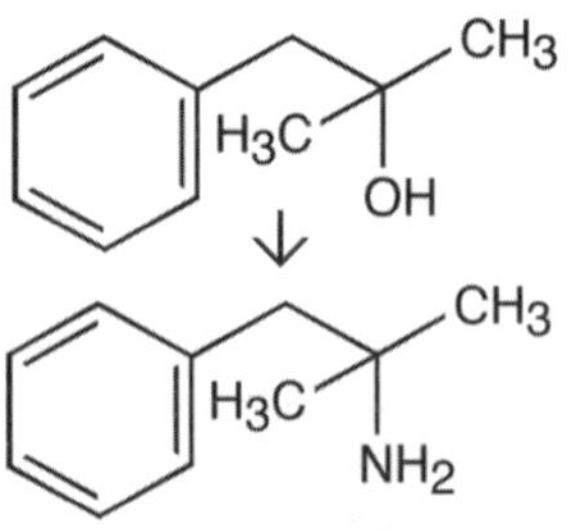

The 1-(phenyl)-2-methyl-2-propylamine hydrochloride is prepared by adding ethanolic hydrogen chloride to an ice-cold solution of the free base in ethanol; the desired salt precipitates and is recrystallized from ethanol. Source: (Fioncchio 1968) exemplified for phentermine preparation. For preparation of alpha, alpha, dimethyl subsitution see Suter 1948 References: (Bruce 1952) (Laing) (Ritter 1948; 1952)

CHAPTER 14: PREPARATION OF MORE PSYCHOSTIMULANTS

Preparation of Methcathinone

by William Merck, Karl Merck, Louis Merck, William Merck, Fritz Merck

...a process for the production of 1-phenyl-2-methylaminopropanone consisting in causing methylamine in aqueous solution to react upon 1-phenyl-1-oxo-2-bromo-propane, with or without addition of an organic solvent which is not miscible with water at temperatures under 50° C., dissolving the resulting 1-phenyl-1-oxo-2-methyl-aminopropane in organic solvents, precipitating as a salt by introducing gaseous hydrogen chloride...

The process... utilizes in its first phase the import knowledge that aqueous solutions of methyl-amine can be caused to react with the bromoketone. A simplification and cheapening is thereby offered as compared with the use of a medium in which both components are present in a dissolved state.

The second part of the present process relates to a new method of isolating the methyl-amino body as the hydrochloride or hydrobromide, which represents a considerable technical improvement as compared with the process given in the literature. The hydrochloride salt, for example, can be obtained with a satisfactory yield and in a high degree of purity by introducing hydrochloric acid gas into a benzene solution of the reaction product from the aqueous methylamine and the bromo-ketone and this as a colourless crystalline powder...

A mixture of 2 molecular proportions of methylamine hydrochloride, 2 molecular proportions of caustic soda in aqueous solution of about 30%, and 1 molecular proportion of bromopropiophenone with the addition of a solvent which is not miscible with water, such as benzene (2 to 10 molecular proportions), is energetically agitated in a horizontal tubular drum, great heating being avoided by cooling, so that the temperature does not increase above 25° C.. The oily product of the reaction separates out and is taken up with benzene (the amount of benzene may be about one half of the volume of the oily product); it is then washed with water and dried. In order to convert the base into the hydrochloride salt, the benzene solution is next treated preferably with alcohol and gaseous hydrogen chloride is introduced, when the hydrochloride of 1-phenyl-2-methylamino-propanone is precipitated in the form of small white crystals, while any oily by-products are kept in solution in the alcohol. The compact crystalline salt is separated by filtering with a filter pump and well washed first with benzene and then with acetone until the crystals are nearly colourless, and dried. It forms a sandy, almost white crystalline powder which, in the pure state, (which is obtained after several recrystallizations with alcohol), melts at 188° C. The hydrobromide salts melts at 144° C. Source: Merck 1929

Preparation of Norpseudoephedrine (Cathine) From Phenylpropanolamine

50 Grams of phenylpropanolamine hydrochloride is mixed with 500 mL of 14% hydrochloric acid. The mixture is refluxed for 12 hours. The solvent is distilled off to leave a residue (49 grams) containing 50% phenylpropanolamine hydrochloride and 50% norpseudo-ephedrine hydrochloride. Reference: (Kanao 1928) (Foder 1948)

Preparation of Norpseudoephedrine (Cathine) From N-Acetyl-Phenylpropanolamine

Method A: 100 Grams of N-acetyl-phenylpropanolamine is mixed with 200 mL of normal hydrochloric acid and refluxed for one hour. The solvent is distilled to leave a residue of norpseudoephedrine hydrochloride. Yields are 70% theoretical.

Method B: 100 Grams of N-acetyl-phenylpropanolamine is mixed with concentrated hydrochloric acid and heated with a small flame until the solution becomes transparent. The solution is then distilled to leave a residue of wet norpseudoephedrine hydrochloride. The hydrochloride salt is then dried in a desiccator over anhydrous Epsom salt. Yields are theoretical. Reference: (Kanao 1928)

Preparation of Methcathinone

(0.10 moles) of bromopropiophenone are dissolved in 20 cc. of alcohol and 19.5 grams of an alcoholic methylamine solution of 33 per cent. strength are added. After standing for several hours, the excess of alcohol is distilled under reduced pressure, the residue is taken up with ethyl acetate and the solution is shaken with dilute hydrochloric acid. The separated hydrochloric acid solution is mixed with a considerable quantity of potassium carbonate, and the oil which separates is taken up in ether. The ethereal solution is dried with sodium sulphate and concentrated. There remains methylamino-propiophenone.
Source: I.G. Farbenindustrie 1932

Preparation of Dialkylaminopropiophenones
by Jandirk Schiitte

1145 grams of *alpha*-bromopropiophenone and 850 grams of diethylamine are combined under stirring and heated on a water bath to boiling. The precipitate is filtered off under suction and washed with benzol. The filtrate is shaken up with aqueous hydrogen chloride, the aqueous solution made alkaline and etherified. The solution freed of the ether is fractionated. The boiling point (6 mm.) is 140° C. and the yield 800 grams. The base is dissolved in acetic ester and precipitated with isopropanolic hydrogen chloride. After suction filtration and washing with ether the yield is found to be 750 grams (80%) and the melting point 168° C

Diethylamine can be replaced with other dialkylamines to produce the appropriate dialkyl substitutions on aminopropiophenone. Source: Schiitte 1961

Preparation of *alpha*-Bromopropiophenone
I.G. Farbenindustrie

(0.2 moles) of propiophenone are dissolved in 250 cc. of methylene chloride and, after addition of 15 grams of calcium carbonate, 32 grams of bromine are introduced drop by drop, while stirring. After about 2 hours the reaction is complete. The precipitate is filtered by suction and the liquid is washed with caustic soda solution and water. The methylene chloride solution separated is dried and concentrated in vacuum (to leave 0.13 mole bromo-propiophenone). Source: I.G. Farbenindustrie 1932

Methanol canbe used in place of methylene chloride Wellcome 1948

Methylaminopropiophenone Compounds Using Sodium Dichromate
By Yvon J. L'Italien, Mildred C. Rebstock

A solution consisting of 0.99 g. of sodium dichromate, 1.32 g. of concentrated sulfuric acid and 4.46 cc. of water is added dropwise with stirring at room temperature to 1.65 g. of *l*-ephedrine dissolved in 4.7 cc. of water and 0.52 cc. of concentrated sulfuric acid. The reaction mixture is stirred at room temperature for 4 to 6 hours, made alkaline with sodium hydroxide solution and the desired free base of *l-alpha*-methylaminopropiophenone extracted from the aqueous solution with ether. The ether extract is dried over anhydrous magnesium sulfate and then the free base of the *l-alpha*-methylaminopropiophenone....

The free base of *l-alpha*-methylpropiophenone are combined, treated with an excess of dry hydrogen chloride and the solvents evaporated. The residual *l-alpha*-methylaminopropiophenone hydrochloride is stirred with petroleum ether, collected and purified by dissolving in ethanol and reprecipitating with ether; M.P. 182°-184° C.; [alpha]D/ 25=-53° (c=1% in water). Source: L'Italien 1957

Product: 2,5-Dimethoxy-*alpha*-methylaminopropiophenone (Morishita 1961). Product: *alpha*-Methylaminopropiophenone (cathinone) (Heinzelman 1953) See also: Bruce, W.F.

ß-Dimethylamino-*alpha*-methyl-propiophenone from Propiophenone, Methylamine HCl and *para*-Formaldehyde

A mixture of 224 grams of propiophenone, 176 grams of dimethylamine hydrochloride, 66 grams of paraformaldehyde, 3.33 mL. of hydrochloric acid and 266 mL. of ethanol is refluxed for two hours. After evaporation of the ethanol, water is added and the water-insoluble material is extracted with ether. The aqueous layer is made basic with aqueous ammonia and the organic base is extracted with ether. The ether is washed, dried and evaporated to yield 149 grams of *beta*-dimethylamino-*alpha*-methyl-propiophenone. Source: CIBA 1961

Cathinone from isoNitrosopropiophenone and Tin Dichloride

14 Grams of... isonitroso-propiophenone are mixed with 38 grams of tin dichloride dissolved in 75 cc. of concentrated hydrochloric acid. The temperature rises rapidly, but it must not exceed 60° C. The tin double salt precipitates. The whole is allowed to stand for about 6 hours, then filtered by suction, dissolved in water and the solution, after removal of the tin, is evaporated to dryness. 10 Grams of... aminopropiophenone hydrochloride are obtained. Source: I.G. Farbenindustrie 1931

Preparation of isoNitrosopropiophenone
by Max Bockmühl, Gustav Ehrhart, and Leonard Stein

23.9 Grams of... propiophenone are dissolved in 250 cc. of ether, mixed with 6.8 grams of finely powdered sodium nitrite and gaseous hydrochloric acid is introduced for 1/2 hour, while stirring. After the whole has been boiled for several hours, the sodium chloride formed is separated by filtering by suction, the residue is absorbed in dilute caustic soda solution. The... isonitrosopropiophenone separates from the alkaline solution by additions of concentrated hydrochloric acid... Source: Bockmühl 1934

Aminorex
(2-amino-5-phenyloxazoline)
Preparation of 3,4,5-Trimethoxyaminorex (TRAX)
by George Ireland Poos

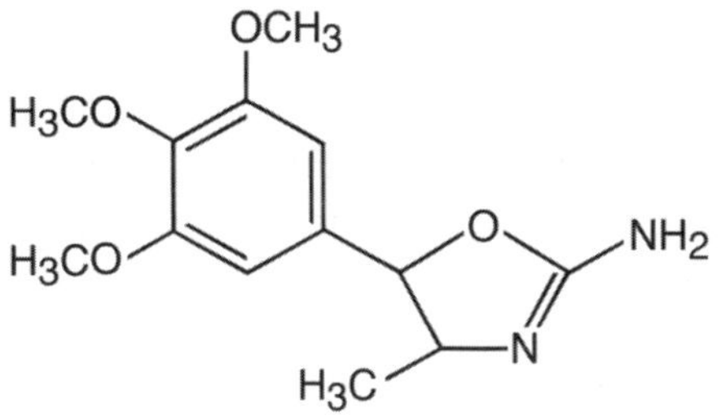

The available compounds possessing central nervous system stimulant activity, such as amphetamine, are subject to defects, particularly the production of side effects which limit their utility. There is therefore a demand for new and unrelated types of compounds which will exhibit such activity without possessing a chemical structure which the known compounds possess and with which their undesirable side effects appear to be connected.

A solution of cyanogen bromide is prepared from 1.58 grams (0.036) of sodium cyanide and 5.7 grams (0.036 mole) of bromine in methanol. To this cyanogen bromide solution (at a temperature of about 5° C.) is added a room temperature solution of 2.98 grams (0.036 mole) of sodium acetate and 7.44 grams (0.03 mole) of α-(aminomethyl)-3,4,5-trimethoxybenzyl alcohol in methyl alcohol. The resulting solution is stirred for one and a half hours at room temperature. It is then made basic by addition of ammonia and concentrated under vacuum. The residue is added about 150 cc. of water and the mixture is made strongly basic by addition of 10% sodium hydroxide. This aqueous alkaline suspension is extracted 3 times with methylene chloride. The combined organic extracts are washed with water, dried over magnesium sulfate, filtered, and concentrated to dryness under vacuum. The residue is slurried in ether and the solid collected and dried, to give 6.04 grams of crude 2-amino-5-(3,4,5-trimethoxy-phenyl)oxazoline. After three recrystallizations from acetone, the purified product melts at 181°-183.5° C.

By using, in the above procedure, the corresponding α-(aminomethyl)-*p*-methoxybenzyl alcohol, α-(aminomethyl)-3,4-dimethoxybenzyl alcohol, α-(aminomethyl)-2,3,4,5-tetramethoxybenzyl alcohol, respectively, the corresponding 2-amino-5-(*p*-methoxyphenyl)oxazoline, 2-amino-5-(3,4-dimethoxyphenyl)oxazoline, 2-amino-5-(2,3,4,5-tetramethoxyphenyl)oxazoline, respectively, are prepared. Source: George Ireland Poos 1964 Check Morishita 1961 for the prepartion of aminoketones from propiophenone and formamide.

CHAPTER 15:
SUBSTITUTED BENZALDEHYDES

Benzaldehydes are used in fragrances, flavorings and in industry. Naturally occurring benzaldehydes can be extracted (e.g. benzaldehyde from oil of bitter almonds, syringic aldehyde from Lilac bark). Most substituted benzaldehydes are produced synthetically because they only occur as trace constituents in natural products. Benzaldehydes are primarily produced by synthetic or semi-synthetic methods.

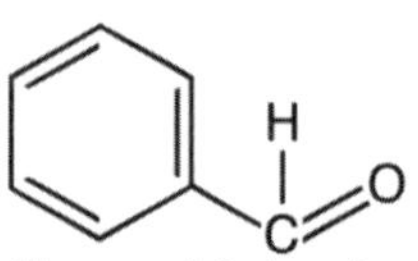

Synthetic substituted benzaldehydes can be made by the following reactions:

Benzaldehyde

1) The partial oxidation of substituted propenylbenzenes (e.g. isosafrole which is 3,4-methylenedioxy-propenylbenzene) transforms them into benzaldehydes (e.g. Piperonal, which is 3,4-methylene-dioxy-benzaldehyde) (Davies 1943) (McLang 1925, 1926). Piperonal can also be prepared by the oxidation of piperic acid (obtained from pepper corns) (Ber 23: 2372).

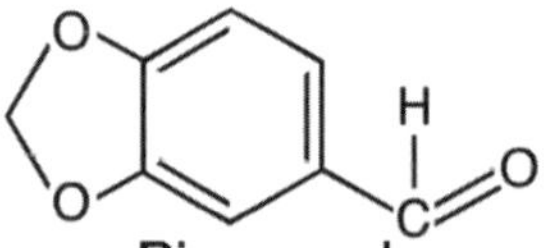

Piperonal

2) The Reimer-Tiemann Reaction creates benzaldehydes from phenols (hydroxy benzenes), chloroform and alkali, such as salicylic aldehyde from phenol; 2-Hydroxy-5-methoxy-benzaldehyde from quinol monomethyl ether (Rubenstein 1925).

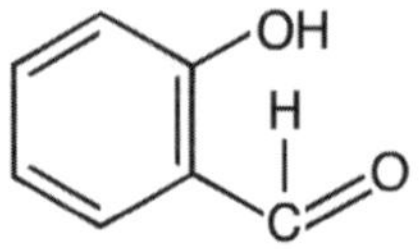

Salicylic Aldehyde

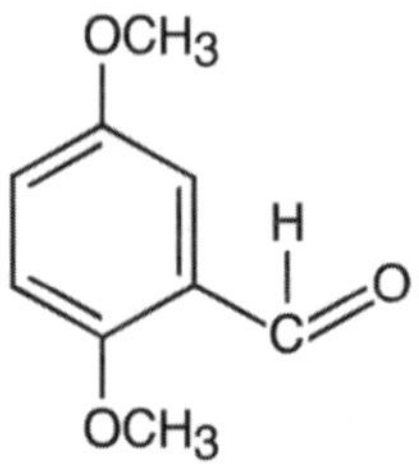

2,5-Dimethoxybenzaldehyde

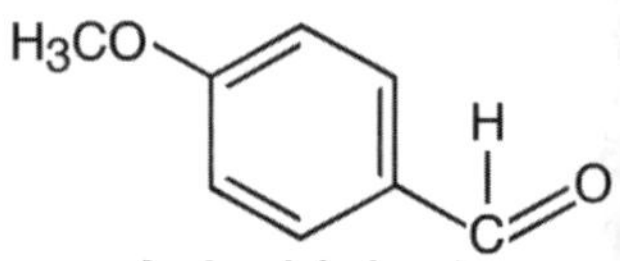

Anisaldehyde

3) The Gattermann Aldehyde Synthesis; from benzenes, cyanide hydrogen chloride and a Lewis Acid (e.g. *p*-anisaldehyde, which is 4-methoxybenzaldehyde can be made from anisole (methoxybenzene) 2,5-dimethoxy-benzaldehyde from *para*-dimethoxybenzene) (Baker 1938 (Niedzielski 1941) (Orinak 1966).

4) The Duff Reaction is used to make ortho-substituted benzaldehydes from substituted phenols with hexamethylenetetramine and an acid catalyst: e.g. 2-hydroxy-benzaldehyde from phenol (hydroxy-benzene); 2-hydroxy-5-methoxybenzaldehyde from *p*-methoxyphenol.

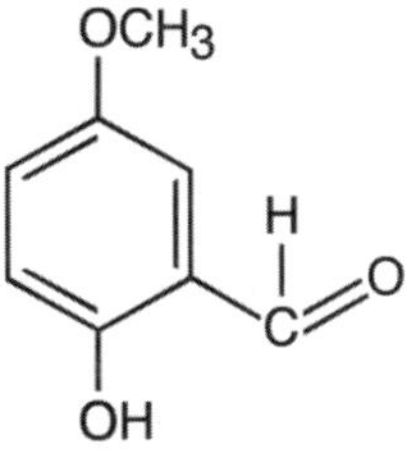

2-Hydroxy-5-methoxybenzaldehyde

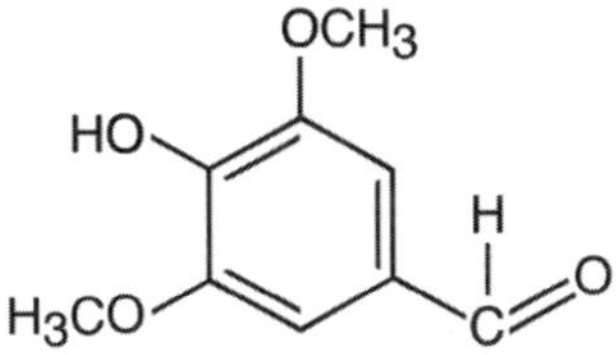

Syringaldehyde

5) Electrolytic reductions can be used to produce substituted benzaldehydes from benzoic acids.

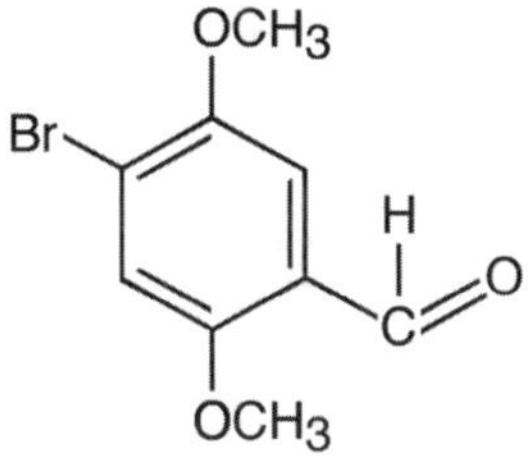

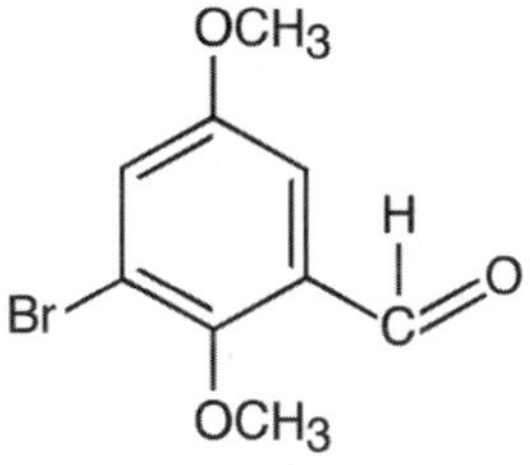

4-Br-2,5-Dimethoxybenzaldehyde   3-Br-2,5-Dimethoxybenzaldehyde

6) Halogenation Reactions are used to create substitutions on benzaldehydes. 4-Br-2,5-Dimethoxybenzaldehyde is created by the bromination of 2,5-dimethoxybenzaldehyde (Nichols 1970). 3-Br-2,5-Dimethoxybenzaldehyde is created by the bromination of 2,5-dimethoxybenzaldehyde (Rubenstein 1925).

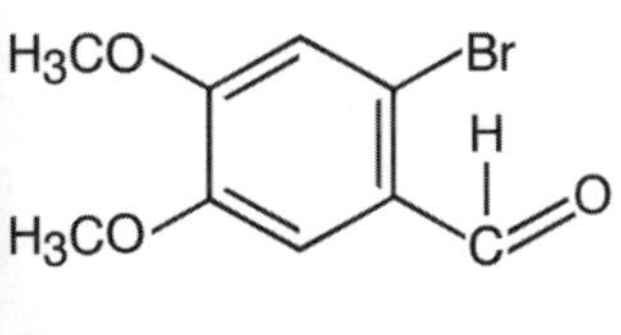

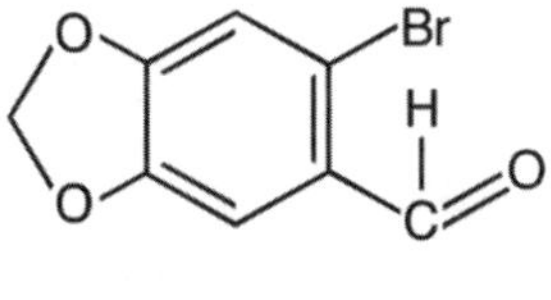

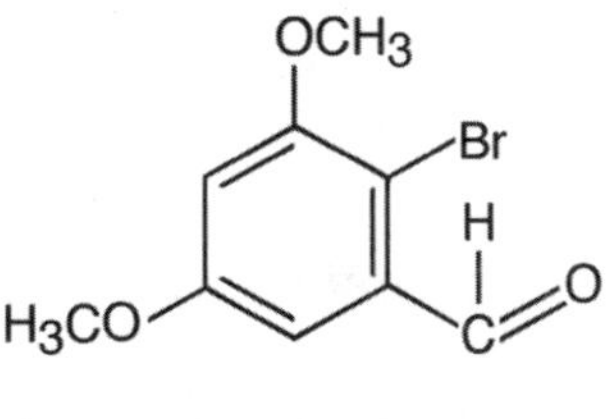

2-Bromo-4,5-dimethoxybenzaldehyde is created by the bromination of 4,5-dimethoxybenzaldehyde (Parijs 1930).

2-Bromo-4,5-methylenedioxybenzaldehyde is created from the bromination of 4,5-methylenedioxybenzaldehyde (Parijs 1930).

5-Bromo-2,4-dimethoxybenzaldehyde is created from the bromination of 2,4-dimethoxybenzaldehyde (Rao 1929).

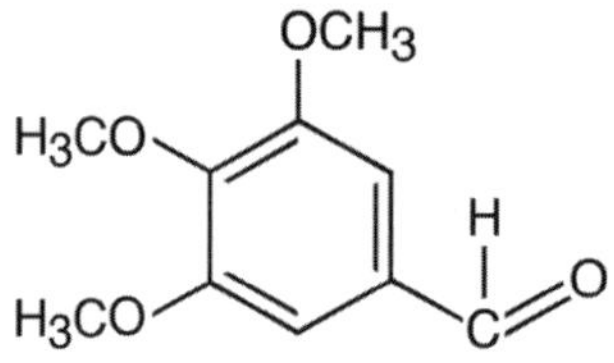

3,4,5-Trimethoxybenzaldehyde

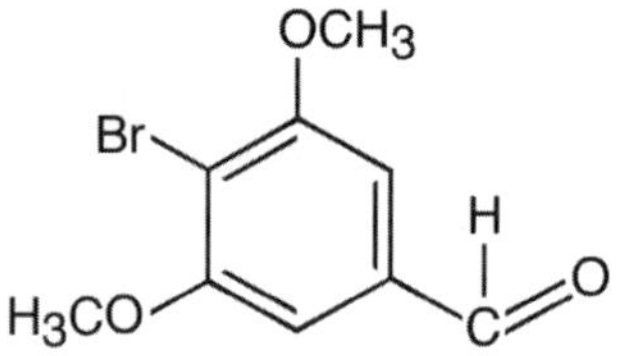

4-Bromo-3,5-dimethoxybenzaldehyde

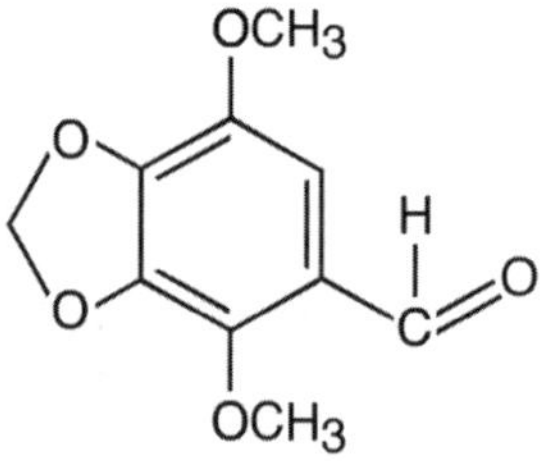

2,5-Dimethoxy-3,4-methylenedioxybenzaldehyde

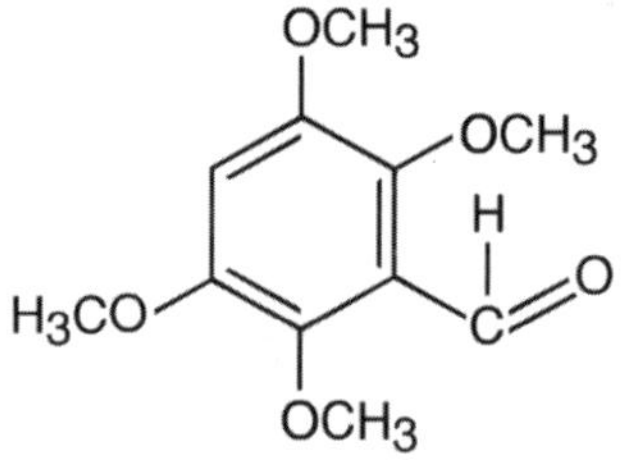

2,3,5,6-Tetramethoxybenzaldehyde

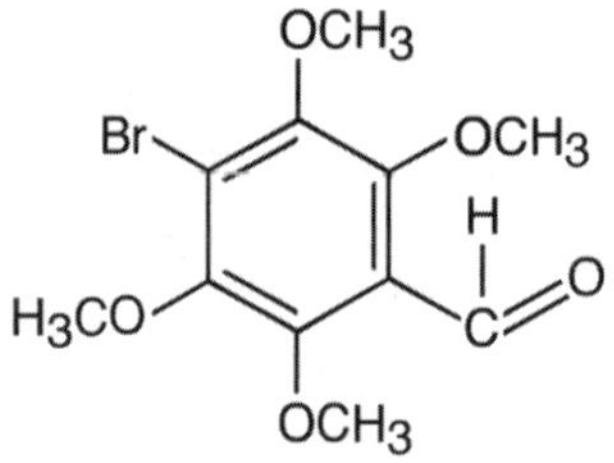

4-Bromo-2,3,5,6-Tetramethoxybenzaldehyde

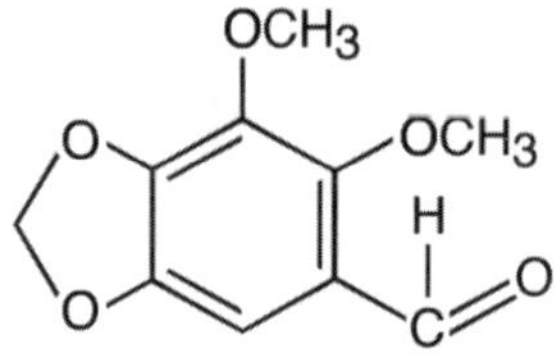

2,3-Dimethoxy-4,5-methylenedioxybenzaldehyde

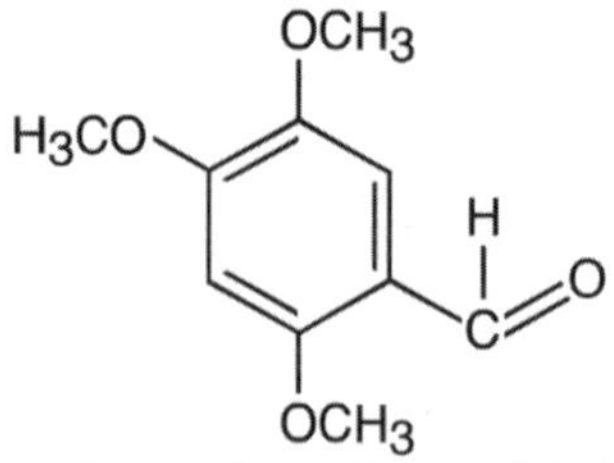

2,4,5-Trimethoxybenzaldehyde

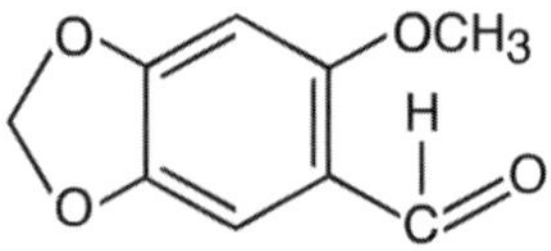

2-Methoxy-4,5-methylenedioxybenzaldehyde

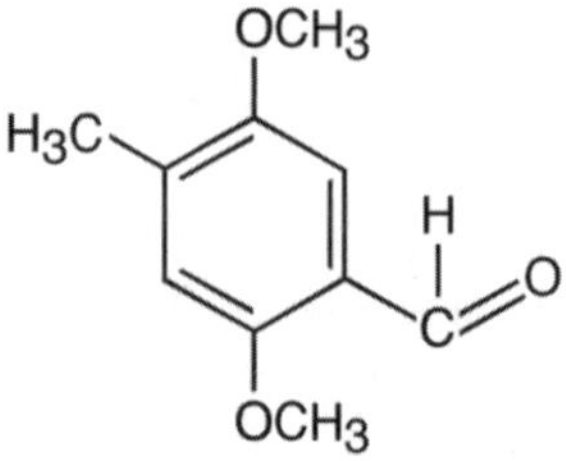

4-Methyl-2,5-Dimethoxybenzaldehyde

Duff Reaction
ortho-Formylation of Phenol

An aldehyde group (formyl group) can be attached *ortho* to the hydroxy group on the benzene ring.

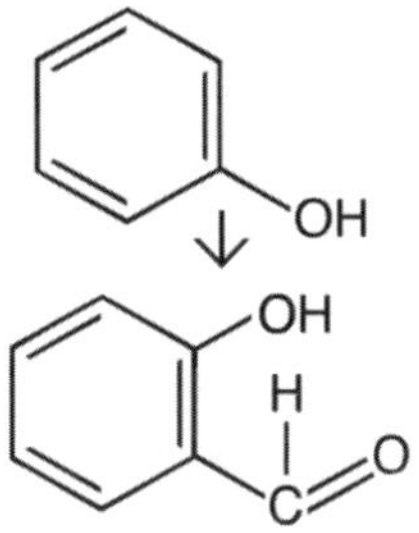

The previous reaction involves the ortho-formylation of phenol. When the *ortho* position is occupied by such groups as methoxy or a carboxylic acid then the formylation takes place on another position on the benzene ring.

A solution of 550 mL glycerine and 160 g. of boric acid is stirred and heated to exactly 170 degrees. The boiling flask is equipped with a downward condenser to distill the water as formed. 120 Grams of hexamine is added and the temperature is allowed to drop to 160 degrees. 0.75 Mole of the phenol is added. The temperature of the solution is raised to 140. The temperature is slowly increased until the reaction becomes exothermic (gives off heat-energy). The temperature of the reaction is kept between 155-160 degrees for 7 minutes while stirring. The temperature is rapidly cooled to 110 degrees.

A solution of 140 mL of concentrated sulfuric acid and 460 mL of water is added to the mixture and stirred for one hour. The mixture is cooled in an ice bath to precipitate the boric acid. The boric acid is suction filtered from the cold solution.

Some of the benzaldehydes can be obtained by steam distillation. Some do not steam distill. Those that are not easily steam distilled can be obtained by extracting with chloroform or appropriate solvent.

The benzaldehyde is extracted from the solvent by mixing with 150 grams of sodium bisulfite. The sodium bisulfite solution is separated and acidified with sulfuric acid.

Sulfur dioxide gas is generated and must be vented.

The aqueous sodium bisulfite solution is heated on a steam bath. When the solution becomes warm, air is then bubbled through the solution until the smell of rotten eggs is not apparent (sulfur dioxide). The solution is cooled to precipitate (as an oil or as crystals) the hydroxy-benzaldehyde.

Starting Molecule: *m*-Cresol
Product: 2-Hydroxy-4-methylbenzaldehyde Reference: (Ono 1973)
Product: 3-Hydroxy-*p*-tolualdehyde Reference: (Duff 1941)

Starting Molecule: *o*-Cresol
Product: 2-Hydroxy-*m*-tolualdehyde Reference: (Duff 1941)

Starting Molecule: *p*-Cresol
Product: 4-Hydroxy-*m*-tolualdehyde Reference: (Duff 1941)

Starting Molecule: *o*-Ethylphenol
Product: 3-Ethyl-salicylaldehyde Reference: (Renz 1947)

Starting Molecule: *p*-Methoxyphenol
Product: 2-Hydroxy-5-methoxybenzaldehyde Reference: (Yakovlev 1950)

Starting Molecule: Phenol
Product: 2-Hydroxy-benzaldehyde Reference: (Duff 1941)

Starting Molecule: Pyrogallol-1,3-dimethyl ether
Product: 4-Hydroxy-3,5-dimethoxybenzaldehyde
Common Name: Syringaldehyde Reference: (Allen 1963)

Elbs Persulfate Oxidation of Benzaldehydes

The oxidation of phenols with potassium persulfate to form
p-dihydroxy molecules is called the Elbs Persulfate Oxidation Reaction.
When the *para* position is occupied, *ortho* substitution will occur.

Starting Molecule: Coumarin
Product: 6-Hydroxy-coumarin
Reference: (Bargellini 1915)

Starting Molecule: Phenol
Product: Quinol   Reference: (Baker 1948)

Starting Molecule (Common Name): Salicylaldehyde
(Chemical Name): 2-Hydroxybenzaldehyde
Product: 2,5-Dihydroxybenzaldehyde
Reference: (Baker 1948) (Hodgson 1927)

Starting Molecule: Vanillin
Prdt.: 3,4-Dihydroxy-5-methoxybenzaldehyde
Reference: (Baker 1948)

Dakin Reaction

0.8 Moles of substituted benzaldehyde is mixed with 350 mL of a sodium hydroxide solution (32 grams of sodium hydroxide). The mixture is stirred to dissolve as nitrogen gas is bubbled into the flask. 1150 mL of 3% hydrogen peroxide solution is added in 50 mL amounts making sure that the temperature of the solution remains between 40-50 degrees. The solution is allowed to cool to 45 degrees after each addition before another 50 mL is added. The entire addition of hydrogen peroxide will take approximately 1 to 2 hours. When all the hydrogen peroxide has been added, the solution is allowed to cool to room temperature and saturated with sodium chloride (salt). The solution is extracted with 800 mL of ether or appropriate water insoluble solvent. The extract is dried and the solvent distilled to leave a residue of the substituted phenol. Yields are approximately 75% theoretical.

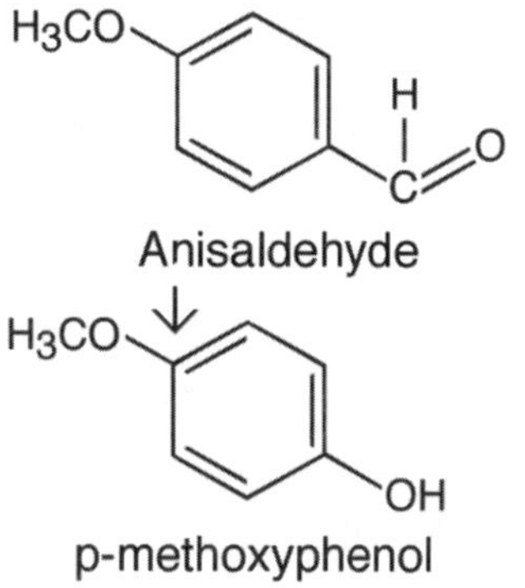

Anisaldehyde

p-methoxyphenol

Starting Molecule: 2-Hydroxy-3-methoxybenzaldehyde
Product: Pyrogallol monomethyl ether Reference: (Surry, *Organic Syntheses*)

METHYLATIONS OF HYDROXYBENZALDEHYDES

0.25 Mole of hydroxybenzaldehyde is melted in a boiling flask equipped with a condenser for reflux. 33 mL of 50% potassium hydroxide solution is added dropwise, with stirring at a rate of 2 to 3 drops per second. 32 mL of dimethyl sulfate is then added at a rate of of 2 to 3 drops per second with stirring. Two hours later the reaction mixture is poured into a beaker, and rapidly cooled (approx. 25 degrees) by pouring onto ice-cold water. The precipitated crystalline mass is suction filtered from the solution (oils are extracted with ether and distilled to leave the methoxybenzaldehyde), ground to powder and mixed with 80 mL of ice-water, suction filtered again and dried over anhydrous magnesium sulfate in a vacuum desiccator or covered casserole dish. Benzaldehydes are highly sensitive to oxidization by air and should be stored in a tightly sealed amber bottle. Yields are 80%+.

References: (Buck; *Organic Syntheses*) (Arthur 1959)

Benzaldehyde from Benzyl Chloride
by Friedrich Brühne

322 grams (2 moles) of benzyl chloride and 750 grams of 25 percent strength hydrochloric acid are heated to the reflux temperature in a 1 liter three-necked flask with a stirrer, reflux condenser, gas inlet tube and thermometer, while stirring vigorously, and the mixture is kept under light reflux for 2 hours. A sump temperature of 106° C. is established. A weak stream of nitrogen is passed through the flask during the reaction. The off-gas escaping from the reflux condenser is absorbed in a washing tower, packed with Raschig rings, with 630 grams of water, which are circulated by means of a pump. After cooling the mixture, 204.0 grams of a light yellow coloured oil which, according to the titrimetric determination, contains 98.1% of benzaldehyde (=200.1 grams pure benzaldehyde) are obtained as the organic phase. This corresponds to a yield of 94.3% theory. Source: Brühne 1980

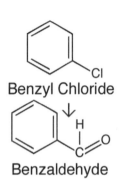

Benzyl Chloride

Benzaldehyde

SUBSTITUTED BENZALDEHYDES FROM SUBSTITUTED PROPENYLBENZENES

Method A can be used with hydroxy, methoxy and methylenedioxy substitutions.

Method A: 1 Mole of substituted propenylbenzene is added to a cupric oxide solution (1900 grams of cupric sulfate pentahydrate, 1070 grams of sodium hydroxide, and 2500 mL of water). The mixture is refluxed for eight hours and filtered of red cuprous oxide. The filtrate is washed with water. The alkaline filtrate and washings are acidified and extracted with ether (or appropriate solvent e.g. benzene, acetone etc.). The acidified solution is mixed for one hour with a solution of 200 grams of sodium bisulfite in 750 mL water. The aqueous layer is separated, washed with appropriate solvent and acidified with a 50% solution of sulfuric acid. The solution is heated on a steam bath for short period and air is bubbled through the solution to remove sulfur dioxide. The substituted benzaldehyde crystallizes from the solution on cooling and is separated by vacuum filtration. Yields are approximately 90%.

Various alkaline copper oxidizing agents (e.g. Fehling's Solution, Benedict's Solution) will produce the same results.

Alkaline copper oxidizing agents are best suited for the oxidization of propenyl group to an aldehyde group. The oxidizing strength of changing a cupric to a cuprous compound is adequate to transform the propenyl to the aldehyde group, but not strong enough to oxidize the benzaldehyde into benzoic acid.

Method B: 1 Mole of substituted propenylbenzene is thoroughly mixed with a solution of 800 grams of 50% sulfuric acid in five liters of water. 200 grams of sodium dichromate in one liter of water is gradually added at 30 to 40 degrees over the period of 30 minutes. The mixture may turn green. Extract the mixture with 3 liters of benzene. Wash the benzene extract with one liter of 5% sodium hydroxide solution and then wash with 3 liters of water. The solvent is distilled from the solution to leave a crude residue of oily 'wet' substituted benzaldehyde which is dried over anhydrous calcium chloride, Epsom salt or appropriate drying agent. The crude product can be purified by dissolving in minimum quantity of hot alcohol, filtered through animal charcoal and concentrated to crystallize the substituted benzaldehyde.

Propenylbenzene

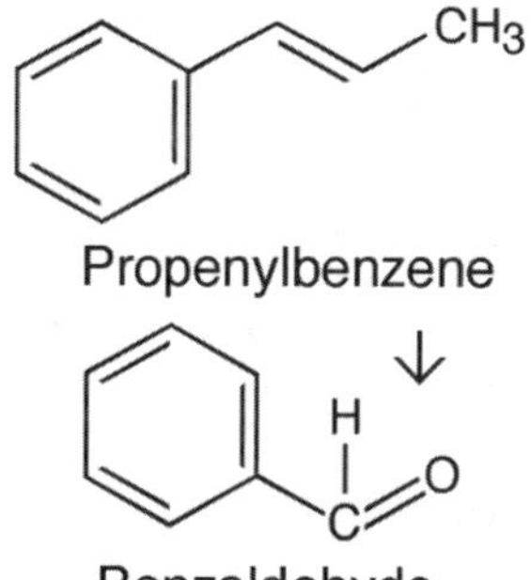

Benzaldehyde

Starting Molecule: 4-Hydroxy-3,5-dimethoxypropenylbenzene
Product: 4-Hydroxy-3,5-dimethoxybenzaldehyde
Common Name: Syringaldehyde
Reference: (Pearl 1950)

Starting Molecule: 3,4-Methylenedioxypropenylbenzene
Product: 3,4-Methylenedioxybenzaldehyde
Common Name: Piperonal
Reference: (Davies 1943)

See also (McLang 1925, 1926)

CHAPTER 16:
ALLY AND PROPENYLBENZENES
FROM NATURAL SOURCES

Substituted phenylpropenes can be obtained by crystallization from commonly available natural essential oils. Essential oils can be obtained by the steam distillation or solvent extraction of many plants, roots, bark and seeds.

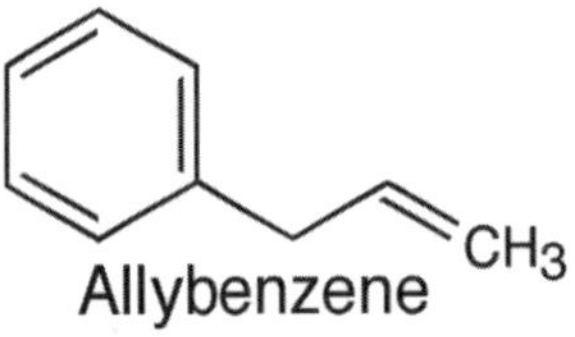

M.F. C9H10
M.W. 118.18
Allybenzene
m.p. -40° b.p. 156°
Propenylbenzene
m.p. -60.5°
b.p. 69° @ 28mm

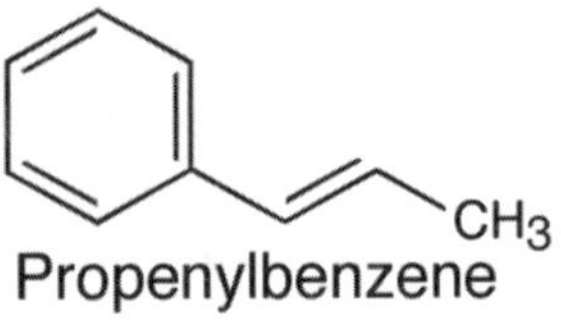

Allybenzene

Propenylbenzene

The best way to obtain the essential oils from botanicals is by steam distillation. The distillate forms two layers. One layer is water and the other layer is the water insoluble essential oil. Another way is to grind the botanical into small granular chunks and do a percolation (or mix the material with the solvent and filter) with a water insoluble solvent such as ether, benzene, toluene, acetone, chloroform etc. The solvent is distilled or evaporated to leave the essential oil.

Essential oils must be kept in a tightly sealed amber bottle and stored in a cool place as phenylpropenes will oxidize with air and poly-merize with light. Synthetic preparation of allybenzene using Grignard Reaction: Hell 1903, 1904; Klages 1902; Tiffeneau 1904.

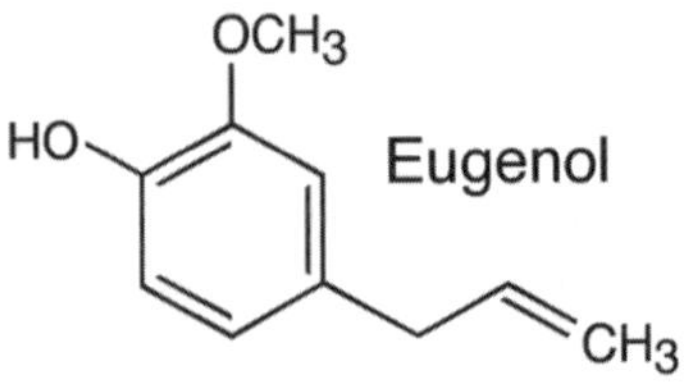

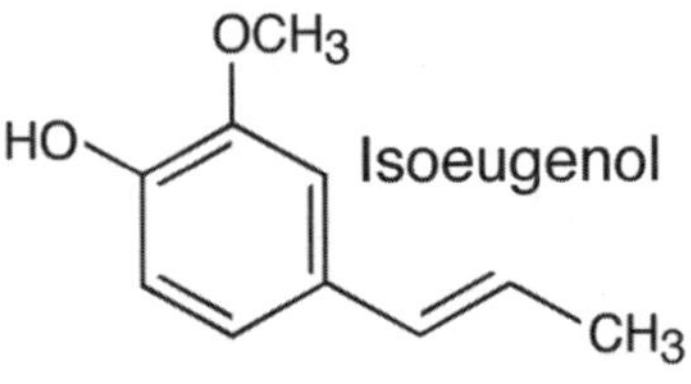

Eugenol

Isoeugenol

The Oil of Clove is obtained by steam distillation. The oil contains approximately 75% eugenol, which is 3-methoxy-4-hydroxy-allybenzene. M.F. C10H12O2 M.W. 164.21 It can be extracted by fractional distilla-tion or crystallization of the oil. Eugenol: m.p. -9.1° b.p. 255°
Isoeugenol: m.p. -10° b.p. 266°

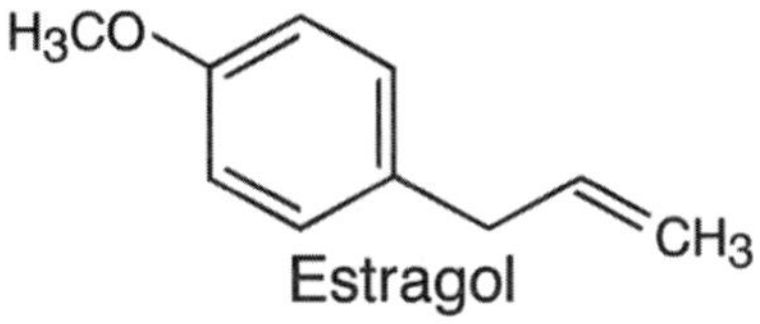

Estragol

Estragol (4-methoxy-allybenzene) can be obtained from Tarragon Oil (*Artemisia dracunculus*) or crude sulfate turpentine. Estragol forms azeotropic (partially dissolves) mixtures with water. (Booth 1968).   b.p. 216° @ 764mm
M.F. C10H12O   M.W. 148.20

Anise seed oil contains 80-90% anethole (4-methoxy-propenyl-benzene). Anethole maybe obtained from the seed oil by placing the oil in a beaker, cooling it in the freezer to crystallize the anethole and suction filtration. Fennel Seed Oil contains approximately 50 to 60% anethole. M.F. C10H12O M.W. 148.20 m.p. 21.4°

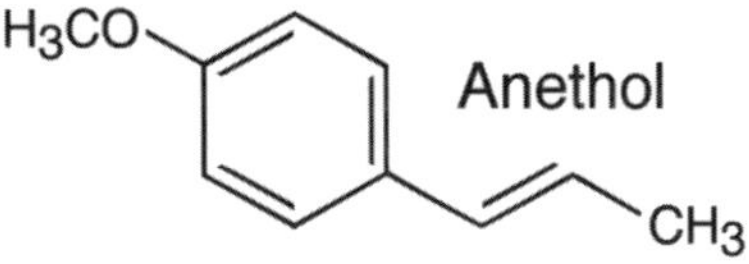

Anethol

Sassafras Root Bark Oil

Sassafras Root Bark Oil is obtained by the steam distillation of the inner bark chips of the Sassafras tree (*Sassafras albidum, S. variifolium and S. albidum*). The distillation of Sassafras bark was an American Industry at one time. It used to be an economic base for Ohio, New Jersey, Indiana, Tennessee, New York and New England during and after the civil war. During the 1940's, Virginia, Maryland and Pennsylvania were the major producers. Today much of the natural Sassafras Oil comes from the exploitation of a tree in the Brazilian rain forest named *Ocotea pretiosa*.

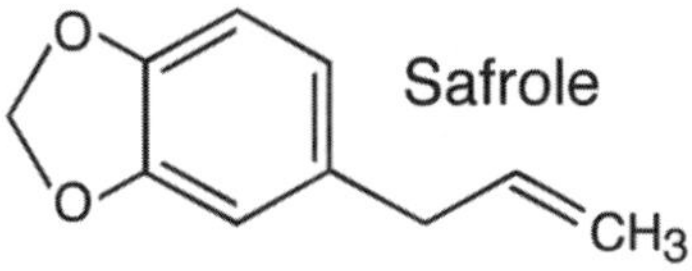

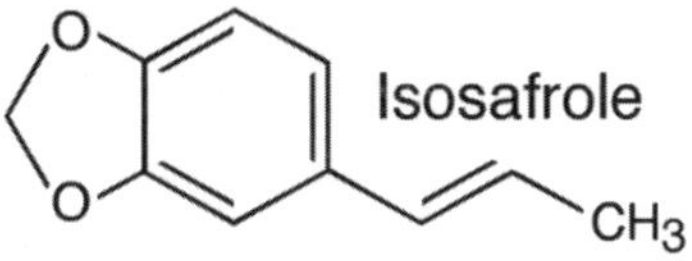

Safrole

Isosafrole

The oil is extracted from the inner bark of the Sassafras tree by steam distillation. The root bark contains between 6 to 9 percent oil. Sassafras oil contains approximately 80% safrole. Safrole can be obtained by fractional crystallization, suction filtration and fractional distillation Synthetic Prep.: (Feugeas 1964; Perkin 1927). Safrole is listed as a carcinogen by the EPA. See: Second Annual Report on Carcinogens (NTP 81-43, Dec. 1981; pgs. 219-220); IARC Monographs (1976) 10: 231-241.
M.F. C10H10O2 M.W. 162.1   Safrol: m.p. -11° b.p. 232°
Isosafrol (3,4-methylenedioxypropenylbenzene): m.p. 8.2° b.p. 253°

2,4,5-Trimethoxyallybenzene

The oil of *Caesulia axillares* contains
2,4,5-trimethoxyallybenzene.
M.F. C12H16O3 M.W. 208.26

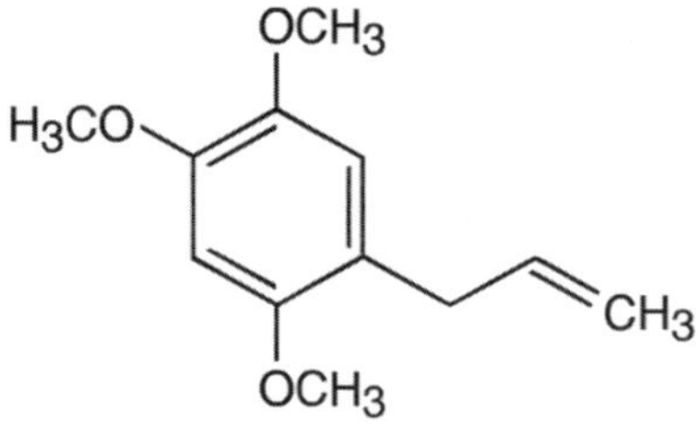

2,4,5-Trimethoxyallybenzene

Asarone

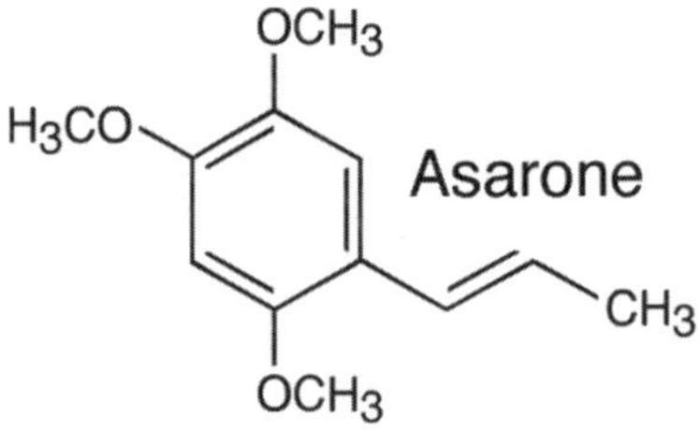

Asarone

Sweet Flag Oil is obtained by the steam distillation of the roots of sweet flag; *Acorus calamus*, and also *Asarum europaeum* and *Asarum arifolium*. The oil contains about 75% 2,4,5-trimethoxy-propenylbenzene; asarone. Asarone can be suction filtered from the crystallized oil that has been exposed to low temperature. Asarone occurs as two isomers in nature. *alpha*-Asarone is also called the *trans* isomer. ß-Asarone is called *beta*-asarone and is the *cis* isomer. The m.p. of asarone is 67°. Synthetic preparation of 2,4,6-Trimethoxy-propenyl-benzene: (Holms 1950). ß-Asarone can also be prepared synthetically (Shulgin 1965) from the decarboxylation of *alpha*-Methyl-ß-2,4,5-trimethoxy-phenylacrylic acid with copper gauze and quinoline (Dandiya 1962).

Apiol (Parsley)

Apiol is the chief constituent of parsley seed oil. Apiol was first obtained from the oil by Stange of Basel, Switzerland in 1823. In 1890 Ciamician and Silber identified the chemical structure of apiol to be 3,4-methylenedioxy-2,5-dimethoxyallybenzene.
Synthetic. Preparation: (Baker 1938)

M.F. C12H14O4 M.W. 222.24

Apiol: m.p. 29.5   b.p. 294
Isoapiol: m.p. 56   b.p. 303-4

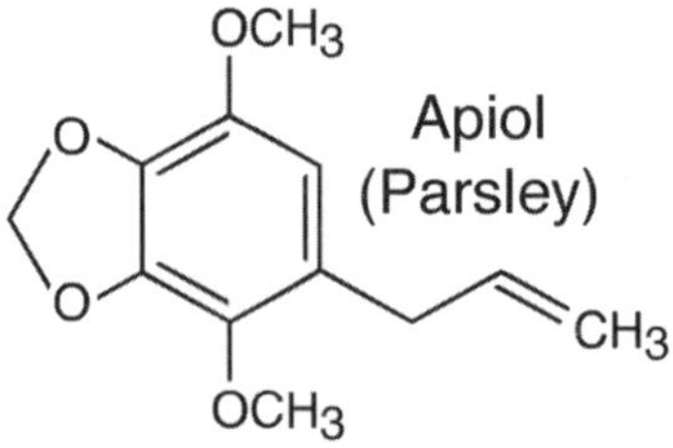

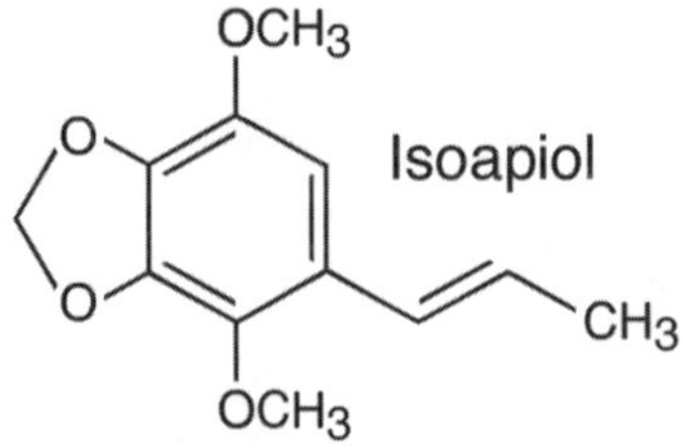

Apiol
(Parsley)

Isoapiol

2,3,5,6-Tetramethoxyallybenzene and Apiol (3,4-methylenedioxy-2,5-dimethoxy-allybenzene) from Parsley Seeds.

Chopped parsley seeds are soaked in ethyl alcohol for two days. The alcohol is filtered from the seeds. The solution is cooled to 10-12 degrees and the crystallized 2,3,5,6-tetramethoxyallybenzene is suction filtered from the solution. Evaporation of the ethanol leaves apiol containing various flavonoglycosides. The solution is washed with water and the non-aqueous layer is refrigerated to crystallize the apiol.

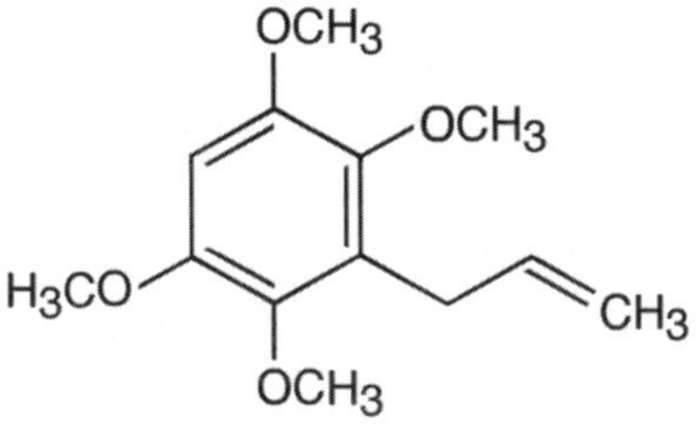

2,3,5,6-Tetramethoxyallybenzene

Apiol occurs as brittle, white, needle shaped crystals, m.p. 30 degrees. (Kolesnikov 1958) 2,3,4,5-Tetramethoxyally-benzene is a constituent of the seed oil of *Apium* species.

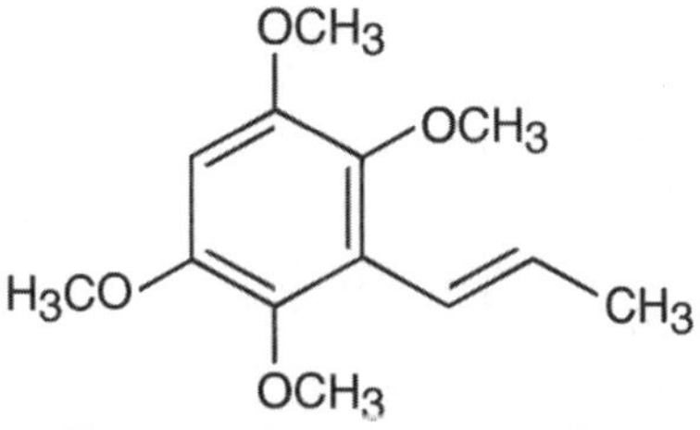

2,3,5,6-Tetramethoxypropenylbenzene

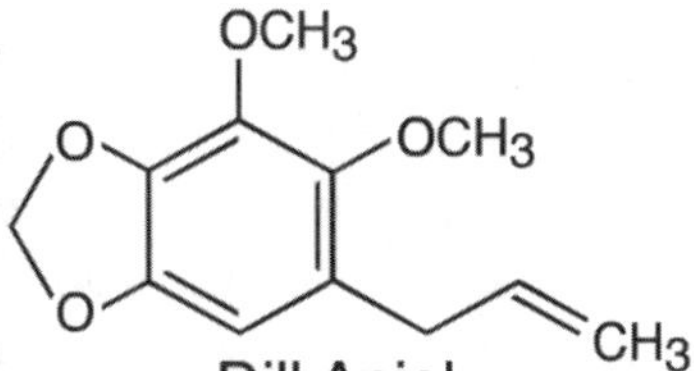

Dill Apiol

Iso Dill Apiol

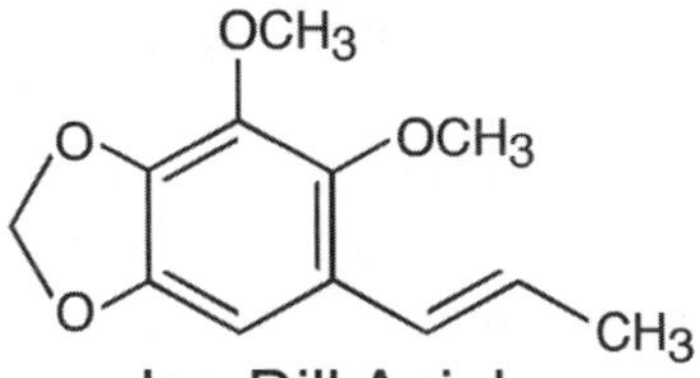

Dill Apiol

The Oil of Dill Seed is obtained by the steam distillation of dill seeds (*Anethum graveolus*). Dill apiol, (2,3-dimethoxy-4,5-methylenedioxy-allybenzene, can be isolated from this oil.

Synthetic Preparation: (Baker 1934) (Dalacker 1969).

M.F. C12H14O4   M.W. 222.24

Dill Apiol: m.p. 29.5 b.p. 285

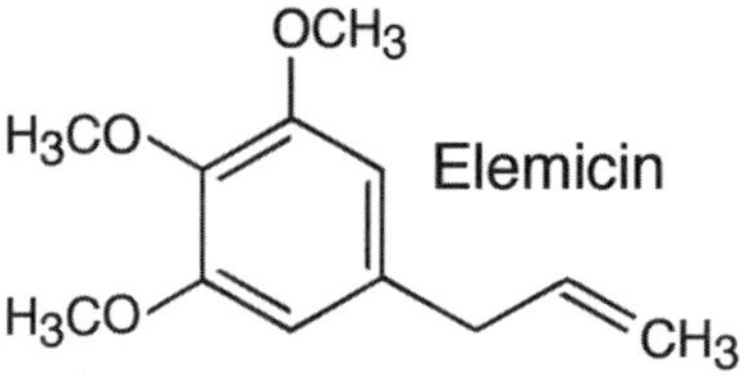

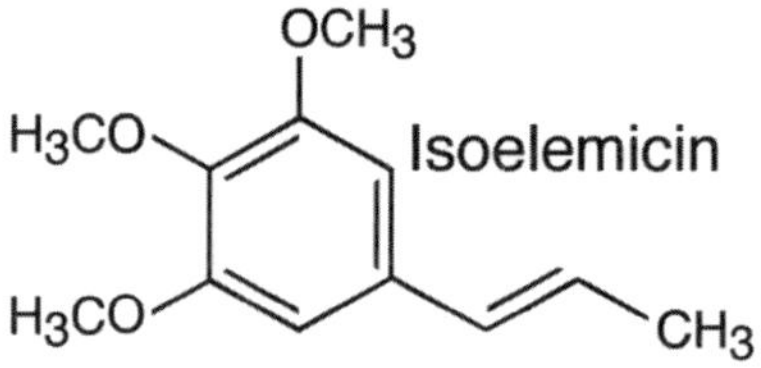

Elemicin

Isoelemicin

Elemicin and Isoelemicin

Elemicin, also called 3,4,5-trimethoxyallybenzene, can be obtained from nutmeg oil (Shulgin 1967) or produced synthetically from eugenol (Dandiya 1962) (Rao 1949) or by Grignard Reaction (Bogert 1914). M.F. C12H16O3 M.W. 208.24 Synthetic Preparation of Myristicin (1-Methoxy-2,3-methylenedioxy-5-allybenzene); Rao 1949; Trikojus 1949.

Carpacin

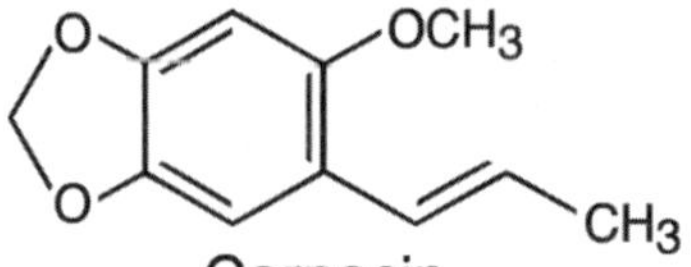

Carpacin

Carpacin, 2-Methoxy-4,5-methylenedioxy-propenylbenzene, is a constituent of Cinnamomum species from Bougainville (Shulgin).

2,5-Dimethoxypropenylbenzene from Asarone

Asarone

2,5,-Dimethoxypropenylbenzene

In a boiling flask; 0.5 mole of the asarone is mixed with 225 mL of ethyl alcohol and 22 grams of selenium dioxide. The solution is refluxed for five hours and then extracted with ether or appropriate solvent. The solvent is distilled under reduced pressure (water aspirator). Two fractions will distill over after distillation of the solvent.
One fraction:
2,5-Dimethoxypropenylbenzene
Other fraction:
2,5-Dimethoxyphenylpropane.
Reference: (Rao 1937)

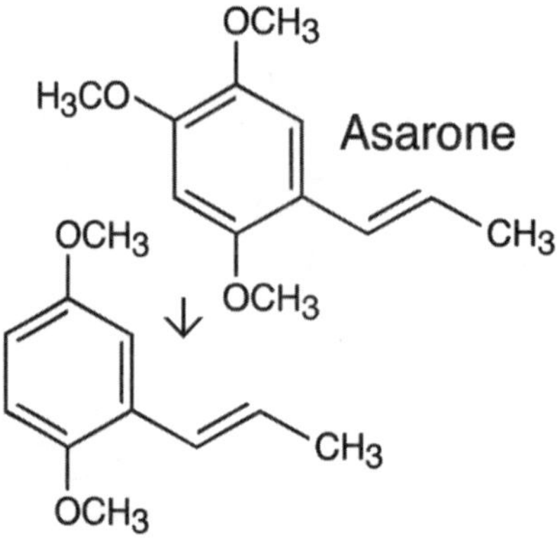

PROPENYLBENZENES FROM PHENYLPROPANOLS

Phenylalkenes such as propenylbenzene can be created by the dehydration of phenyl-1-propanols. This reaction is carried out by heating 1-phenyl-1-propanol with alumina (aluminum oxide) or vermiculite. 3-Phenyl-1-propanol will produce allybenzenes.

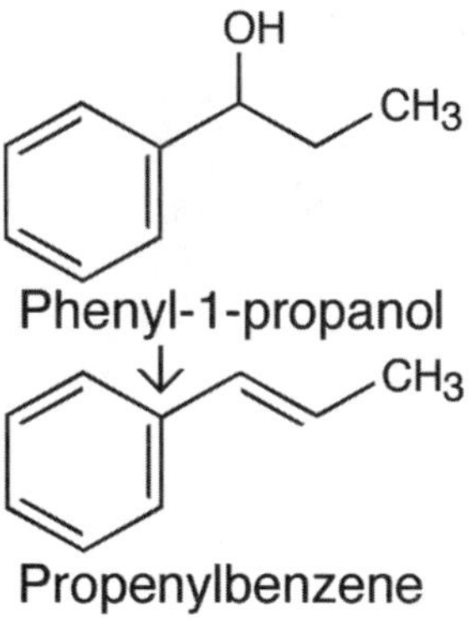

Phenyl-1-propanol

Propenylbenzene

Propenylbenzene from Phenyl-1-propanol

A) By Boiling with Alumina:

1-Phenyl-1-propanol (0.25 moles) is mixed in a distillation apparatus with 75 g. alumina and a pinch of hydroquinone (*p*-dihydroxybenzene) or pyrogallol (inhibitor). The mixture is heated under a vacuum for 1 hour at 150 degrees. The mixture is washed, in a separatory funnel with a dilute solution of sodium hydroxide and then water. The water insoluble layer is dried over anhydrous calcium chloride, sodium sulfate or magnesium sulfate. 85% yields of propenylbenzene are obtained.

Starting Molecule: 1-(4-Methoxyphenyl)-1-propanol
Product: Anethole; (4-Methoxypropenylbenzene)
Reference: (Müller 1957)

B) By Heating With Vermiculite:

0.25 Mole of 1-phenyl-1-propanol is heated at 90 degrees for five minutes (under reduced pressure) with 3 mL of concentrated sulfuric acid on 8 grams of vermiculite. The mixture is cooled and washed with a dilute solution of sodium hydroxide and water. The water insoluble layer is dried.

Starting Molecule: 1,1-Dimethyl-2-hydroxy-2-(*p*-methoxyphenyl)ethane
Product: 1,1-Dimethyl-2-(*p*-methoxyphenyl)ethene
Reference: (Bruce 1952)

C) By Heating With Potassium Bisulfate:

Starting Molecule: 1-(1,3-Benzodioxol-5-yl)butan-1-ol
Product: 1-(1,3-Benzodioxol-5-yl)butene
Reference: (Nichols 1985)

Allybenzene From 3-Phenyl-1-propanol By Thermal Dehydration

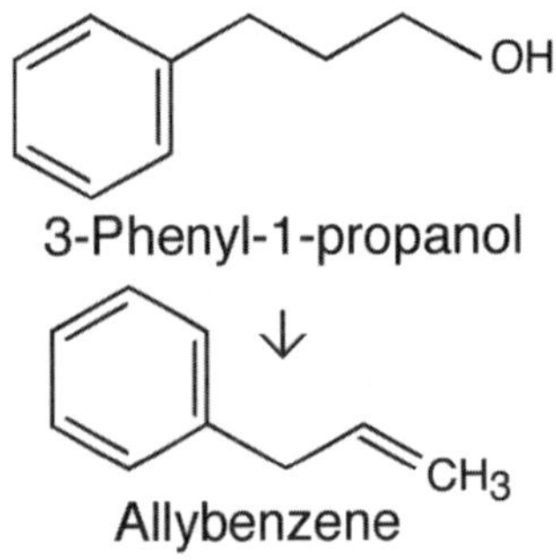

3-Phenyl-1-propanol

Allybenzene

Pyrolysis Apparatus

A quartz or high temperature Pyrex tube (e.g. combustion tubing), approximately 2 mm thickness, 20 mm in diameter, one foot long is used in this apparatus. Ten inches of the tube is filled with activated alumina (8 to 14 mesh) which is held in place with wire gauze and a metal spring. An iron-constant thermocouple lead is placed in a glass tube which is positioned half way up on the outside of the tube. The entire tube is heated by a Nichrome wire or heating tape wrapped around it and regulated by a variable transformer.

The receiving flask is connected to a vacuum outlet and is immersed in a Dry Ice-alcohol bath. One mole of the propanol containing a pinch of pyrogallol (inhibitor) is placed in a dropping funnel at the top of the column and slowly dripped into the column at a rate of one drop per second. The temperature is maintained at 300 degrees under a vacuum of 20-25 mm. (water aspirator).

The reaction may be carried out at atmospheric pressure, but the top of the column must be closed to force the vapors down the column. A yellow liquid separates from the water formed during the dehydration. The yellow liquid is washed with dilute sodium hydroxide and water or aqueous sodium carbonate to remove any adhering inhibitor. The product is then dried over anhydrous calcium chloride or magnesium sulfate. Yields 80 to 85%.

References: Fort 1955, 1955; Overburger 1951, 1954)

Propenylbenzenes From Allybenzenes

One mole of allybenzene is mixed with a small amount pyrogallol (inhibitor) and passed dropwise through the column. The temperature is maintained at 300 degrees at 20-25 mm. The resulting light yellow liquid is washed with a dilute sodium hydroxide solution then water and dried over anhydrous calcium chloride. Yields are over 80%.

Starting Molecule: Allybenzene Product: 1-Propenylbenzene
Reference: (Frisch 1959)

Propenylbenzenes from Allybenzenes

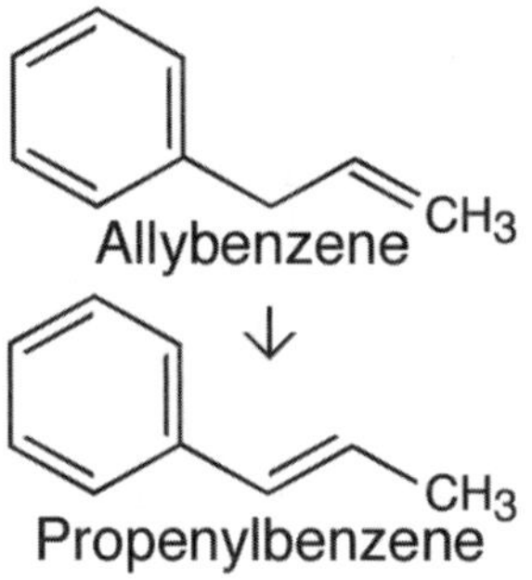

Allybenzene CH3

Propenylbenzene CH3

50 grams of allybenzene is mixed with 50 grams of anhydrous alcohol. 175 grams of potassium hydroxide flakes are added and the solution is refluxed for 24 hours with occasional stirring. The reaction is quelled with excess water and then extracted with ether or appropriate solvent. The solvent is distilled under reduced pressure to leave propenylbenzene. 75-95% yields approx.

Product: 3-Methoxy-4,5-methylenedioxypropenylbenzene Ref.: (Trikojus 1949) Product: 2,3,4-Trimethoxypropenyl-benzene Ref.: (Shulgin 1965) Product: 2,3,5-Trimethoxypropenylbenzene Ref.: (Shulgin 1965) Product: 2,4,6-Trimethoxypropenylbenzene Reference: (Holmes 1950) (Shulgin 1965)

Quelet Reaction
Preparation of Para-substituted Propenylbenzenes From Para-substituted Benzenes

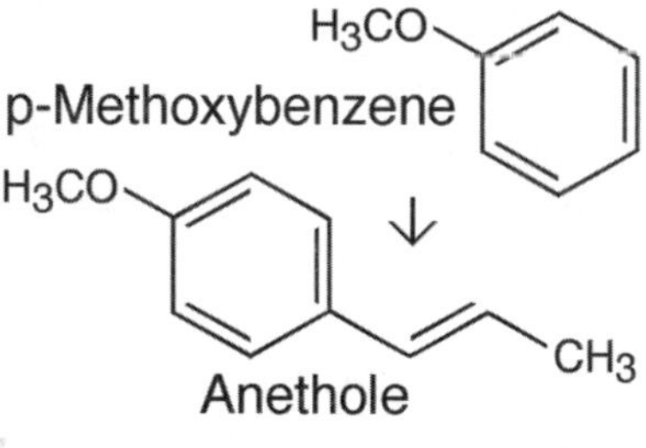

3 Moles of *p*-methoxybenzene is mixed with 3 moles of propionaldehyde, 250 mL of concentrated hydrochloric acid and 75 grams of phosphoric acid. This solution is placed in a tall graduated cylinder. The flask is equipped with a magnetic stirrer and a two hole stopper. One glass tube is run from a hydrogen chloride gas source through the stopper and to the bottom of the glass cylinder (above the stir bar). A gas diffusion stone, made of an inert material such as a glass filter, is attached at the end of the glass tubing. Another glass tube is attached to the other hole on the stopper. This tube is run through several traps containing water to absorb hydrogen chloride gas that exits the apparatus.

p-Methoxybenzene

Anethole

The solution is cooled to 5 degrees and saturated with anhydrous hydrogen chloride gas for 2.5 hours with stirring. The solution is then poured on ice and extracted with petroleum ether. The *p*-methoxy-1-phenyl-1-chloropropane) should not be distilled as the material will decompose to form phenylpropene, polymerized products and hydrochloric acid). The petroleum ether extract contains the crude p-methoxy-1-(phenyl-1-chloropropane) (approximate 25 to 50% theoretical yields).

300 grams of pyridine is mixed with the petroleum ether extract of crude p-methoxy-1-(phenyl-1-chloropropane). The petroleum ether is distilled off the solution. The pyridine containing the p-methoxy-1-(phenyl-1-chloropropane) is heated at 115 degrees for 6 hours. The solution is composed of 50% p-methoxypropenylbenzene and 50% 1,1-bis(p-methoxypropenyl-benzene). The p-methoxy-propenylbenzene is obtained from the solution by:

1) being acidified with dilute hydrochloric acid, and is fractionally distilled.

2) in some propenylbenzenes (such as anethole) can be crystalized from the solution by exposing the solution to a cold temperature (the freezer). Yields are 50% theoretical.

This reaction is called the Quelet Reaction. It was primarily designed to produce para and methoxy substituted styrenes from methoxy benzene (anisole). Various phenylalkenes can be produced using this reaction. Chain lengths can be shortened or lengthened. If the propionaldehyde is replaced with equal molar amounts of paraldehyde, styrenes will result. If butanal replaces the propionaldehyde, butenylbenzenes will result. Substitutions on the benzene ring should be obtained by replacement of the benzene with equal molar amounts of substituted benzene to produce substituted phenyl-alkenes.

para-Dimethoxybenzene has been reported in one study not to form 2,5-dimethoxypropenylbenzene. As this reaction has not been fully studied, (zinc chloride might be used in place of phosphoric acid, see Blanc Reaction), I speculate that there is much that can be done to increase yields by a more intensive study of chloroalkylation of substituted benzenes. Readers should also review the Blanc (chloromethylation) Reaction.   Refs.: (Quelet 1936, 1940, 1943)

Starting Molecule: Anisole (methoxybenzene)
Product: Anethole (4-methoxypropenylbenzene)

Phenyl-1-Propanols Using the Grignard Reagent

The Grignard reaction was originally observed by Barbier in 1899. The reaction was identified as being composed of two stages by Grignard in 1900. The reaction is used to produce a very diversified series of products. In the following, I will only be describing the synthesis of phenyl-1-propanols. I would suggest to any reader that a more explicit description of this reaction will be found in any organic chemistry text.

The reaction includes formation of the Grignard Reagent. It is created by the addition of magnesium to an organo halide forming RMgX. This is done in a solution of ether or appropriate solvent which is non-reactive to the the reagent. Oxygen, water, etc. must be excluded from the reaction as the reaction will occur very rapidly; much too rapidly for the safety of the chemist. Ketones (eg. acetophenone) maybe used in place of the aldehyde (eg. benzaldehyde).

Benzaldehyde

Phenyl-1-propanol

A Grignard reagent is prepared: 0.75 moles of magnesium turnings is mixed with 250 mL of dry ether. One gram of ethyl bromide is added to initiate formation of reagent. More ethyl bromide (in 250 mL dry ether) is added to a total bromoalkane of 0.75 moles. The mixture is refluxed with stirring until the magnesium has disappeared.

750 mL of dry ether is mixed with 0.5 moles of benzaldehyde and added dropwise with stirring under reflux for a total of four hours. The solution is cooled to 0 degrees and the reaction complex is decomposed with the slow addition of an aqueous solution of ammonium chloride. The aqueous layer is separated and extracted with benzene. The benzene extract is combined with the organic (non-aqueous) layers, dried with Epson salts and evaporated to leave the phenyl-1-propanol.

Starting Molecules: Anisaldehyde & Isopropyl chloride
Product: 1,1-Dimethyl-2-hydroxy-2-(p-methoxyphenyl)ethane
Reference: (Bruce 1952)

Starting Molecule: 3,5-Dimethoxybenzaldehyde
Reagent: n-Hexylmagnesium bromide
Product: 1-(3,5-Dimethoxyphenyl)heptan-1-ol Reference: (McOmie 1966)

Starting Molecules: 3,5-Dimethoxybenzaldehyde Reagent: Lauryl magnesium bromide
Product: 3,5-Dimethoxyphenyl(dodecyl)methanol Reference: (Ridley 1968)

Starting Molecules: 3,5-Dimethoxybenzaldehyde
Reagent: Tetradecyl magnesium bromide
Product: 3,5-Dimethoxy-(1'-hydroxypentadecyl)-benzene
Reference: (Wasserman 1948)

Starting Molecules: 3,4-Methylenedioxybenzaldehyde Reagent: 1-Bromopropane
Product: 1-(1,3-Benzodioxol-5-yl)butan-1-ol Reference: (Nichols 1986)

Starting Molecules: Syringaldehyde Reagent: Ethyl magnesium bromide
Product: 3,5-Dimethoxy-4-hydroxyphenyl-1-propanol
References: Pepper 1964 ; *J.A.C.S.* 72: 5760 (1950)

Starting Molecule: 3,4,5-Trimethoxybenzaldehyde Reagent: Alkyl magnesium bromide
Product: 3,4,5-Trimethoxyphenylalkylcarbinols Reference: (Bailey 1974)

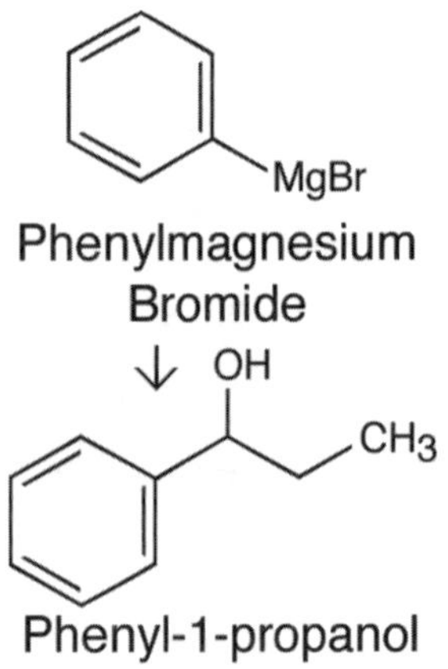

Phenylmagnesium Bromide

↓ OH

Phenyl-1-propanol

Starting Molecule:
3,4-Methylenedioxybenzene magnesium bromide
Reagent: Acetaldehyde
Product: 3,4-Methylenedioxyphenyl-1-propanol
Reference: (Freugeas 1964)

4-Bromo-1,2-methylenedioxybenzene can be prepared in acetic acid by the bromination of 1,2-methylenedioxybenzene (Jones 1917).

5-Bromo-1,2,4-trimethoxybenzene can be prepared by the bromination of 1,2,4-trimethoxybenzene (Baker 1938).

Phenyl-1-Propanol
By Reduction of Propiophenone

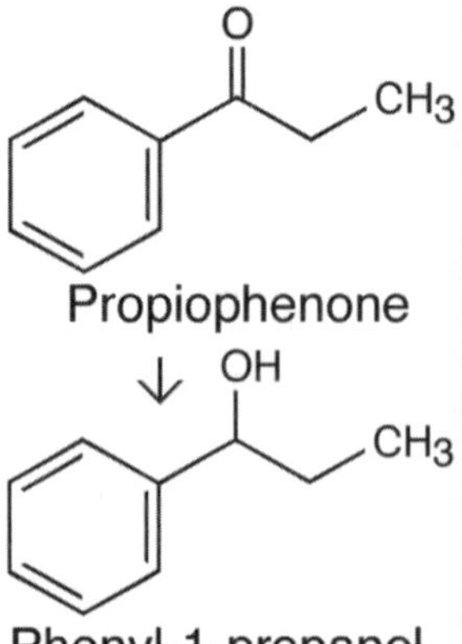

Propiophenone

↓ OH

Phenyl-1-propanol

A mixture of 225 mL of ethanol, 70 grams of potassium hydroxide and 0.25 mole of ketone is heated at 200 to 220 degrees in a rocking autoclave for 6 hours. The mixture is mixed with 475 mL of water and the ethanol is distilled. The aqueous solution is extracted with ether; the ether solution is then washed with 10% potassium hydroxide. The alkaline solution is then acidified and extracted with ether. The ether is distilled and the residue is fractionally distilled to obtain the phenyl-1-propanol.

Methoxy groups also crack to form hydroxy groups.

Starting Molecule: Anisyl-3-hexanone-4 References: (Rubin 1944)
Products: 50% *p*-Hydroxyphenyl-3-hexanol-4; 25% *p*-Methoxyphenyl-3-hexanol-4

Preparation of Propenylbenzene from Chloroephedrine

10 grams of sodium carbonate are mixed with 10 grams of chloroephedrine in 40 mL. of ether. 60 mL. of water are added with stirring. The solution is then washed rapidly with ether. The ether extracts are combined, dried with anhydrous magnesium sulfate, filtered and evaporated. 10 grams of zinc are added and the reaction was allowed to reach a rapid boil under reflux. The reaction was contained by cooling and allowed to continue. The yield of the yellow propenylbenzene (8-8.5 grams) is approximately 80%.

Ref: Gero 1951

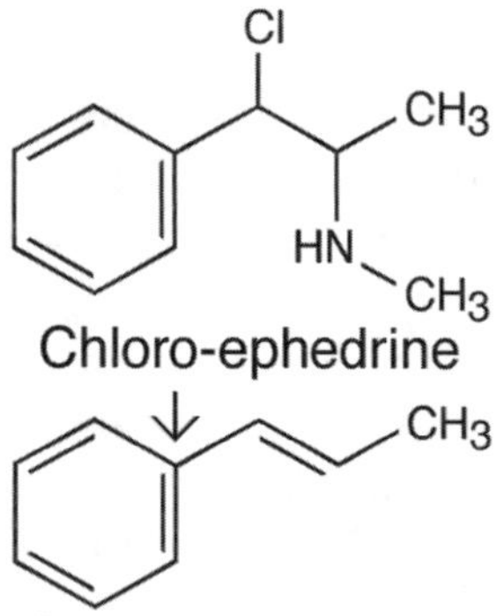

Chloro-ephedrine

Propenylbenzene

CHAPTER 17
PREPARATION OF NITROALKANES
FROM ALKANES

Nitroalkanes, (nitroparaffins), are used in synthetic fuels (e.g. funny car fuel and model airplane fuel) in octane boosters for automobiles, motorcycles, big rigs, in organic synthesis, solvents for lacquers and use in explosives. Nitroalkanes are generally produced by the vapor phase nitration of alkanes (paraffins).

Nitromethane is explosive with difficulty. Attempts to explode nitroethane or higher homologs have been unsuccessful. No. 8 blasting caps failed to detonate nitroethane; so have attempts with red hot wire coils and burning. The vapor phase nitration has been reported to produce explosions if fuming nitric acid is used or the alkane gas is allowed to stop bubbling through the hot acid.

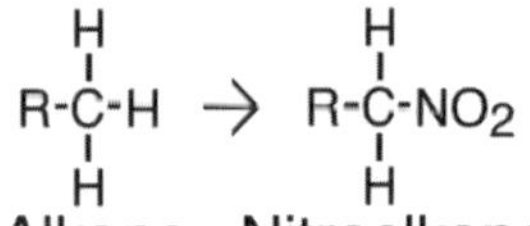

In 1872 a person by the name of Meyer first produced nitroparaffins. Little research was conducted on the preparation of nitroalkanes during the first quarter of the 1900's. In 1930 Hass, Hodge and Vanderbilt began studying the vapor phase production of nitroalkanes.

$$R\text{-}\underset{\underset{H}{|}}{\overset{\overset{H}{|}}{C}}\text{-H} \rightarrow R\text{-}\underset{\underset{H}{|}}{\overset{\overset{H}{|}}{C}}\text{-NO}_2$$

Alkane   Nitroalkane

Manufacture of Nitroalkanes

by Henry B. Hass, Edward B. Hodge and Byron M. Vanderbilt

In nitrating these saturated aliphatic hydrocarbons which have secondary and/or tertiary carbon atoms, and of which isobutane is taken as an example, we may carry out the process either in batches or in continuous process. In using isobutane as an example, we do so with no intent to limit the invention; for it is applicable without charge to other instance as n-butane, propane, etc., as already noted.

The apparatus for doing this is illustrated in the accompanying drawings. Fig. 1 shows an apparatus for carrying out our process in batches; Fig. 2 is a sectional view of a water-cooled bomb which is especially suitable for the batch method of Fig. 1...

A reaction vessel or bomb 10, constructed of material which is resistant to dilute nitric acid, such for instance as Allegheny metal, and capable of withstanding high pressure, is filled with a mixture of liquid (alkane) and dilute nitric acid-one mole of nitric acid to two moles of (alkane). We prefer to make the mixture within the bomb by putting in

Process of Nitrating Paraffin Hydrocarbons

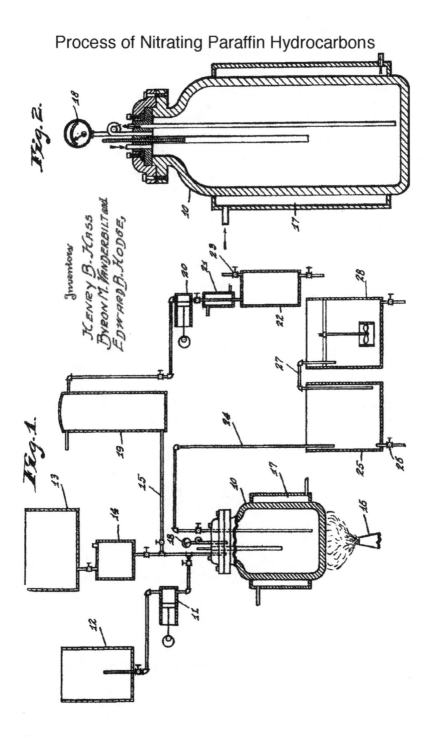

Fig.2.

Fig.1.

Inventors
KENEY B. JASS
BYRON M. VANDERBILT and
EDWARD B. HODGE,

35% nitric acid in sufficient amount to give the desired molar proportion to the (alkane) used and then run in the (alkane) in sufficient quantity to fill the bomb to the extent of 5-20%. The (alkane) maybe supplied by a pump 11 from an (alkane) storage tank 12, and the nitric acid from a nitric-acid storage reservoir 13 by way of a measuring tank 14, all suitably connected to the bomb by suitable valved piping 15 shown diagrammatically. The bomb is then closed, and gradually heated by a burner 16 until abundant reaction starts, which is at about 135° C. This temperature is above the critical temperature of (alkane) for such critical temperature (eg. isobutane is 134° C.), but with some hydrocarbons abundant reaction starts below the critical temperature although with the reagents in the gas or vapor phase. The reaction develops a pressure with the bomb of the order of 600 to 2400 pounds per square inch-fuller the bomb the greater the pressure-; but in spite of the increased pressure, the hydrocarbon remains in the gas or vapor phase by the increase in temperature produced by the heat of the reaction, and the nitric acid is at least partly in vapor phase. Thus the reaction is practically wholly between gases or vapors.

As the reaction is exothermic, it tends to become very violent once it has started, and hence we provide means for cooling the bomb, as by circulating water through an outside jacket 17 with which it is provided as shown in Fig. 2.

When the reaction has substantially ceased, by using up of the nitric acid, the pressure substantially stops rising and the bomb is cooled to room temperature. We prefer to have a suitable manometer 18 connected with the bomb, for indicating the pressure within it.

When the bomb has been cooled to room temperature, and the pressure sufficiently lowered, the gasses therefrom are released through the valved piping 15 into a scrubbing tower 19, and there scrubbed with some reagent with removes nitric-acid vapor from them, such as sodium carbonate. The gases leaving the tower 19 are compressed by means of a compressor 20 and cooled by a condenser 21. A sufficient pressure is produced to condense substantially all of the (alkane), which is removed from the gaseous reaction products in a separator 22. The uncondensed gases are vented from a valve 23 on the separator 22, and the condensed (alkane) is recycled or sent to storage. If desired the oxides of nitrogen may be converted to nitric acid in known manner.

The tertiary (nitroalkane) may be removed from the contents of the reaction vessel 10 by the following procedure. Such contents are removed by piping 24 from the reaction vessel or bomb 10 to a separating tank 25. The spent acid, which forms a lower layer, is removed form the separating tank 25 through a drain-valve 26. The crude tertiary nitro-(alkane) which remains is transferred by piping 27 to a washing tank 28; where it is agitated with concentrated sodium hydroxide to dissolve any primary nitro-(alkane), and the alkali is allowed to settle and is drawn off. The tertiary nitro-(alkane) is then further purified by rectification. If desired it may be still further purified by crystallization. Source: Hass 1934

Preparation of Nitroethane

Nitroethane can be prepared in small quantities by the nitration of diethyl sulfate.

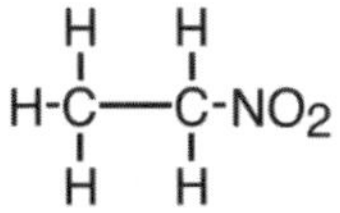

125 Grams of diethyl sulfate, 190 grams of sodium nitrite and 240 mL of water are mixed in a separatory funnel. The funnel stopper is clamped so as not to leak and mechanically shaken for 21 hours. Occasionally the funnel is opened to release pressure and then continued to be shaken. After being mechanically shaken for 21 hours the funnel is allowed to set. Two layers form. The top layer is dried with calcium chloride or appropriate drying agent and poured into a distillation apparatus. The solution is distilled under reduced pressure (14 mm.) until the temperature reaches 60 degrees. The residue is diethyl sulfate and can be reused. The distillate is factionally distilled at atmospheric pressure. The 114-116 degree fraction is the nitroethane.

The nitroethane is washed with water, dried and redistilled at atmospheric pressure. The 114-115.5 degree fraction is collected. Nitroethane is a clear liquid that mildly smells like chloroform. Yields are approximately 50% theoretical. References: (McCombie 1944)

The setup and vapor phase production of nitroalkanes is not for amateurs, but maybe of interest to the readers. Check citations in the reference section. The nitration of ethane produces approximately 15% nitromethane and 85% nitroethane. The nitration of propane produces approximately 10% nitromethane, 25% nitroethane, 3% 1-nitropropane and 30% 2-nitropropane. References: (Bachman 1954) (Hass 1934; 1936; 1947; 1949) (McCleary 1938) (Reidel 1956)

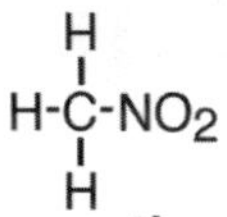

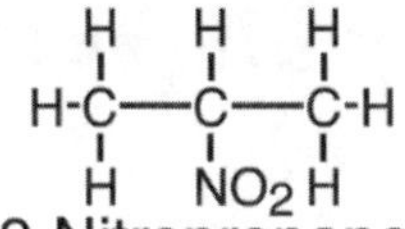

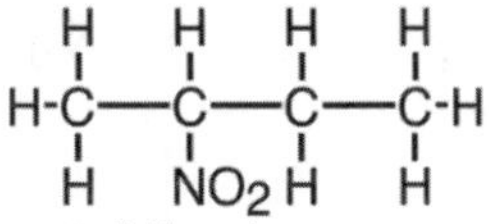

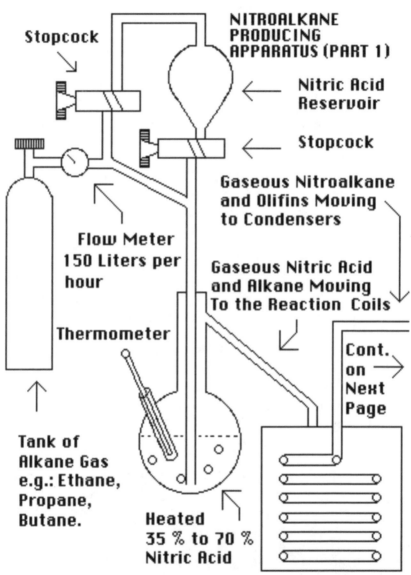

Stopcock

NITROALKANE PRODUCING APPARATUS (PART 1)

← Nitric Acid Reservoir

← Stopcock

Gaseous Nitroalkane and Olifins Moving to Condensers

Flow Meter 150 Liters per hour

Gaseous Nitric Acid and Alkane Moving To the Reaction Coils

Thermometer

Cont. on Next Page

Tank of Alkane Gas e.g.: Ethane, Propane, Butane.

Heated 35 % to 70 % Nitric Acid

Reaction Coils Immersed in a heated mixture of Granular Sodium Nitrite and Potassium Nitrite

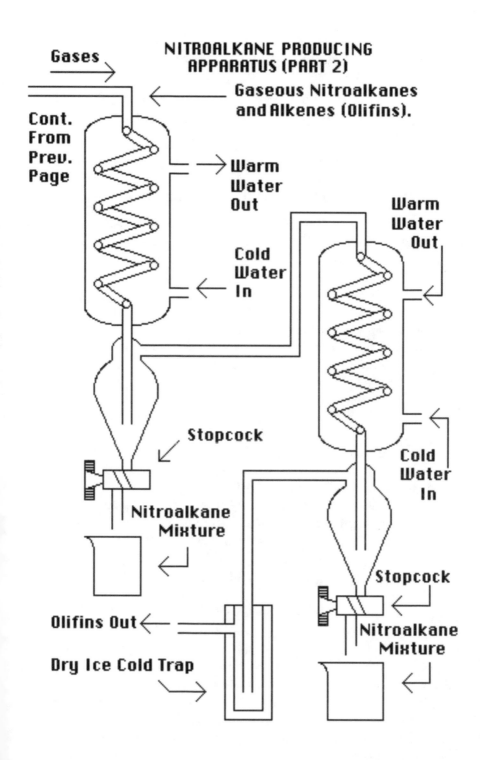

NITROALKANE PRODUCING
APPARATUS (PART 2)

CHAPTER 18:
SEPARATION OF OPTICAL ISOMERS

Dextrorotatory and Levorotatory isomers are optical isomers. A chemical composed of 50% dextro isomer and 50% levo isomer is called a racemic chemical.

Examples: *d*-amphetamine is the dextro isomer of amphetamine.
l-amphetamine is the levo isomer of amphetamine.
d,l-amphetamine is the racemic mixture.

Dextrorotatory (Latin: dexter, right) means that the chemical rotates light to the right. Levorotatory (Latin: laevus, left) means that the chemical rotates light to the left. Racemic mixtures do not rotate light as the mixture of dextrorotatory and levorotatory neutralize the bending of the light.

The instrument that is used to determine the specific rotation to the plane of polarized light is called a polarimeter. The device is composed of a light, a tube (e.g. a small card board tube) to hold the substance being analyzed and two polarized lens (e.g. Polaroid or Nicol) at the ends of the tube, which can be turned.

The polarimeter is pointed towards the light and the lens is turned so that the maximum amount of light is being passed through the polarimeter. The substance is placed in the tube and the polarimeter is pointed towards the light again. The lens closest to the light is called the polarizer; the lens closest to the eye is called the analyzer. The analyzer lens is rotated. If the light does not dim as the lens is being rotated either clockwise or counter clockwise the substance is optically inactive. If the light dims when the analyzer lens is turned then the material is considered optically active. The degree of rotation can also be determined.

The Discovery of Optical Activity and Stereochemistry

In 1815 a physicist by the name of Jean-Baptiste Biot discovered that some chemicals had optical activity. In 1848 Louis Pasteur was repeating an experiment that had been done by another scientist. Previous to this Pasteur had received his baccalaurent es sciences this university and was considered mediocre in chemistry. He wanted to learn more about crystallography. While crystallizing an optically inactive substance, sodium ammonium tartrate, he noticed that the some of the crystals were of different shape and carefully separated the crystals with tweezers and a magnifying glass into two piles. Then he checked them with the polarimeter.

The crystals of each pile were optically active. The original mixture was optically inactive and yet the two separate crystals were optically active (Jarowski 1943) (Pfanz 1956) (Witkop 1957). The specific rotations of each set of crystals was equal, but opposite in sign (e.g. +, -). The two piles of crystals were the same chemical, the only difference being that they rotated the plane of polarized light in opposite directions. Louis Pasteur had discovered stereochemistry.

The Stereochemistry of Amphetamine

Amphetamine exists as two isomers, the dextrorotatory and the levorotatory. They rotate the plane of polarized light in two equal, but opposite directions. They are mirror images of each other. Mirror images can be depicted on paper like this:

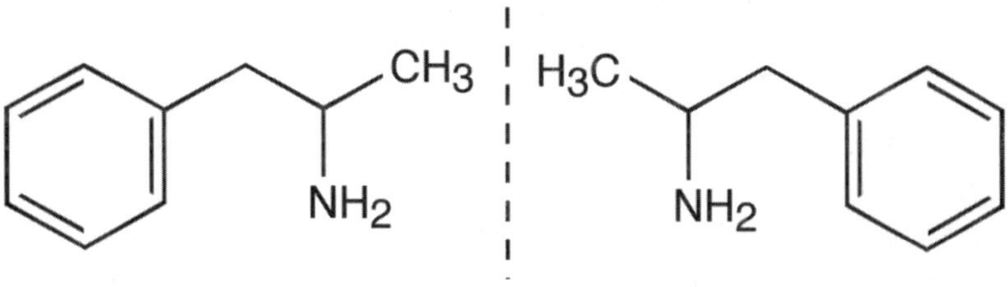

The amphetamine molecule is drawn on the left. The imaginary mirror image is then drawn on the right. In order to determine if they are isomers we try to superimpose the image on the left with the image on the right.

The rules are that we can spin the molecules around so long as we don't lift them off the paper. We can see that they are not superimposable. This means that they are isomers. Mirror images are called enantiomers.

Chirality

Molecules who's mirror images are not superimposable are called chiral molecules. The understanding of chirality helps to determine if isomers are enantiomers. This is done by finding the chiral center of the molecule. The chiral center is determined by finding a carbon atom that has four different groups of atoms attached to it.

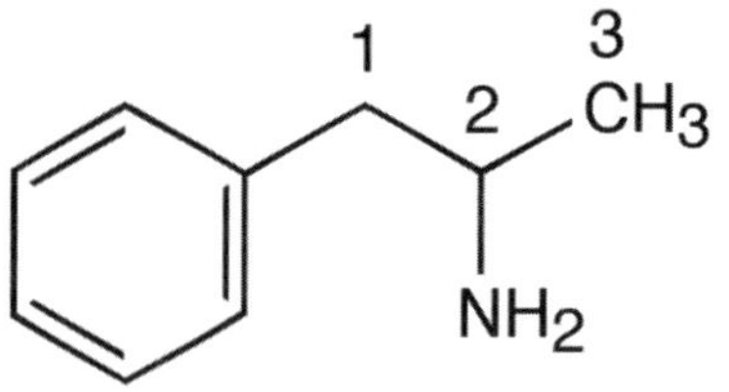

Carbon 1 can not be chiral because it has two hydrogen atoms attached to it. Carbon 3 can not be the the chiral carbon because it has three hydrogen atoms attached to it. Carbon 2 is the chiral center because it has four groups (groups of atoms) attached to it that are not the same. To the right is a methyl group (CH3). Above it is a hydrogen atom. To the left of it is a benzyl group (C7H7). Underneath the chiral carbon is an amino group (NH2).

I will review:

The mirror image of the amphetamine molecule is not superimposable. The two mirror images are optical isomers called enantiomers. (If the mirror image of a molecule can be superimposed then the molecule is not an isomer). There exists a chiral center. The chiral center is carbon 2 because the four groups attached to the carbon are not the same.

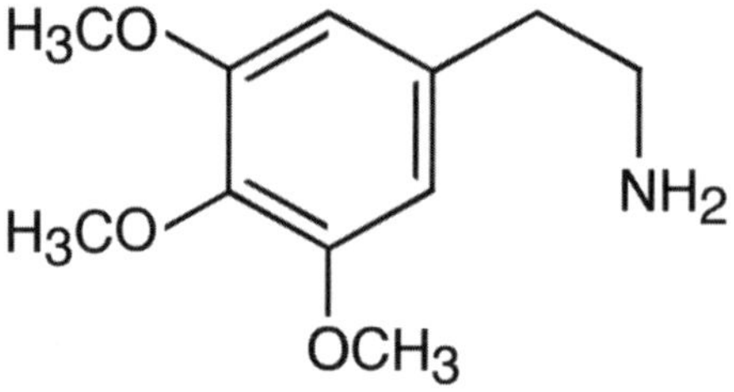

The mescaline molecule is not chiral. Each carbon atom is attached to two of the same type of atoms.

Separation of Dextro-Phenylpropanolamine

30 Grams of *d,l*-phenylpropanolamine is mixed with 45 grams of *d*-tartaric acid and dissolved into 1350 mL of boiling alcohol. The solution is then filtered and refrigerated to precipitate 50 grams of *d*-phenylpropanolamine-*d*-bitartrate.

Evaporation of the solution leaves *l*-phenylpropanolamine.

The *d*-phenylpropanolamine-d-bitartrate can be transformed into the hydrochloride by dissolving into warm acetone, cooling in an ice bath and adding an equal molar amount of hydrochloric acid. The precipitated *d*-phenylpropanolamine hydrochloride is collected by suction filtration.

The resolution of racemic amphetamine can be done by the same procedure.

References: (Flassig 1956) (Fodor 1948) (Heizelman, 1953) (Jatung 1931). (Johns, 1938)

CHAPTER 19
HALLUCINOGENIC DRUGS
SEROTONIN RECEPTORS
DOPAMINE AND NEUROTOXICITY

Many psychoactive (psychotropic, hallucinogenic, antidepressant) drugs have been found to bind to serotonin receptors. Amphetamine type psychoactives bind to serotonin subtype (5-HT2) auto receptors (presynaptic receptors) (Battaglia 1988) (Lyon 1978). In small dosages, many of these psychoactives exhibit mood elevation effects, in larger dosages they produce hallucinations. There are many molecules which bind to this receptor in varying degrees.

Many of the amphetamine and phenylethylamine series of molecules have been found to be neurotoxic to serotonergic axions causing long term reductions in brain serotonin levels and reductions of spinal fluid 5-hydroxyindoleacetic acid (Stone 1986). Psychotropic drugs such as imipramine, amitriptyline and nortriptyline also cause reductions in 5-hydroxy-indoleacetic acid (Maas 1977). Reductions in spinal fluid 5-hydroxyindoleacetic acid have been noticed in suicide victims and violent aggression in laboratory animals (Brown 1986).

The neurotoxicity of amphetamines has been linked to a metabolic reaction following the ingestion these molecules (Heikkila 1971). This neurotoxicity can be blocked by pre and/or post ingestion of specific serotonin reuptake inhibitor (eg. fluoxetine, etc.) before the amphetamine molecule metabolizes (approximately six hours).

Serotonin reuptake blocking molecules cause super sensitivity of the presynaptic receptors. (Check Serotonin Syndrome.) Amitriptyline and imipramine cause super sensitivity of serotonin receptors to 5-methoxy-N,N-dimethyl-tryptamine (Friedman 1979) (De Montigany 1978). Adverse reactions in bipolar patients such as mood swings have been noted in not only with iminodibenzyl (tricyclic antidepressants) molecules (eg. nortriptyline) but also Serotonin Specific Reuptake Inhibitors (SSRI) such as fluoxetine. It is important that patients who are receiving antidepressants be monitored by the practitioner to make sure the drug is not aggravating a condition.

Imipramine blocks the neurotoxicity of *p*-chloroamphetamine imipramine does not increase receptor affinities of 5-HT2 receptors. Fluoxetine and other SSRI's (Serotonin Specific Reuptake Inhibitors) have been found to block the neurotoxicity of MDMA (Battaglia 1988a)

(Sanders-Bush 1978) (Schmidt 1987) (Steranka 1978). GABA-transaminase inhibitors also block neurotoxicity (Stone 1987).

Serotonin Neurotoxins

p-Bromomethamphetamine; p-Chloroamphetamine;
p-Chloromethamphetamine; N-Hydroxy-p-chloroamphetamine
Fenfluramine; Norfenfluramine (m-trifluromethyl-amphetamine)
3,4-Methylenedioxyamphetamine (MDA)
3,4-Methylenedioxy-N-methylamphetamine (MDMA)
3,4-Methylenedioxy-N-ethylamphetamine (MDEA)

N-Ethyl-p-chloroamphetamine, N-isopropyl-p-chloro-amphetamine, and N,N-dimethyl-p-chloroamphetamine all metabolize into p-chloroamphetamine and are neurotoxic. p-Fluoroamphetamine is also neurotoxic, but depletes serotonin for a shorter time than the previously listed molecules. There is an increase in brain concentrations of 5,6-dihydroxytryptamine (endogenous neurotoxin) in rats following the administration of p-chloroamphetamine.

6-Hydroxydopamine (2,4,5-trihyroxyphenylethylamine) and 6-aminodopamine (2-amino-4,5-dihyroxyphenylethylamine) are both neurotoxic to dopamine receptors (Saner 1970) (Lundstrom 1973).

It has been speculated that superoxide and peroxide groups are responsible. If this is so. Superoxide dimutase elevation in the brain may also prevent this oxidation reaction.

The study of phenylethylamines has lead to major breakthroughs in the understanding of brain mechanisms. The activity and mechanisms of action of these molecules are very diversified and can not be predetermined in any one theory. A simple addition of a 6-hydroxy group on the neurotransmitter, dopamine, results in a molecule which is neurotoxic. Phenylethylamine is a trace amine/neurotransmitter in the brain. By a methyl addition on to the *alpha* carbon results in the psychostimulant amphetamine which is neurotoxic.

The hydroxy addition on the *beta* carbon of methamphetamine results in the formation of norephedrine which has been found not to be neurotoxic (Smith 1974). p-Chloroephedrine has also be reported not to be neurotoxic.

The study of phenylethylamines and related molecules begins with the building of altered structures from a parent structure (template) of known neurotransmitter molecular structures.

para-Bromination
of Substituted Phenylalkylamines

para-Bromination (addition of Br to the 4th position on the benzene ring) of substituted phenylalkylamines can activate inactive molecules or increase the potency of the parent psychoactive. It also increases the duration of action and generally produces an empathogenic effect at small to moderate dosages. This reaction will work with any phenylalkylamine which does not have a substitution on the *para* position.

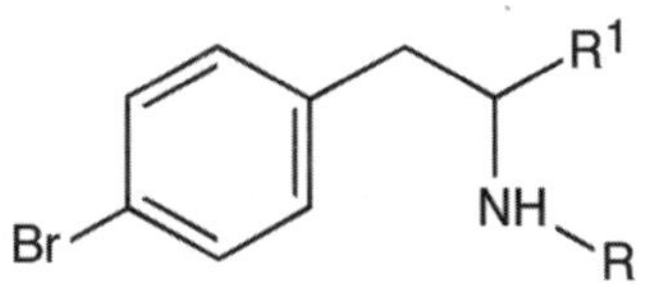

4-Bromo Phenylalkylamine Hydrobromide Salt
From Phenylalkylamine (Free Base)

Solution A: 0.6 Mole of substituted phenylalkylamine (free base) is mixed with 45 mL of glacial acetic acid.

Solution B: Solution B is added to solution A over a period of 15 minutes and stirred for approximately 24 hours.

Precipitation and Purification of Crude
4-Bromo-Substituted
Phenylalkylamine Hydrobromide

The mixture is evaporated to leave a residue. The residue is dissolved in a minimum quantity of warm isopropyl alcohol, ether or acetone and refrigerated to precipitate the 4-bromo-substituted phenylalkylamine hydrobromide salt. The precipitated hydrobromide salt is collected by suction filtration and washed of impurities with cold ether or acetone. Yields are 50 to 60% theoretical.

Starting Molecule: 2,5-Dimethoxyamphetamine
Product: 4-Bromo-2,5-dimethoxyamphetamine
References: (Harley-Mason 1953) (Nichols 1973; 1974)(Sepulveda 1972)

4-*Para*-Chlorination of Substituted Phenylalkylamine

The *para*-chlorination (addition of Cl to the 4th position on the benzene ring) of substituted phenylalkylamines also increases the potency of the parent psychoactive comparable to the *para*-bromination.

4-Chloro-Phenylalkylamine Hydrochloride Salt From Phenylalkylamine (Free Base)

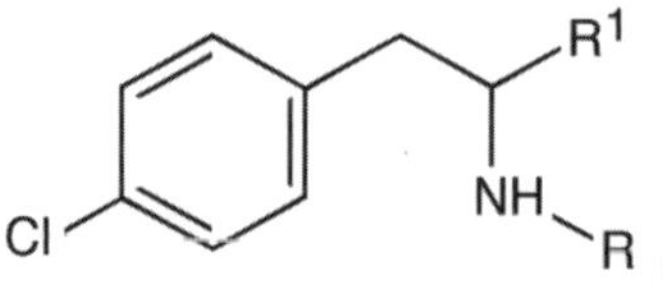

To a solution of 0.6 mole of phenylalkylamine (free base) in 65 mL glacial acetic acid, chlorine gas is bubbled until 2 grams of chlorine are absorbed. At 0 to 5 degrees is added to a solution of 3.8 grams of chlorine in 65 mL of glacial acetic acid. The mixture is stirred for 6 hours and evaporated. The residue is dissolved in a minimum quantity of warm isopropyl alcohol, ether or acetone and refrigerated to precipitate the 4-chloro-phenylalkylamine hydrochloride salt which is collected by suction filtration. Yields are 40% theoretical.

Starting Molecule: 2,5-Dimethoxyamphetamine
Product: 4-Chloro-2,5-dimethoxyamphetamine
Reference: (Nichols 1974)

Scientific Inquiry

Scientific inquiry follows a course of building on parent molecule to identify structural activity relationships (SAR). A psychotropic substance called MDMA was being testing in clinical settings for use as an adjunct to psychotherapy. Many proponents of this molecule found it to be particularly useful in assisting couples seeking marriage counseling and maybe useful in the treatment of PTSD. MDMA belongs to a class of molecules which were originally described as empathogens. These molecules produce feelings of empathy and a lessening of fears in the psychotherapeutic process. Today, these molecules are called entactogens.

In 1986 this molecule was recommended, by those who were familiar with its uses and actions, that it be placed on schedule 3 so that further development could take place. MDMA is non-patentable as it was created in 1912. This creates a problem for all those who might have something to gain from it; pharmaceutical companies will not develop a non-patentable drug that they can not monopolize on. They would rather have someone else put in all the money for the development of a breakthrough drug. They in turn develop a chemical analog to the patent medication; Piggy Back Pharmacology.

Entactogens are a new therapeutic class of molecules. The most familiar molecule is N-Methyl-1-(1,3-benzodioxol-5-yl)-2-butanamine.

"(N-Methyl-1-(1,3-benzodioxol-5-yl)-2-butanamine) represents a novel type of psychoactive compound that is not hallucinogenic, but rather facilitates communication and introspective states. We propose to designate this compound as representative of a new therapeutic class to be called "entactogens". This derived from the Greek roots "en" for within or inside and "gen" to produce or originate and the Latin root "tactus" for touch. Hence, the connotation of this word is that for producing a "touching within"' (Nichols 1986).

"(N-Methyl-1-(1,3-benzodioxol-5-yl)-2-butanamine) instills new CNS properties termed entactogen and provides a compound devoid of hallucinogenic activity with little or no stimulant effect remaining." (Dal Cason 1990)

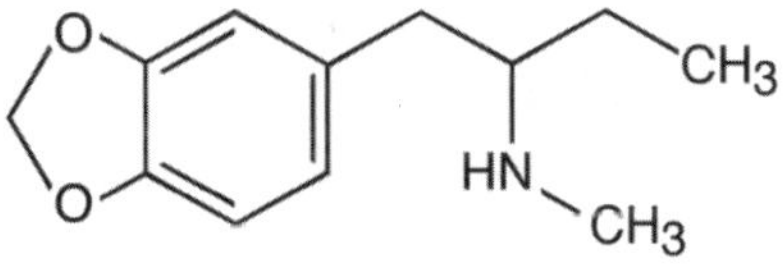

N-Methyl-1-(1,3-benzodioxol-5-yl)-2-butanamine is relatively easy to produce by conventional syntheses. It has not appeared as a drug of abuse.

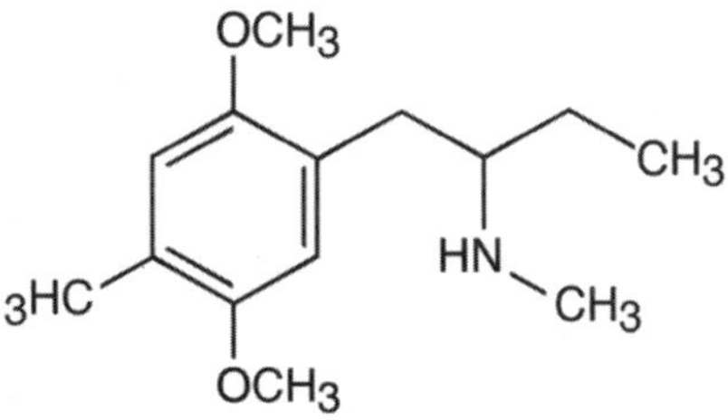

2-Amino-1-(2,5-dimethoxy-4-methyl-phenyl)butane is a short acting mood elevator and anorexic (Standridge 1976) with no stimulant or hallucinogenic action (Winter 1980).

The public must have easy access to literature on scientific research and statistical analyses to determine the viability of substances for therapeutic use. Freedom of choice comes down to benefit/risk comparisons and not whether a substance or drug has been approved or not by the FDA.

Freedom of choice is our right to survival.

Anyone who has experienced or witnessed a major illness realizes the inadequacies of the medical-pharmaceutical communities and yet there are no ceilings to cost or protections for the unknowing consumer. The dilemma of drug and or medical development in this nation is much like what has happened to the automobile, electronic, steel and other industries. Simultaneously congress is being highly lobbied with money from domestic pharmaceutical and medical interests which neutralize efforts for reform of the medical-pharmaceutical system.

The Decade of the Brain has herald in a national and international renaissance of researching and understanding of the brain. The brain weighs approximately three pounds and is the most highly developed multiprocessing biological computer that has evolved on the planet. Enclosed with in it are all the happiness, joy, sadness, depression, love, laughter; everything. Composed with in it are the creative geniuses of Thomas Jefferson, Albert Einstein, Thomas Edison, Louis Pasteur, the Wright Brothers, Charles Goodyear, Albert Hofmann, Patrick Henry, Benjamin Franklin, Linus Pauling, Alexander Shulgin, Alexander Fleming and Edward Salk to name a few.

Cradled within the mind are the foundations of democracy, science, freedom, truth, justice, love, compassion, understanding, discovery, all rational thought and the ability to discover its own mechanisms.

We are the dawn of a new age. An age where scientists and researchers are deciphering the neurochemistry of the brain and unlocking the mysteries of the mind. Throughout the world neurochemists and organic chemists are being funded to continue the great exploration. Pioneers in the brain race will continue making breakthroughs as long as there is a national commitment in the development and application of new technologies. The interest and input of new minds from the private sector will guarantee that new paradigms will continue to be dynamic, visionary and progressive.

"I know of no depository of the ultimate powers of society but the people themselves ..." Thomas Jefferson.

LD-50's OF CONVENTIONAL PSYCHOATIVES

LD 50 is a term used in research which means the minimum lethal dosage of a substance in 50 out of 100 animals. Generally rats or mice are used. The following is a list of substances with their LD 50's, which appears in Psychotropic Drugs and Related Compounds (NIMH Edition) and various other sources. Least toxic are those at the top. Most toxic are at the bottom of the chart.

Drug	LD 50 per kilogram intravenous in mice	LD 50 per kilogram intravenous in rats.
Psilocybin:	285 mg.	280 mg.
Mescaline:	157 mg.	157 mg.
Chlordiazepoxide:	95 mg.	165 mg.
Flurazepam:	84 mg.	
LSD-25:	65 mg.	16.5 mg.
Thioridazine:	51 mg.	71 mg.
Delta 9-THC:	42 mg.	29 mg.
Promethazine:	40 mg.	50 mg.
MDMA:		49 mg.
Protriptyline:	37 mg.	
Imipramine:	35 mg.	22 mg.
Nortriptyline:	28 mg.	22 mg.
Mesoridazine:	26 mg.	
Desipramine:	22 mg.	19 mg.
Amitriptyline:	21 mg.	14 mg.
Cocaine:	17.5 mg.	
Doxepin:	15-19 mg.	13-19 mg.
Chlorpromazine:	6 mg.	25 mg.
Haloperidol:	5 mg.	22 mg.
D-Methamphetamine:	9 mg.	
Nicotine:	0.3 mg.	

SUGGESTED READINGS

A Decade of DAWN: Benzodiazepine-Related Cases 1976-1985,
DHHS Publication No. (ADM) 88-1575

A Man Against Insanity; De Kruif, P.; Grove Press, Inc. (1957)

A National Plan for Schizophrenia Research; Report of the National Advisory Mental Health Council, 1988; DHHS Publication No. (ADM) 88-157

A Killing Cure, Walker, E.; Young, P.D.;
Henry Holt and Company, (1986) ISBN: 0-03-069906-1

Advances in Substance Abuse: Behavioral and Biological Research Vol. 1,
Mello, (Ed.); JAI Press

Amphetamines and Related Compounds; Costa, E.; Garattini, S.;
Raven Press (1970) LC: 77-84114

Amphetamine Manifesto, Cohen; The Olympia Press Inc, (1972)

An Introduction to Modern Experimental Organic Chemistry, Roberts R.M.;
Gilbert, J.C.; Rodewald, L.B.; Wingrove, A.S.; Hold, Rinehart and Winston, Inc., (1974) ISBN: 0-03-091555-4

Anorectic Agents; Mechanisms of Aciton and Tolerance; Garattini, S.; Samanin,
R., (Eds.); Raven Press (1981) ISBN: 0-89004-640-9

Backstage Passes: Life on the Wild Side with David Bowie, Bowie, A. with Carr,
P.; G.P. Putnam's Sons; ISBN:0-399-13764-5 (1993)

Biochemistry of S-Adenosylmethionine and Related Compounds; *Proceedings of a Conference held at the Lake of the Ozarks (Missouri) on October 26-29, 1981*; Usdin, E.;
Borchardt, R.T.; Creveling, C.R., (Eds.); 1982; MacMillan Press; ISBN: 0-333-33059-5

Biology of Suicide; Maris, R., (Ed.); Guilford Press;1986;ISBN:0-89862-578-5

Broca's Brain; Sagan, C.; 1974; Ballantine Books; ISBN: 0-345-33689-5

Chemical Calculations, Benson; John Wiley & Sons, 1966, LC: 63-12218

Chemical Principles, Masterton, W.L.; Slowinski, E.J.; Saunders Golden Series,
1973, ISBN: 0-7216-6172-6

Choline and Lecithin in Brain Disorders; Raven Press (1979)
ISBN:0-89004-366-3

Cholinesterase, Whittaker, M.; Karger Publishing (1986)

Confessions of a Medical Heretic, Mendelsohn, M.D.; Warner Books (1979)

Controlled Substances! Chemical & Legal Guide to the Federal Drug Laws
Shulgin, A.T.; Ronin Publishing (1990) ISBN: 0-91417-50-x

Daughters at Risk, Fenichell & Charfoos; Doubleday & Co, (1981),
ISBN: 0-385-17154-4

Designer Drugs Serial No. 73, May 1, 1986, Hearing Before the Subcommittee on Crime

The Dispensatory of the United States of America 24th Ed.; (1947);
Osol, A.; Farrar, G.E.; J.B. Lippincott Company

Dr. Caligari's Psychiatric Drugs, pub. by NAPA

Drug Interactions in Psychiatry; Fisher, M.G.; Eckhart, C., Eds.; Williams &
Wilkins; (1989) ISBN: 0-683-01943-0

Ecstasy: The Clinical, Pharmacological, and Neurotoxicological Effects of the Drug Mdma (Topics in the Neurosciences, No. 9) by Peroutka, Stephen J. (Editor); Kluwer Academic Publishers; ISBN: 0792303059; (1990)

Ecstasy: The Complete Guide: A Comprehensive Look at the Risks and Benefits of MDMA; Holland, J. (Ed.), Julie Holland M.D.; Inner Traditions Intl Ltd; ISBN: 0892818573; (2001)

Ecstasy: The Clinical Pharmacological & Neurotoxicological Effects of the Drug MDMA, Peroutka; S.J., (Ed.).; Kluwer Academic (1989) ISBN: 0-7923-0305-9

Ecstasy: Dance, Trance and Transformation; Saunders, N.; Doblin, R.; Quick American (1996) ISBN: 0-932551-20-3

Ecstasy: The MDMA Story, Eisner, B.; Ronin Publishing, (1994) ISBN: 0-914171-68-2

Exercizes in General Chemistry; Deming, H, G.; Arenson, S.B.; John Wiley & Sons, Inc.; (1924)

The Extra Pharmacopoeia (29th ed), The Pharmaceutical Press, ISBN: 0-85369-210-6

Federal Code of Regulations 21: 1300 to end.

Hallucinogens: An Update; Lin, G.C.; Glennon, R.A.; NIDA Research Monograph 146 (1994); NIH Publication Number 146: 94-3872

Handbook of Chemistry and Physics 55th Edition, Weast, R.C., (Ed.); Chemical Rubber Pub. Co., CRC Press

The Harvard Guide to Modern Psychiatry; Nicholi, A.M. Jr., (Ed.); Belknap Press; (1980) ISBN: 0-674-37566-1

The Healing Journey, New Approaches to Consciousness, Naranjo, C.; Pantheon Books 1973; ISBN:0-394-48826-1

Healing Nutrients, Quillin, P.; Vintage Books, (1989) ISBN: 0-679-72187-8

Laboratory Experiments in Organic Chemistry, Adams, R.; Johnson, J.R.; Wilcox, C.F. Jr.; MacMillan Company, 1971, LC: 70-87890

Maximizing Human Potential, Decade of the Brain 1990-2000, Administrative publication.

MDMA: A New Psychotropic Compound and Its Effects in Humans; Greer, G., M.D. (1983)

MDMA (Methylenedioxy-Methamphetamine) (Neuropsychobiology); Parrott, A. C.; (Editor) Publisher: S. Karger Publishing; ISBN: 3805571100; Bilingual edition (2000)

Merck Index 10 th Ed., Merck & Co., 1983, ISBN: 911910-27-1

Methamphetamine Abuse: Epidemiologic Issues and Implications, Miller, M.A.; Kozel, N.J.; NIDA Research Monograph 115 (1991); DHHS pub. no. (ADM) 91-1836; ISBN: 0-16-035810-8; The National Advisory Mental Helath Council Report to Congress on the Decade of the Brain, DHHS Pub. no. (ADM) 89-1580

The Neuroleptic Malignant Syndrome and Related Condtions, Lazarus, A.; Mann, S.C.; Caroff, S.N.; Amer. Psychiatric Press (1989) ISBN: 0-88048-134-X

Neuropsychiatric Side-Effects of Drugs in the Elderly; Laraus, A.; Raven Press (1979) ISBN: 0-89004-285-3

Nutrition and Mental Illness: An Orthomolecular Approach to Balancing the Body Chemistry, Pfeiffer; Healing Arts Press (1987)

Opiods In Mental Illness: Theories, Clinical Observations, and Treatment Possibilities, Vereby, K.; N.Y. Academy of Sciences; (1981) ISBN: 0-89766-186-9

Organic Chemistry, R.C.; Snyder, H.R.; John Wiley & Sons, Inc. (N.Y.)

Organic Chemistry, Morrison, R.T.; Boyd, R.N.; Allyn & Bacon, Inc. (1975) LC: 72-91904

The Organic Chemistry Lab Survival Manual: A Student Guide to Techniques by Zubrick, James W. ; Publisher: John Wiley & Sons; ISBN: 0471387320; 5th edition (2000)

Organic Experiments, Fieser, L.F.; Williamson, K.L.; D.C. Heath & Co., (1979), ISBN: 0-669-01688-8

Organic Synthesis; Ireland, R.E. Jr. (Ed.); Prentice-Hall, Inc.; (1969) LC: 73-76870

Pharmacology and Toxicology of Amphetamine and Related Designer Drugs, Asghar, K.; De Souza, E.; Eds.; NIDA, DHHS Pub. no. (ADM) 89-1640 (1989)

Physician's Guide to Rare Diseases, Thoene, J.G. (Ed.); Dowden Publishing Co. (1992) ISBN: 0-9628716-0-5

PIHKAL: A Chemical Love Story, Shulgin, A.T. & Shulgin, A.; Transform Press (1991) ISBN: 0-9630096-0-5

Post-Traumatic Stress Disorder; A Victim's Guide to Healing and Recovery; Flannery, R.B.; The Crossroad Publishing Company (1992) ISBN: 0-8245-1194-9

The Premenstral Syndromes, Gise, L.H.; Churchill Livingstone Inc., 1985, ISBN: 0-443-08537-4

Principles and Cases of the Law of Arrest, Search, and Seizure; by Gardner, T.J.; Manian, V.; McGraw-Hill Book Company; (1974) ISBN: 0-07-022837-X

Problems of Drug Dependence 1989, Research Monogram 95; NIDA; DHHS Publication Number (ADM)90-1663

Psychedelics Encyclopedia, Stafford, P.; Ronin Publishing (1993) ISBN: 0-914171-51-8

Psychiatric Drugs, Hazards to the Brain, Breggin, P.; Springer Publishing Co. (1983) ISBN: 0-8261-2930-7

Psychopharmacology; A Generation of Progress, Lipton, M.A.; DeMascio, A.; Killam, K.F. (Eds.); Raven Press (1978) ISBN: 0-89004-191-1

Psychopharmacology of Hallucinogens, Stillman & Willette (Eds.); NIDA, Pergamon Press, 1978, ISBN:0-08-021938-1

Psychopharmacology of the Limbic System; Trimble, M.R; Zarifian, E. (Eds.); (1984); Oxford University Press

Psychotropic Drugs and Related Compounds, 2nd Ed., Efron, D.E.; Usdid, E.; eds.; U.S. Department of Health, Eduction and Welfare; NIMH

Pursuit of Ecstacy: The MDMA Experience; Beck, J.; Rosenbaum, M.; SUNY Press (1994) ISBN: 0-7914-1818-9

'QuaSAR' Research Monograph No. 22; Barnett, G.; Trsic, M.; Willette, R. Eds.; NIDA (1978)

Quinolinic Acid and the Kynurenines, Stone, T. Jr. (Ed.), CRC Press (1989) ISBN 0-8493-6592-9

Reduction, Techniques and Applications; Augustine, R. L. (Ed.); (1968) Marcel Dekker Inc. N.Y.

Rethinking Psychiatry, From Cultural Category to Personal Experience; Kleinman, A.; The Free Press (1988) ISBN: 0-02-917442-2

The Secret Chief: Conversations With a Pioneer of the Underground Psychedelic Therapy Movement; Stolaroff, Myron J. ; published by MAPS; ISBN: 0966001915; (1997)
Selective 5-HT Reuptake Inhibitors: Novel or Commonplace Agents?, pub. by Karger (1988) ISBN: 3-8055-4776-5
Serotonin Neurotoxins, Jocby, J.H.; Lytle, L.D. (Eds.) New York Academy of Sciences (1978) Vol. 305, ISBN: 0-89072-078-9
The Serotonin Receptor; Saunders-Bush, Elaine; Humana Press (1988) ISBN: 0-89603-142-X
Solving Problems in Chemistry; Himes, G.K.; Charles E. Merrill Publishing (1971) ISBN: 0-675-07447-9
Special Report: Schizophrenia 1987; Reprint from *Schizophrenia Bulletin* 13 (1) (1987); NIMH publication.
Testing for Abuse Liability of Drugs in Humans, Fischman, M.W.; Mello, N.K.; eds.; NIDA, Research Monograph 92 (1989)
Thanatos to Eros: 35 Years of Psychedelic Exploration; Stolaroff, M.; Thanatos Press (1994) ISBN: 3-86135-453-5
Through The Gateway of the Heart, Adamson, S. (Ed.); Four Trees, 1985, ISBN: 0-936329-00-9
TIHKAL; The Continuation; Shulgin, A.; Shulgin, A.; Joy, D. (Ed.) Transform Press; (1997); ISBN: 0-9630096-9-9
Toxic Psychiatry; Breggin, P.; (1994) St. Martin's Press
You Must Be Dreaming, Noël, B. *et al.* (1992); ISBN: 0-671-74153-5

REFERENCES

Abbott, L.D, Jr.; Smith, J.D.; Chemical Preparation of Homogentisic Acid; *Journal of Biological Chemistry*; (1949) 179: 365-368

Adams, R.; Kamm, O.; Organic Chemical Reagents. I. Dimethylgloxime; *Journal of the American Chemical Society* (1918) 40: 1281-1289.

Adams, R.; Thal, F.; Kamm, O.; Matthews. A.O; Benzyl Cyanide: *Organic Syntheses*, Volume 2 (1922) pgs. 9-11

Adams, R.; Thal, F.; Kamm, O.; Matthews, A.O; Phenyl Acetic Acid: *Organic Syntheses*, Volume 2 (1922) pgs. 63-65

Adams; *Journal of the American Chemical Society* (1924) 46: 1889

Aghajanian, G.K.; Wang, R.Y.; Physiology and Pharmacology of Central Serotonergic Neurons; In *Psychopharmacology; A Generation of Progress*, (1978)

Air Force (1944) March U.S. War Dept. Cir. Letter No. 58 2/23/1943

Albert, H.E.; Kibler, R.W.; Alkali Spitting of Secondary and Tertiary Formamides; (1956) *US 2,773,097*

Aldous, F.A.B.; Barrass, B.C.; Brewster, K.; Buxton, D.A., Green, D.M.; Pinder, R.M.; Rich, P.; Skeels, M.; Tutt, K.J.; Structure-Activity Relationships in Psychotomimetic Phenylalkylamines; *Journal of Medicinal Chemistry* (1974) 17 (10): 1100-1111

Allen, C.F.H.; Leubner, G.W.; Syringic Aldehyde; *Organic Syntheses* (1963) *Coll. IV*: 866-869

Allen, A.C.; Cantrell, T.S.: Synthetic Reductions in Clandestine Amphetamine and Methamphetamine Laboratories; *Forensic Sciences International* (1989) 42:183-199.

Allen, A.C.; Kiser, W.O.; Methamphetamine From Ephedrine:1. Chloroephedrines and Aziridines; *Journal of Forensic Sciences* (1987) 32: 953-962.

Allen, A.C.; Stevenson, M.L.; Nakamura, S.M.; Ely, R.A.; Differentiation of Illicit Phenyl-2-Propanone Synthesized from Phenylacetic Acid with Acetic Anhydride Versus Lead (III) Acetate; *Journal of Forensic Sciences* (1992) 37 (1): 301-322.

Alles, Gordon A.; Salts of 1-Phenyl-2-aminopropane; *U.S. Patent 1,879,003*

Alles, Gordon A.; *dl*-Beta-Phenylisopropylamines; *Journal of the American Chemical Society*; (1932) 54: 271-274

Alles, G.A.; 1-(Paramethoxyphenyl)-2-formylaminopropane and Method of Preparing Same; (1935) *US 2,011,790.*

Alles, G.A.; 1-(Paramethoxyphenyl)-2-methylaminopropane and its Acid Addition Salts; (1935) *US 2,015,578.*

Alles, G.A.; Metamethoxybenzylmethylcarbinamines and Medicinal Preparations Comprising the Same; (1935) *US 2,361,372.*

Alles, G.A.; Fairchild, M.D.; Jensen, M.; Chemical Pharmacology of *Catha Edulis*; *J. Med. Pharm. Chem.* (1961) 3: 323-352; *CA* (1961) 55: 14825

Angrist, B.M.; Schweitzer, J.W.; Friedhoff, A.J.; Gershon, S.; Investigation of *p*-Methoxyamphetamine Excretion in Amphetamine Induced Psychosis; *Nature* (1970) 225: 651-652

Arthur, H.R.; Ng, Y.L.; Syntheses of the four Dimethoxy-N-methylphthalimides; *Journal of the Chemical Society* (1959) 3094.

Austin, Paul R.; Johnson, John R.; Abnormal Reactions of Benzylmagnesium Chloride; *Journal of the American Chemical Society* (1932) 54; 655.

Bachman, G.B.; Pollack, M.; Vapor Phase Nitration. Factors Affecting Degration to Lower Nitroparaffins; *Industrial and Engineering Chemistry* (1954) 46 (4): 713-718

Bailey, K.; A Synthesis of 1-Alkyl-3,5-dimethoxybenzenes; *Canadian Journal of Chemistry* (1974) 52: 2136-2138

Bakalar, J.B.; Ginspoon, L.; Testing Psychotherapies and Drug Therapies: The Case of Psychedelic Drugs; In *Ecstasy: The Clinical Pharmacological & Neurotoxicological Effects of the Drug MDMA* (1990)

Baker, W.; Brown, N.C.; Elbs Persulfate Oxidation of Phenols and its Adaptation to the Preparation of Monoalkyl Ethers of Quinols; *Journal of the Chemical Society* (1948) 2303-2307; *Chemical Abstracts* (1949) 43: 3386-3387

Baker, W.; Evans, C.; Derivatives of 1,2,3,4-Tetrahydroxybenzne. Part IV. Attempted Syntheses; *Journal of the Chemical Society* (1938) 372-375

Baker, W.; Jukes, E.H.T.; Subrahmanyam, C.A; Derivatives of 1,2,3,4-Tetrahydroxybenzene. Part 111. The Synthesis of Dill Apiole, and the Extension of the Dakin Reaction; *Journal of the Chemical Society* (1934) 1681-1684

Baker, W.; Savage, R.I.; Derivatives of 1,2,3,4-Tetrahydroxybenzene. Part V. The Synthesis of Parsley Apiole and Derivatives; *Journal of the Chemical Society* (1938) 1602-1607

Baltzly, R.; de Beer, E.; Buck, J.S.; (Burroughs Wellcome & Co.); ß-(2,5-Dimethoxyphenyl)-ß-hydroxyisopropylamine; (1944) *U.S. Pat. 2,359,707*

Baltzly, R.; Buck, J.S.; (Burroughs Wellcome & Co. Contribution); Amines Related to 2,5-Dimethoxyphenylethylamine 1.; *Journal of the American Chemical Society* (1940a) 62: 161-164

Baltzly, R.; Buck, J.S.; (Burroughs Wellcome & Co. Contribution); Amines Related to 2,5-Dimethoxyphenylethylamine 2; *J. of the American Chem. Soc.* (1940b) 62: 164-67

Baltzly, R.; Buck, J.S.; Ide, W.S.; (Burroughs Wellcome & Co. Contribution); Amines Related to 2,5-Dimethoxyphenylethylamine V; *Journal of the American Chemical Society* (1950) 72: 382-384.

Ban, Yoshio; Preparation of 3,4,-Dimethoxyphenethylamine; *Journal of the Pharmaceutical Society of Japan* (1954) 74: 212-213; *CA* 49: 1610 d-f.

Barfknecht, C.F.; Caputo, J.F.; Tobin, M.B.; Dyer, D.C.; Standridge, R.T.; Howell, H.G.; Goodwin, W.R.; Partyka, R.A.; Gylys, J.A.; Cavanagh, R.L.; Congeners of DOM; Effect of Distribution of the Evaluation of Pharmacologic Data; In *'QuaSAR'* pgs. 16-26

Barfknecht, C.F.; Nichols, D.E.; Potental Psychotomimetics. Bromomethoxy-amphetamines; *Journal of Medicinal Chemistry* (1971) 14(4); 370-372

Bargellini; Monti; *Gazzetta* (1915) 45:90

Battaglia, G.; Brooks, B.P.; Kulsakdinun and De Souza, E.B.; Pharmacologic Profile of MDMA (3,4-Methylenedioxy-methamphetamine) at Various Brain Recognition Sites; *European Journal of Pharmacology* (1988) 149: 159-163

Battaglia, G.; Yeh, S.H.; DeSouza, E.B; MDMA - Induced Neurotoxicity: Parameters of Degeneration and Recovery of Brain Serotonin Neurons; *Pharmacology Biochemistry and Behaviour* (1988a) 29: 269-274

Baum, R.M.; New Variety of Street Drugs Poses Growing Problem; *Chemical & Engineering News*; 9/9/85; pgs. 7-16

Beckett, A.H.; Brookes, L.G.; The Effect of Chain and Ring Substitution on the Metabolism, Distribution and Biological Action of Amphetamines; In *Amphetamines and Related Compounds* (1970)

Beers, M.; Avorn, J.; Soumerai, S.B.; Everitt, D.E.; Sherman, D.S.; Salem; Psychoactive Medication Use in Intermediate-Care Facility Residents; *Journal of the American Medical Association* (1988) 260 (20) 3016-3020

Benington, F.; Morin, R.D.; Clark, L.C.; Mescaline Analogs. 1; *Journal of Organic Chemistry* (1954) 11-

Benington, F.; Morin, R.D.; Clark, L.C.; Mescaline Analogs. 2. Tetra- and Penta-Methoxy-beta-Phenylethylamines; *J. of Organic Chemistry* (1955) 20: 102-108

Benington, F. et al.; *Journal of Organic Chemistry* (1958) 23: 1979

Bennett, J.P. Jr.; Snyder, S.H.; Stereospecific Binding of *d*-Lysergic Acid Diethylamide (LSD) to Brain Membranes: Relationship to Serotonin Receptors; *Brain Research* (1975) 94: 523-544

Beregi, L.G.; Hugon, P.; Le Douarec, J.C.; Laubie, M.; Duhault, J.; Structure-Activity Relationships in CF3 Substituted Phenylethylamines; In *Amphetamines and Related Compounds* (1970)

Besson, H.; Sur les properietes vaso-motrices de la R-pseudo-norephedrine; *Compt. rend Societe de Biologie* (1936) 122: 40-42; *Chemical Abstracts* 30: 5299

Biel, John. H.; Structure-Activity Relationships of Amphetamine And Derivatives; In *Amphetamines and Related Compounds* (1970)

Biniecki, S.; Krajewski, E.; (Akad. Med. Warsaw); Preparation of *d,l*-1-(3,4-Methylenedioxyphenyl)-2-(methylamino)propane and *d,l*-1-(3,4-Dimethoxyphenyl)-2-(methyl-amino)propane; *Acta Polon Pharm* (1960) 17: 421-425 (in Polish). *Chemical Abstracts* (1961) 14350 e-g

Birch, A.J.; Reductions by Dissolving Metals Part II; *Journal of the Chemical Society* (1945) 809-813

Bobranskii, B.R.; Ya. V. Drabik; *J. Applied Chem (USSR)* (1941) 14: 410-414; *Chemical Abstracts* 36: 2532

Brockmühl, M.; Ehrhart, G.; Stein, L.; Process of Preparing Compounds of the 1-Pheny-2-aminoalcohols-1 Series Hydroxylated in the Phenyl Nucleus; (1934) *US 1,948,162*

Bogert; Davidson; *J. of the American Chemical Society* (1932) 54: 334

Bogert, M.; Isham, R.M.; Preparation and Properties of Certan Methoxylated Carbinols, Olefines and Ketones from Trimethylgallic acid; *J. Amer. Chem. Soc.* (1914) 36: 314-530; *Chemical Abstracts* 8: 1577, 3789.

Bollinger, W.; Sletzinger M.; Merck & Co. Inc.; (1962) Phenylalanine Deriviatives; *Chemical Abstracts* (1963) 59:1753d

Boissier, J.R.; Hirtz, J.; Dumont, C.; Gerardin, A.; Some Aspects of the Metabolism of Anorexic Phenylisopropylamines in the Rat; in *Amphetamines and Related Compounds* 1970.

Booth, A.B.; Method of Obtaining Essentially Pure Estragole; *US Patent 3,408,405* (1968)

Braun, U.; Braun, G.; Jacob III, P.; Nichols, D.E.; Shulgin, A.T.; Centrally Active N-substituted Analogs of 3,4-Methylenedioxypheylisopropylamine (3,4-Methylenedioxyamphetamine); *Journal of Pharmaceutical Sciences*; (1980) 69(2): 192-195

Braun, U.; Braun, G., Jacob III, P.; Nichols, D.E.; Shulgin, A.T.; Mescaline Analogs: Substitutions at the 4-Position; In *'QuaSAR'* (1978) Research Monograph 22, Pages 27-37

Briody, R.G.; Cuevas, E.A.; Aluminum Amalgam Preparation; (1971) *US 3,619,176*

Brown, G.L.; Goodwin, F.K.; Cerebrospinal Fluid Correlates of Suicide Attempts and Aggression; *Annals of the New York Acadamy of Sciences* (1986) 487: 175-188

Bruce, W.F.; Cholestanone; *Organic Syntheses Collective II*: 139-140.

Bruce, W.F.; Szabo, J.L.; Hill, D.; Tubis, S.; (Wyeth Inc.); N-Alkylaminomethyl-phenyl-propane and Method of Preparing Same; *U.S. Patent 2,597,445*; *Chemical Abstracts* (1953) 47: 2771

Bruce, W.F. (Wyeth Inc.) (1952a); Tertiary Butyl Secondary Amines and Method of Preparing Same; *US Patent 2,597,446* (1952); *Chemical Abstracts* (1953) 47: 2771-2772

Brücke, F.T. von; Central Stimulating Action of the Alkaloid Cathine; *Arch. exptl. Path. Pharmakol.* (1941) 198: 100-146; *Chemical Abstracts* 38: 4683.

Bruckner, V.V.; Über das Pseudonitrosit des Asarons; *J. prakt. Chem.* (1933) 138: 268-274

Buck, J.S.; Veratraldehyde; *Organic Syntheses* 619-621

Burton, B.T.; Heavy Metal and Organic Contaminants Associated with Illicit Methamphetamine Production; In *Methamphetamine Abuse: Epidemiologic Issues and Implications*

Buu-Hoi, NG. Ph.; Welsh, M.; Dechamps, G.; Le Bihan, H.; Binon, F.; Xuong, NG. D.; Some Tuberculostatic Thiosemicarbazones; *Journal of Organic Chemistry* (1952) 18: 121-126

Butler, E.A.; Peters, D.G.; Swift, E.H.; Hydrolysis Reactions of Thioacetamide in Aqueous Solutions; *Analytical Chemistry* (1958) 30 (8): 1379-1383

Canter, F.W.; Curd, F.H.; Robertson, A.; Hydroxy-carbonyl Compounds. Part II. The Benzoylation of Ketones Derived From Phloroglucinol; *Journal of the Chemical Society* (1931) 1245-1255

Cantor, F.C.; Perry, M.A.; Conversion of Aldehydes to Ketones; (1968) *US 3,384,668.*

Cantrell, T.S.; John, B.; Johnson, L.; Allen; A.C.; A Study of Impurities Found in Methamphetamine Synthesized From Ephedrine; *For. Sci. Int.* (1988) 39: 39-53

Carmack, M.; DeTar, DeLos F.; The Willgerodt and Kindler Reactions. III. Amides from Acetylenes and Olefins; Studies Relating to the Reaction Mechanisms; *Journal of the American Chemical Society* (1946) 68: 2029-2033

Carter. H.E.; *Journal of Biological Chemistry* (1935) 106: 619

Chalk, A.J.; Magennis, S.A.; Process for the Preparation of Aryl Substituted Aldehydes, Ketones and Alcohols; (1978) *US 4,070,374.*

Chen, K.K.; Wu, Chang-Keng; Henriksen E.; Relationship Between the Pharmacological Action and the Chemical Constitution and Configuration of the Optical Isomers of Ephedrine and Related Compounds; *J. Pharmacol.* (1929) 36: 363-400; *Chemical Abstracts* (1930) 24: 2198-99

Chenevert, R. Fortier, G.; Rhlid, R. B.; *Tetrahedron* (1992) 48:6769-6776.

Chretien, A,; Longi, Y.; The Preparation of Organic Nitrites by Means of the Hydrolysis of Aluminum Nitrite; *Compt. rend.* (1945) 220: 746-747

Chretien, A.; Longi, Y.; Nitrosation by the Method of Chretien and Longi; *Bull. soc. chim. France* (1957) 337-338

CIBA; Tertiary Amines and Process for Their Manufacture; (1961) *GB 885,801*

Commins & Seiden; *Brain Res.* (1986) 365: 15-20

Cook, C.E.; Pyrolytic Characteristics, Pharmacokinetics, and Bioavailability of Smoked Heroin, Cocaine, Phencyclidine, and Methamphetmaine; In *Methamphetamine Abuse: Epidemiologic Issues and Implications*; NIDA Research Monograph 115

Cooke, W.T.; The Laboratory Preparation of Sodium Nitrite; *Austrialian Chem. Inst. J. & Proc.* (1944) 11: 49-51. *Chemical Abstracts* (1944) 3561

Coppen, A.; Rowsell, A.R.; Turner, P.; Padgham, C.; 5-Hydroxytryptamine (5-HT) in the Whole-Blood of Patients With Depressive Illness; *Postgraduate Medical Journal* (1976) 52: 156-158

Cooper, D.A.; Allen, A.C.; Synthetic Cocaine Impurities; *Journal of Forensic Sciences* (1984) 29 (4); 1045-1055

Cooper, S.R.; Resacetophenone; *Organic Synth.* (1941) 21: 103-104

Costa, E.A.; Groppetti, A.; Revuelta, A.; *British Journal of Pharmacology* (1971) 41: 57-64.

Coughlin, R.W.; Mahmoud, W.M.; El-Sayed, A.H.; Enhanced bioconversion of toxic substance (1992) *US 5,173,413*.

Coutts, R.T. and J.L. Malicky; The Synthesis of Some Analogs of the Hallucinogen 1-(2,5-Dimethoxy-4-methylphenyl)-2-aminopropane (DOM); *Canadian Journal of Chemistry* (1973) 51: 1402-1409.

Cowan, D.M.; Jeffery, G.H.; Vogel, A.I.; Physical Properties and Chemical Constitution. Part V. Alkyl Ketones; *Journal of the Chemical Society* (194)) 62: 171-176.

Dal Cason, T; An Evaluation of the Potential for Clandestine Manufacture of 3,4-Methylenedioxyamphetamine (MDA) Analogs and Homologs;
Journal of Forensic Sciences (May 1990) 35 (3); 675-697

Dal Cason, T.A; Angelos, S.A.; Raney, J.K.; A Clandestine Approach to the Synthesis of Phenyl-2-propanone From Phenylpropenes;
Journal of Forensic Sciences (1984) 29(4): 1187-1208

Dallacker, F.; Derivatives of Methylenedioxybenzene. XXVII. Synthesis of Allyldimethoxy(methylenedioxy)benzenes. *Chem. Ber.* (1969) 102(8): 2663-2676; *Chemical Abstracts* (1969) 71: # 90987v

Dandiya, P.C.; Sharma, P.K.; Menon, M.K.; Studies on The Central Nervous System Depressants Part IV. Structure-Activity Relationship of Some Locally Synthesized Trimethoxy Benzene Dervatives; *Indian J. of Med. Research* (1962) 50: 750-753; CA 59: 5067c-h

Davies, R.R; Hodgson, H.H.; The Preparation of Aldehydes by the Ruptive Oxidation of the Ethylene Linkage; June 1943 Pages 90-92

Davis, C.H.; Carmack, M.; The Willgerodt Reaction. V. Substituted Acetamides From ß-Substituted Acrylic Acids; ??? pgs. 76-78

De Montigany, C.; Aghajanian, G.K.; Tricyclic Antidepressants: Long-Term Treatment Increases Responsivity of Rat Forebrain Neurons to Serotonin;
Science (1978) 202(22): 1303-1306

Desseigne, Giral; *Mem. Poudres* (1952) 34:49-53

Dessi, P.; Preparation of 3,4,5-Trimethoxybenzaldehyde and 1-(4-Methoxyphenyl)-2-methylaminopropane; *Arch. ital. sci. farmacol.* (1952) 2 (3) 376-383 *Chemical Abstracts* 50: 3314-3315.

DeTar, DeLos F.; Carmack, M.; The Willgerodt Reaction. II. A Study of Reaction Conditions with Acetophenone and Other Ketones; *Journal of the American Chemical Society* (1946) 68: 2025-2029.

Dev., Sukh; Sesquiterpenes. III. Synthesis of Homocadalenes; *Journal of the Indian Chemical Society* (1948) 25: 315-322; see *Chemical Abstracts* 1949; 43: 2606 e-h.

Dikstein, S.; Segal, M.; Stimulant; Dec. 6, 1983; *US 4,419,367*

Drefahl, G.; Grahmer, H.; Thomas, W.; A New Synthesis of *dl-threo*-1-Hydroxy-1-phenyl-2-aminopropane; *Chem. Ber.* 91:282-283 (1958); *Chemcial Abstracts* 52: 16419 g-i

Duff, J.C.; A New General Method for the Preparation of *o*-Hydroxyaldehydes from Phenols and Hexamethylenetetramine; *Journal of the Chemical Society* (1941) 547-550

Edeleano, L.; Ueber einige Derivate der Phenylmethacrylsäure und der Phenylisobuttersäure; *Ber.* (1887) 20: 616-622.

Elks, J.; Hey, D.H.; ß-3,4-Methylenedioxyphenyisopropylamine; *Journal of the Chemical Society* (1943) 15-16

Ellinwood; *American Journal of Psychiatry* (1975) 127: 1170-1175

Ely, R.A.; McGrath, D.C.; Lithium-Ammonia Reduction of Ephedrine to Methamphetamine; An Unusual Clandestine Synthesis; *Journal of Forensic Sciences* (1990) 35(3): 720-723

I.G. Farbenindustrie; Manufacture of 1-Phenyl-2-alkylaminopropanols (1) Hydroxylated in the Phenyl nucleus; (1932) *GB 367, 951*

Fackelmann, K.A.; Birth Defect Linked to Decongestant Drug; *Science News* (1995) 141: 262

Feugeas, C.; Synthesis in the 1,2-Methylenedioxybenzene Series (Safrole, Piperonal and Piperine).; *Bull. Soc. Chim. France* (1964) 8: 1892-1895; *Chemical Abstracts* (1964) 61: 16001 a-e

Fioncchio, D.V.; Huebner, C.F.; The Suppression of Appetite with 1(o-Chlorophenyl)-2-methyl-2-propylamine and Acid-addition Salts Thereof; (1968) *US 3,415,937*

Fishbein et. al.; *Bio. Chemistry* (1989) 25 (8):1049-1066

Flassig, E.; Resolution of *dl*-Norephedrine; *Osterr. Chemiker-Ztg* (1956) 57: 308; *Chemical Abstracts* (1958) 15838 e-f

Fleischer, J.C.; Reynolds, J.W.; Young, H.S.; Catalytic Synthesis of Ketones from Aldehydes; (1968) *US 3,410,909.*

Fleischmajer, S.; Hyman, A.B.; Clinical Significance of Derangements of Tryptophan Metabolism; A Review of Pellagra, Carcinoid and Hartnup Disease; *Arch. Dermatol.* 84: 563- (1961)

Flemenbaum, A.; Does Lithium Block the Effects of Amphetamine? A Report of Three Cases; *American Journal of Psychiatry* (1974) 131 (7): 820-821.

Fodor, G.; Kiss, J.; Separation of *dl*-Norephedrine from *dl*-Nor-pseudoephedrine.; *Acta Univ. Szegediensis, Pars Phys. et Chem. Sci. Nat. Acta Phys. et Chem.* 1, No 1/4, 3-7 (in English); *Chemical Abstracts* 50: 15451-15452

Fodor, G.; Bruckner, V.; Kiss, J.; Ohegyi, G.; Use of Acyl Migration in Separating Diastereoisomeric Amino Alcohols; ???? (1948) 337-345

Fort, A.W.; Roberts, J.D.; The Reactions of 3-Phenyl-1-propylamine-1-14C and 3-(*p*-Methoxyphenyl)-1-propylamine-1-14C with Nitrous Acid; *Journal of the American Chemical Society* (1955) 78: 584-590

Frank, R.S.; The Clandestine Drug Laboratory Situation in the United States; *Journal of Forensic Sciences* (1983) 28(1): 18-31

Frisch, K.C.; The Synthesis of Aromatic Divinylogs and Aromatic Halogenated Vinylogs; *Journal of Polymer Science* (1959) XLI; 359-367

Fujisawa, Shunro; Methyl(2-phenylisopropyl)amine; *Japan 173,746* Sept., 27, 1946; *Chemical Abstracts* 46: 2432 a-b

Fujisawa, T.; Okada, M.; Deguchi, Y.; 1-(ß-Diethylaminoethoxyphenyl)-3-methyl-3,4-dihydro-6,7-methylenedioxyisoquinoline; *Japan 8673 ('56); Chemical Abstracts* (1958) 52: 11965 b-f

Fusco, R.; Caggianelli, G.; Sympathomimetic Substances. I. Synthesis of Some (*p*-Hydroxyphenyl)isopropylalkylamines; *Farm. Sci. e tec (Pavia)* (1948) 3:125-36; *Chemical Abstracts* (1949) 43: 1741 c-h

Fuller, R.W.; Recommendations for Future Research on Amphetamines and Related Designer Drugs; In *Pharmacology and Toxicology of Amphetamine and Related Designer Drugs*, (1989)

Fuller, R.W.; (Lilly Research Laboratories); Structure Activity Relationships Among the Halogenated Amphetamines; In *Serotonin Neurotoxins* (1978)

Gaday, S.; Harris, S.R.; Studies of Falvin Adenine Dinucleotide - Requiring Enzymes and Phenothiazines. I. Interaction of Chlorpromazine and D-amino Acid Oxidase; *Biochem. Pharmacol* (1965) 14: 7-21

Gairaud, C.B.; Lappin, G.R.; The Synthesis of Nitrostyrenes; *Journal of Organic Chemistry* (1952) 18: 1-3

Gal, E.M.; Sherman, A.D.; Cerebral Metabolism of Some Serotonin Depletors; In *Serotonin Neurotoxins*

Galizin, M.A.; Moret, C.; Verzier, B.; Langer, S.Z.; Interaction Between Tricyclic and Nontricyclic 5-Hydroxytryptamine Uptake Inhibitors and the Presynaptic Inhibitory Autoreceptors in the Rat Hypothalmus; *The Journal of Pharmacology and Experimental Therapeutics* (1985) 235(1): 200-211

Gardos, G.; Cole, J.O.; Tarsy, D.; Withdrawl Syndromes Associated with Antipsychotic Drugs; *American Journal of Psychiatry* (1978) 135 (11) 1321-1324

Garrard, J.; Makris, L.; Dunham, T.; Heston, L.L.; Copper, S.; Ratner, E.; Zelterman, D.; Kane; Evaluation of Neuroleptic Drug Use by Nursing Home Elderly Under Proposed Medicare and Medicaid Regulations; *Journal of the American Medical Association* (1991) 265 (4); 463-467

Geis et al.; *Soc. Neurosci Abst* (1985) 11: 49

Gero, A.; Some Reactions of 1-Phenyl-chloro-2-methylaminepropane. I. Reaction with Metals and with Hydrogen; *Journal of Organic Chemistry* (1951) 16: 1731-1735

Giudiclli, Don P.R.L.; Sous-Bois, Fontenay; Najer, Henry (1978) Phenylethylamine Derivatives; *US 4,129,598*

Giudiclli, Don P.R.L.; Sous-Bois, Fontenay; Najer, Henry (1976) Phenyl Propanones: *US 3,965,190*

Giudiclli, Don P.R.L.; Sous-Bois, Fontenay; Najer, Henry (1979); 1-(3'-Trifluromethylthiophenyl)-2-ethylaminopropane Pharmaceutical Composition and Method for Treating Obesity; *US 4,148,923*

Glassman, A.H.; Carino, J.S.; Roose, S.P.; Adverse Effects of Tricyclic Antidepressants: Focus on the Elderly; *Adv. Biochem. Psychopharmacol* (1984) 39: 391-398

Glennon, R.A.; Stimulus Properties of Hallucinogenic Phenylalkylamines and Related Designer Drugs; Formulation of Structure-Activity Relationships; in *Pharmacology and Toxicology of Amphetamine and Related Designer Drugs*; pgs 43-67

Glennon, R.A.; Yousif, M.; Naiman, N.; Kalix, P.; Methcathinone: A New and Potent Amphetamine-Like Agent; *Pharmacology Biochemistry & Behavior* (1987) 26: 547-551

Goldstone, M.S.;(letter) ; 'Cat' - Methcathinone - A New Drug of Abuse; *Journal of the American Medical Association* (1993) 269(19):2508

Giffith, J.D.; Cavanaugh, J.H.; Held, J.; Oates, J.A.; Experimental Psychosis Induced by the Administration of *d*-Amphetamine; In *Amphetamines and Related Compounds* (1970)

Greer, G.R.; *MDMA: A New Psychotropic Compound and Its Effects in Humans* (1983)

Greer, G.R.; Tolbert, R.; Subjective Reports of the Effects of MDMA in a Clinical Setting; *Journal of Psychoactive Drugs* (1986) 18 (4): 319-327

Greer, G.R.; Tolbert, R.; The Therapeutic Use of MDMA; In *Ecstasy: The Clinical Pharmacological & Neurotoxicological Effects of the Drug MDMA* (1990)

Grignard, V.; Chambret, F.; Ketonic Fission of Tertiary Alcohols; *Compt. rend.* 182, 299-302; *Chemical Abstracts* (1926) 20: 1602.

Grinspoon v. Drug Enforcement Administration, 828F.2d881(1st Cir. 1987)

Groger, D., Schmander, H. P. and Mothes, K. *Z. Allg. Mikrobol.*, (1966) 6:275

Gyogyszer, Chinoin; New Aralkylamines and their Preparation; *GB 1,031,425* (1963)

Hall, J.N.; Broderick, P.M.; Communitiy Networks for Response to Abuse Outbreaks of Methamphetamine and Its Analogs; In *Methamphetamine Abuse: Epidemiologic Issues and Implications*

Hall, S.S.; Lipsky, S.D.; Small, G.H.; Selective Lithium-Ammonia Reduction of Aromatic Ketones and Benzyl Alcohols: Mechanistic Implications; *Tetrahedron Letters* (1971) 21: 1853-1854.

Hall, S.S.; Lipsky, S.D.; Alkylation-Reduction of Aromatic Ketones and Aldehydes: A Convenient Synthesis of Aromatic Hydrocarbons; *Journal of the American Chemical Society (Chem. Trans.)* (1971) 1242-1243.

Hamada, K.; *et al.*; Phenylacetone; *Japan 4367* (1950) December 16;*Chem. Abstracts* (1953) 47: 3347 i

Hambourger; *JAMA* (1939) 112: 1340

Hargis, C.W.;Young, H.S.; Reynolds, J.W.; Catalytic Synthesis of Ketones from Aldehydes; (1969) *US 3,453,331.*

Harley-Mason, J.; *Journal of the Chemical Society* (1953) 200

Hart, M.C.; Woodruff, E.H.; Alkyl Phenols. I. The 4-n-Alkyl-pyrogallols; *Journal of the American Chemical Society* (1936) 58: 1957-1959

Hartung W.H.; Munch, J.C.; Amino alcohols; VI. The Preparation and Pharmacodynamic Activity of Four Isomeric Phenylpropylamines; *Journal of the American Chemical Society* (1931) 53: 1875-1879

Hass, H.B., Alexander, L.G.; Oxygen-Induced Vapor-Phase Nitration of Paraffins; *Industrial and Engineering Chemistry* (1949) 41 (10); 2266-2270

Hass, H.B.; Hodge, E.B.; Vanderbilt, B.M.; Nitration of Gaseous Paraffins; *Industrial and Engineering Chemistry* (1936) 28 (3): 339-344

Hass, H.B. & H. Shechter; Vapor-Phase Nitration of Saturated Hydrocarbons; *Industrial and Engineering Chemistry* (1947) 39 (7); 817-821

Hass, H.B.; Susie, A.G.; Heider, R.L.; Nitro Alkene Derivatives; *Journal of Organic Chemistry* (1950) 15: 8-12

Hass, H.B.; Vanderbilt, B.M.; Hodge, E.B.; Process of Nitrating Paraffin Hydrocarbons and Product Thereof; *U.S. Patent 1,967,667*

Heacock, R.A.; Hutzinger, O.; Synthesis of Metanephrine and Normetanephrine; *Chemistry and Industry* (161) 595

Heacock, R.A.; Hutzinger, O.; Nerenberg, C.; A Note on the Preparation of Some 1-Phenyl-2-nitroethanol Derivatives; *Canadian Journal of Chemistry* (1961) 39: 1143-1147

Hecht, A.; Tranquilizers: Use, Abuse, and Dependence, HHS Publication No. (FDA)

Heidelberger, Michael; Chloroacetone; 1923; In *An Advanced Laboratory Manual of Organic Chemistry*; J.J. Little & Ives Company

Heinzelman, R.V.; o-Methoxyphenylacetone; *Organic Syntheses* 4: 573-576

Heinzelman, R.V.; Physiologically Active Secondary Amines. *Beta-(-o-*Methoxyphenyl)-isopropyl-N-methylamine and Related Compounds; *Journal of the American Chemical Society* (1953) 75: 921-927

Heischober, B.; Miller, M.; Methamphetamine Abuse in California; In *Methamphetamine Abuse: Epidemiologic Issues and Implications*

Hell, C.; Bauer, H.; Aromatic propene derivatives,; *Ber.* (1903) 36: 204-208; *J. Chem. Soc.* (1903) I, 242; *Ber.* (1903) 1184-1192; *Ber.* (1904) 37: 230-233; IV Isoeugenol ethyl ether. *Ber* (1904) 1128-1132; *J. Chem. Soc* (1904) I: 241-242.

Herbst, R.M.: Manske, R.H.; *Organic Syntheses* (1943) *Collective Vol. II*: 389-391

Hey, D.H.; *dl*-ß-Phenylisopropylamine and Related Compounds; *Journal of the Chemical Society* (1930) 18-21

Higgitt *et al.*; *Br. Med. J.* (1985) 291: 688

Hildebrandt, G.; Klavdhn, W.; Manufacture of *Levo*-1-Phenyl-2-Methylamino-propanol-1 (1931); *GB 360,334*

Hildebrandt; Gustav (1939); Preparation of *beta-p*-Hydroxyphenylisopropyl-methylamine; *US 2,146,474*

Hildebrandt, G.; Klavdhn, W.; Manufacture of Levo-1-Phenyl-2-Methylaminopropanol-1 (1934) *US 1.956,950*

Hildebrandt, Gustav (1944); Preparation of *beta-(meta*-hydroxyphenyl)-isopropylmethylamines; *US 2,344,356*

Ho, Beng T.; Tansey, W.; Balster, R.L.; An, R.; McIsaac, W.M.; Harris, R.T.; Amphetamine Analogs. 2. Methylated Phenylethylamines; *Journal of Medicinal Chemistry* (1970) 13: 134-135

Ho, T.; Wong, C.M.; Synthesis of Desoxybenzoins. Deoxygenation with the Red Phosphoris/Iodine System; *Synthesis* (1975) 161.

Hodgson, H.H.; Beard, H.G.; The Preparation of 2,5-Dihydroxy-benzaldehyde (Gentisaldehyde); ????? (1927) 2339-2340

Hoelderich, W.; Merger, F.; Mross, W.D.; Fischer, R.; Preparation of Ketones by Isomerization of Aldehydes; (1987) *US 4,694,107.*

Hoffer, A.: Nicotinic Acid: An Adjunct in the Treatment of Schizophrenia; *American Journal of Psychiatry* (1963) 120: 171

Hofmann, H.; Opitz, K.; Schnelle; Action of Nor-pseudoephedrine; *Arzneimittel-Forsch.* (1955) 5: 367-370; *Chemical Abstracts* 49: 16232 f-g

Hoffmeister, F.; Wuttke, W.; *Pharmacol. Rev.* (1975) 27: 419-428

Holmes, P.; White, D.E.; Wilson, I.H.; Allybenzene Compounds. II. 2,4,6-Timethoxyallybenzene; *Journal of the Chemical Society*; (1950) 2810-2811; *Chemical Abstracts* (1951) 45: 3346-3347

Hoover, F.W.; H.B. Hass; Synthesis of 2-Amino-1-Phenyl-1-Propanol and its Methylated Dervatives; *Journal of Organic Chemistry* (1947) 12: 506-509

Horii. Z.; Tsuji, J.; Inoi, T.; Syntheses of Arylalkylamines. 1. Syntheses of *alpha*-Methyl-2-methoxyphenethylamines; *Yakugaku Zasshi* (1957) 77: 248-451; 2. Syntheses of 1-(2-Methoxyphenyl)-2-propanone; *Yakugaku Zasshi* (1957) 77: 252-255. 3. Syntheses of *alpha*-Methyl-2-methoxy-phenethylamines; *Yakugaku Zasshi* (1957) 77: 256-258; *Chemical Abstracts* (1957) 51: 8671-8672

Horst-Myer, H. zur; Influence of the Appetite Inhibitors Cyclohexylmethyl Aminopropane (Obesine) and Pseudo-nor-ephedrin (E50) on the Carbohydrate Metabolism of Healthy Persons; *Deutsche Zeitschrift fur Verdauungs und Stoffwechselkrankh* (1959) 19: 148-151; *Chemical Abstracts* 10142

Hyort, A.M.; Randall, L.O.; De Beer, E.J.; Pharmacology of Compounds Related to ß-2,5-Dimethoxy-phenethyamine. 1. The Ethyl, Isopropyl, and Propyl Derivatives; *J. Pharmacol Exptl. Therap.* (1948) 92: 283-290

Ide, W.S.; Buck, J.S.; 3-Methyl-3,4-dihydroisoquinolines and 3-Methyl-1,2,3,4-tetrahydroisoquinolines; *Journal of the American Chemical Society* (1940) 62: 425-428

Ingersoll, A.W.; Brown, J.H.; Kim, C.K.; Beauchamp, W.D.; Jennings, G.; Extensions of the Leuckart Synthesis of Amines; *Journal of the American Chemical Society* (1936) 58: 1808-1812

Ingersoll, A.W.; Bircher, L.J.; Brubacker, M.M.; Semicarbazide Sulfate; *Organic Syntheses* 5: 93-97

Ingersoll, A.W.; Hydrocinnamic Acid; *Organic Syntheses* 9: 42-45

Ingersoll, A.W.; Hydrocinnamic Acid; *Organic Syntheses Coll.* 1: 311-314 (1941)

Inoi, T.; Okamoto, T.; Aromatic carbonyl compounds; *Japan Patent 69 09,892; Chemical Abstracts* (1969) 71: 61016x

Irvine, G.D.; Chin, L.; The Environmental Impact and Adverse Health Effects of the Clandestine Manufacture of Methamphetamine; In *Methamphetamine Abuse: Epidemiologic Issues and Implications*

Jackson & Short; *Journal of the Chemical Society* (1937) 513-516

Jacob, P.T.; Shulgin, A.T.; Structure-Activity Relationships of the Classical Hallucinogens and Their Analogs; In *Hallucinogens: An Update*; Lin, G.C.; Glennon, R.A.; NIDA Research Monograph 146 (1994); NIH Publication Number 146: 94-3872

Jacob, T.A.; Bachman, G.B.; Hass, H.B.; Synthesis of 1,1-Bis(alkoxyaryl)-2-nitroalkanes for Insecticidal Evaluation; *Journal of Organic Chemistry* 16: 1572-1576

Jarowski, C.; Hartung, W.H.; Amino Alcohols; XII. Optical Isomers in the Ephedrine Series of Compounds (1); ??? *Journal of Organic Chemistry* (1943) 564-571

Jew, S.; Kim, H.; Cho, Y.; Cook, C.; A Practical Preparation of Conjuncted Nitroalkenes; *Chemistry Letters* (1986) 1747-1748

Johns, I.B.; Burch, J.M.; The Synthesis and Resolution of *alpha-o*-Chlorobenzylethylamine; *Journal of the American Chemical Society* (1938) 60: 919-20

Jones, H.I., Wheatley, R.; The Preparation of Methylamine; *Journal of the American Chemical Society* (1918) 40: 1411-1415.

Jones, T.G.H.; Robinson, R.; *Journal of the Chemical Society* (1917) 111: 918

Jönsson, L.E.; Gunne, L.M.; Clinical Studies of Amphetamine Psychosis; In *Amphetamines and Related Compounds* (1970)

218 AMPHETAMINE SYNTHESES: OVERVIEW & REFERENCE

Kalvekhn, W.; Manufacture of 1-Phenyl-2-methylamino-1-propanol; (1929) *GB 336,412*

Kamlet, J.; Preparation of Arylnitroalkanols; (1939) *US 2,151,517*

Kanao, S.; Nor- and Nor-pseudo-ephedrine; *Journal of the Pharmaceutical Society (Japan)* (1928) 48: 947-948; *Chemical Abstracts* (1929) 23: 22431-2432; Also check, *Journal of the Pharmaceutical Society (Japan)* (1927) 47: 102

Kanao, S.; Nor- and Nor-pseudo-ephedrine. II.; *Journal of the Pharmaceutical Society (Japan)* (1928) 48: 1070-1081; *Chemical Abstracts* (1929) 23: 2705; *Chemical Abstracts* 46: 3980 d-e

Kanao, S.; Constituents of the Chinese Drug "Ma Huang." VII. *l*-Norephedrine; *Ber.* (1930) 63B: 95-98; *Chemical Abstracts* (1930) 24: 2545; see also *Chemical Abstracts* 23: 1472

Kanao, S.; Alkamines III.;*Journal of the Pharmaceutical Society (Japan)* (1929) 49: 238-46; *Chemical Abstracts* (1929) 23: 5162

Kefalas; Appetite-reducing Compositions Comprising Amino-phenyl-propane Derivatives; *GB 906,331*; *Chem. Abs.* 58: 6654c

King, J.A.; McMillan, F.H.; Studies on the Willgerodt Reaction. I. Some Extensions of the Reaction; *Journal of the American Chemical Society* (1946) 68: 525-526

King, J.A.; McMillan, F.H.; The Decarboxylative Acylation of Arylacetic Acids; *Journal of the American Chemical Society* (1951) 73: 4922-4915.

Klages, A.; Styrenes II; *Ber.* (1902) 35: 2633-2646; *J. Chem. Soc.* (1902) I, 666.

Knoll A.-G. (1937a); A Process for the preparation of *Beta-(p*-Oxyphenyl)-Isopropylmethylamine; (1937) *GB 482,414*

Knoll A.-G.(1937b); A Process for the preparation of *Beta-(p*-Oxyphenyl)-Isopropylmethylamine; *GB 482,180* (1937)

Knoll, J.; Psychotomimetic Effects of Amphetamines; In *Amphetamines and Related Compounds* (1970)

Knoll, József; Ecsery, Zoltán; Hermann née Vörös, Judit; Török, Zoltán; Somfai, Éva; Bernáth, Gábor; Szeged; N,N-Disubstitued-2-furylethylamines; *US 4,162,327* (1979)

Kolesnikov, D.G.; Maksyutina, N.P.; Bezruk, P.I.; Spasmotic Substances Present in the Seeds of *Petroselinum Sativum*; *Aptechnoe Delo* (1958) 7 (4): 27-30; *Chemical Abstracts* (1960) 54: 12491

Konao, T.; Shinozaki,Y.; Ishii, S; Preparation of ß-Phenylethylamine Derivatives (Synthesis of 3-Methoxy-4-ethoxy-1-[ß-aminoethyl] benzene); *J. Pharm. Soc. (Japan)* (1928) 48: 1070-1081; *Chemical Abstracts* (1929) 23: 2951

Krami, A.; Bruckner, V.; Use of Pseudonitrosites of Propenyl-Containing Phenyl Ethers for the Synthesis of alpha-Arylated ß-hydroxylamino and ß-amino-propanols. New Consideration on Acyl Wandering 3. Anethole Derivatives; *J. Prakt. Chem.* (1937) 148: 117-125; *Chemical Abstracts* (1937) 31: 4296-4297

Krassner, M.B.; Brain Chemistry; *Chemical & Engineering News* 8/29/83; pgs 22-33

Laboratoires Amido; Aralkyl Amines; (1954) *Fr. M2782*; *Chemical Abstracts* (1965) 5227-5228;

Langer, G.; Schoenbeck, G.; Koinig, G. *et al.*; Hyperactivity of Hypothalamic-Pituitary-Adrenal Axis in Endogenous Depression; *Lancet* (1979) 2: 524

Laing, R.R.; Dawson, B.; The Ritter Reaction Using Safrole: An Encounter In Two Clandestine Labs; Health Protection Branch, Drug Analytical Service, Health Canada, 3155 Willingdon Green, Burnaby, B.C., V5G 4P2

Leuenberger, H.G.W.; Matzinger, P.K.; Seebach, D.; Zueger, M.F.; Process to produce *alpha*-substituted derivatives of 3-hydroxypropionic acid; (1988) *US 4,734,367*

Leccese & Lyness; *Soc. Neurosci Abst* (1983) 9: 1146

Les Usines De Melle; Process for the Production of Aldehydes and Ketones; (1946) *GB 615,543*.

Linstid, H.C.; Koermer, G.S.; Isomerization of Branched Aldehydes to Ketones; (1985) *US 4,537,995*.

L'Italien, Yvon J.; Rebstock, Mildred C.; Methylaminopropiophenone Compounds and Methods for Produceing the Same; (1957) *US 2,802,865* see also Parke Davis 1957

Long, A., James, P. and Ward, O. P.; *Biotechnol. Bioeng.*, (1989) 33:657-660

Loomis, Chauncey C.; Process of Chlorinating Toluene; (1918) *US 1,280,612*

Lyness et al.; *Pharmacol.Biochem.Behav.*(1983)18:721-724

Lyon and Titeler; Pharmacology and Biochemistry of the 5-HT2 Receptor; Chapter 3 (5). 5-HT2 Receptor: Site of Action of Hallucinogenic Drugs; In *Serotonin Neurotoxins*

Maas, J.W.; The Effects of Psychopharmacological Agents on Central Nervous System Amine Metabolism in Man; *Annu. Rev. Pharmacol. Toxicol.* (1977) 17: 411-424

Magidson, O.Yu.; Garkusha, G.A.; The Synthesis of 2-Phenylisopropylamine (phenamine); *J. Gen. Chem. (USSR)* (1941) 11: 339-343 *Chemical Abstracts* (1941) 35: 5868

Manske, R.H.F.; Johnson, T.B.; Synthesis of Ephedrine and Structurally Similar Compounds. I. A New Synthesis of Ephedrine; *J. Amer. Chem. Soci.* (1929) 51: 580-582

Martin, E.L.; (E.I. du Pont de Nemours and Company, Inc.); The Clemmensen Reduction; *Chemical Reviews* ? Chapter 7, pgs 155-168

Marvel, C.B.; Hager, F.D.; Caudle, E.C.; Diphenylacetic Acid; *Organic Syntheses Collective Vol.* 1: 224-225.

Mason, J. P.; Terry L.I.; Preparation of Phenylacetone; *Journal of the American Chemical Society* 62: 1622

McClain, H., Jr.; Sapienza, F.; The Role of Abuse Liability Testing in Drug Control Procedures; In *Testing for Abuse Liability of Drugs in Humans*, (1989).

McCleary R.F.; Degering, E.F.; Reaction Mechanism for Nitrating Paraffin Hydrocarbons; *Ind. & Engineering Chem.* (1938) 30 (1): 64-69

McCombie, H.; Saunder, B.C.; Wild, F.; Preparation of Nitroethane; *Journal of the Chemical Society* (1944) 24-25

McKenna, D.J., Guan, X.M.; Shulgin, A.T.; 3,4-Methylenedioxy-amphetamine (MDA) Analogues Exhibit Differential Effects on Synaptosomal Release of 3H-Dopamine and 3H-5-Hydroxytryptamine; *Pharmacology Biochemistry & Behavior* (1991) 38: 505-512

McLang, J.; The Manufacture of Vanillin; Production From Oil of Cloves; *The Chemical Trade Journal and Chemical Engineer*; July, 3, 1925; pgs. 3-4

McLang, J.; The Aromatic Aldehydes; The Manufacture of Heliotropin; *The Chemical Trade Journal and Chemical Engineer*; Sept. 24, 1926; pgs. 359-361

McOmie, J.F.W.; Turner, A.B.; Tute, M.S.; The Structure of Pulvilloric Acid; *Journal of the Chemical Society (C) Org.* (1966) 18: 1608-13; *Chemical Abstracts* 65: 15307g (1966)

Meadows, G.G., Huff, M.R.; Fredericks, S.; Amitrptyline-Related Peripheral Neuropathy Relieved During Pyridoxine Hydrochloride Administartion; *Drug Intelligence an Clinical Pharmacology* (1982) 16: 876-877

Mellor, J.W.; (1928).-*Treatise on Inorg. and Theor. Chem.*, Vol. VIII, p.477.

E. Merck (1912) Verfahren zur Darstellung von Alkyloxyaryl-, Dialkyloxyaryl- und Alkylendioxyarylamino-propanen bzw. deren am Stichstoff monoalkylierten Derivaten; *DE 274350*

Merck, W.; Merck, K., Merck, L.; Merck, W.; Merck, F.; Process for the Preparation of 1-Phenyl-2-methylaminopropanol-1; (1929) *GB 284,644*

Merck & Co., Inc. (1962); Phenylalanine Deriviatives; *Chemical Abstracts* (1968) 69: 3416 Chemical No. 36445n

Messing, R.B.; Fisher, L.A.; Phebus, L.; Lytle, L.D.; Interaction of Diet and Drugs in the Regulation of Brain 5-Hydroxyindoles and the Response to Painful Electic Shock; *Life Sciences*; (1976) 18: 707-714

Messing, R.B.; Pettibone, D.J.; Kaufman, N.; Lytle, L.D.; Behavioral Efffects of Serotonin Neurotoxins; An Overview; In *Serotonin Neurotoxins* (1978)

Metzger, H.; Bases of the 1-Phenyl-2-aminopropane Series; *Chemical Abstracts* 1960: 54: 7654 a-c

Miczek, K.A.; Tidey, J.W.; Amphetamines: Aggressive and Social Behavior; In *Pharmacology and Toxicology of Amphetamine and Related Designer Drugs*, (1989)

Morgan, G.T.; The Manufacture of Sodium Nitrite; *Journal of the Society of the Chemical Industry* (1908) 27: 483-485 *Chemical Abstracts* 2287 (1909?)

Morishita, H.; Satoda; Kusuda, F., Omoto, T.; 1-(2,5-Dialkoxyphenyl)-1-hydroxy-2-aminopropane and its Salts; *Japan. 2176 (1961)* March 28; *Chemcial Abstracts* (1961) 24681-24682

Murahashi, S.; Haniwara, N.; Hirao, I.; Phenylacetone; *Japan 3616* (1950), October 19; *Chemical Abstracts* (1953) 47: 3347

Müller, E.; Rösscheisen, G.; A Variation of the Wurtz Synthesis. I Catalyzed Reactions of Benzyl and Allyl Halides with Alkali Metals; *Chem. Ber.* (1957) 90: 543-553; *Chemical Abstracts* (1957) 51: 15469

Murphy, D.L.; Campbell, I.; Costa, J.L.; Current Status of the Indoleamine Hypothesis of the Affective Disorders; in *Psychopharmacology; A Generation of Progress*, (1978)

Nabenbauer, F.P.; Substituted benzyl carbinamines; *GB 447,792*; *CA* 30: 7467.

Nagayoshi, Nagai (1918); Improvements in and Relating to Synthetic Drugs; *GB 120,936*

Nagai, W.N.; Synthetically-Compounded Drug Product and Method of Producing The Same; (19??) *US 1,399,144*

Nagai, W.N.; Mydriatic and Method of Producing The Same; (19??) *U.S. Patent 1,356,877*

Nagai, W.; Kanao, S.; Constituents of Chinese Drug "Ma Huang." VI; *Journal of the Pharmaceutical Society (Japan)* (1928) 48: 845-851; *Chemical Abstracts* 23: 1472

Nagai, A.; Process of Synthetically Producing Ephedrine Homologue and its Salts; (1934) *US 1,973,647*

Nagai, W.; Kanao, S.; Synthesis of Isometric Ephedrines and Their Homologs; Ann. (1929) 470: 157-182; *Chemical Abstracts* 23: 3689-3690; *Chemical Abstracts* 23: 1472

Naranjo, C.: Shulgin, A.T.; Sargent, T.; Evaluation of 3,4-Methylene-dioxyamphetamine (MDA) as an Adjunct to Psychotherapy; *Med. Pharmacol. Exp.* (1967) 17: 359-364

Nencini, P.; Ahmed, A.M.; Elmi, A.S.; Subjective Effects of Khat Chewing in Humans; *Drug and Alcohol Dependence* (1986) 18: 97-105

Neuberg, C.; Hirsch, J.; Uber ein Kohlenstoffketten knüpfendes Ferment (Carboligase); *Biochem. Z.*, (1921) 115:282-310

Neuberg, C. and Ohle, H.; Zur Kenntnis der Carboligase; *Biochem. Z.*, (1922) 128:610-618.

New York Times (Article); August 11, 1983; see also *Popular Science* October 1983 under Science & Chemistry.

Newton, P.; Pickering, M.V.; High Performance Liquid Chromatography and the Mystery of L-Tryptophan; *LC-GC* 9 (2) 208-213

Nichols, D.E.; Barfknecht, C.F.; Rusterholz, D.B.; Benington, F.B.; Morin, R.D.; Asymmetric Synthesis of Psychotomimetic Phenylisopropylamines; *Journal of Medicinal Chemistry* (1973) 16(5): 480-483

Nichols, D.E.; Hoffman, A.J.; Oberlender, R.A.; Jacob, P. III; Shulgin, A.T.; Derivatives of 1-(1,3-Benzodioxol-5-yl)-2-butanamine: Representatives of a Novel Therapeutic Class; *Journal of Medicinal Chemistry* (1986) 29: 2009-2015

Nichols, D.E.; Oberlender, R.; Structure-Activity Relationships of MDMA-Like Substances; In *Pharmacology and Toxicology of Amphetamine and Related Designer Drugs;* (1989) pgs. 1-29

Nichols, D.E.; Oberlender, R,; Structure-Activity Relationships of MDMA and Related Compounds: A New Class of Psychoactive Agents?; In *Ecstasy: The Clinical Pharmacological & Neurotoxicological Effects of the Drug MDMA* (1990)

Niedzielski, E.L.; Nord, F.F.; On the Mechanism of the Gatterman Aldehyde *Synthesis.* 1; (1941) 63: 1462-1463

Noller, C.R.; Adams, R.; The Use of Aliphatic Acid Anhydrides in the Preparation of Ketones By The Friedel and Crafts Reaction; *Journal of the American Chemical Society* (1924) 46: 1889-1896.

Norris, J.F.; *Experimental Organic Chemistry*; McGraw-Hill Book Co. 1924

Okeda, H., Taniguchi, K.; Enoki, K.; Taniguchi, T.; Kaji, A.; **Abe, K.; Sakimoto, R.**; Sulfisoxazole. 1. Syntheses of methyl *alpha*-Chloroethyl ketone and *alpha*-Acetylpropionitrile; *J. Pharm. Soc. Japan* (1956) 76: 60-62

Odinak, A. et al; Upjohn Co.;*GB*1069409; 2,5-Dialkoxybenzaldehydes; *CA* (1966)

Ogata, I.; Kawabata, Y.; Process for Preparation of Aldehydes; (1980) *US 4,229,381.*

Ogren, S.O.; Fuxe, K.; Agnate, L.F.; Gustafsson, J.A.; Jonsson, G.; Holm, A.C.; Reevaluation of the Indolemine Hypothesis of Depression. Evidence for a Reduction of Functional Activity of Central 5-HT Systems by Antidepressant Drugs; *Journal of Neural Transmission* (1979) 46: 85-103

Ono, Masako; Shimamine, M.; Kazunori, T.; Hallucinogens. IV. Synthesis of 2,5-Dimethoxy-4-methylamphetamine; *Eisei Shikenjo Hokoku* (1973) 41(4): 91; (1974) 80: pges 379-380; Chem. No. 108090 v

Orndorff, W.R.; *A Laboratory Manual of Organic Chemistry*; 1913; D.C. Heath & Co.

Oswald, M.; (1914).-*Ann. Chimie*, (9) 1:74.

Overberger, C.G.; Fischman, A.; Roberts, C.W.; Arond, L.H.; Lal, J.; Monomers containing Large Alkyl Groups. III. The Synthesis of 2-Alkyl-1,3-butadienes; *Journal of the American Chemical Society* (1951) 73: 2540-2543

Overberger, C.G.; Tanner, D.; Ionic Polymerzation. A Convenient Synthesis of *alpha* and ß-Alkylstyrenes. The Effect of an *alpha*-Alkyl Group on the Ultraviolet Absorption Spectra; *Journal of the American Chemical Association* (1955) 77: 369-373

Parke, Davis & Co.; Aminoketones; *Chemical Abstracts* (1957) 51: 15552 g-i; *GB 768,772*

Pacholczyk, T.; Blakely, R.D.; Amara, S.G.; Expression Cloning of a Cocaine and Antidepressant - Sensitive Human Noradrenaline Transporter; *Nature* (1991) 350: 350-354

Parijs, A.H; Recl. *Trav. Chim. Pays-Bas* (1930) 49: 1

Patrick, T.M. Jr.; McBee, E.T.; Hass, H.B.; Synthesis of Arylpropylamines. I. From Ally Chloride; *Journal of the American Chemical Society* (1946) 68: 1009-1011

Pearl, I.A.; (Sulphite Products Corp.); Method of Synthesizing Syringaldehyde; *U.S. Patent 2,516,412*

Pearl, I.A., Beyer, D.L.; Reaction of Vanillin and its Derived Compounds. XII. Benzyl Methyl Ketones Derived From Vanillin and its Related Compounds; ???? (1950) 221-224

Pelet; Corni; Industrial Preparation of Alkali Nitrites; *Chemical Abstracts* 2: 1330

Pepper, J.M.; Saha, M.; The Synthesis of Aroyl Methyl Ketones as Lignin Model Substances; *Canadian Journal of Chemistry* (1964) 42: 113-120

Percy, L.J.; Oliver, J.J.; *Organic Syntheses Collective Vol.* 2: 391-392.

Perkin, W.H.; Trikojus; V.M.; CCXII A Synthesis of Safrole and o-Safrole; 1663-1666

Peterson, D.W.; Maitai, C.K.; Sparber, S.B.; Relative Potencies of Two Phenylalkylamines Found in the Abused Plant *Catha Edulis*, Khat; *Life Sciences* (1980) 27: 2143-2147

Pfanz, H.; Wieduwilt, H.; Rearrangements in the Arylpropanolamine Series; (1955) 288: 563-582; *Chemical Abstracts* (1956) 50: 7082-7084

Pfister, K. III; Stein, G.V.; Merck & Co. Inc.; *alpha* Methyl Phenylalanines; *US 2,868,818*

Poos, George Ireland; 2-Amino-5-aryloxazoline Products; (1964) *US 3,161,650*

Potapov, V.M.; Terent'ev, A.P.; Stereochemical Studies. IV Schiff bases from optically active *alpha*-benzylethylamine; *Zhur. Obshchei Khim.* (1958) 28: 3323-3328; *CA* 53: (1959) 53:14028 (h-i) - 14029 (a-d).

Potts, K.T.; Some *alpha*-Methylamino-Acids; *Journal of the American Chemical Society* (1955) 1632-1634

Pradhan, S.N.; Battachargya, A.K.; Pradhan, S.; Serotoninergic Manipulation of the Behavioral Effets of Cocaine in Rats; *Community Psychopharmacology* (1978) 2: 481-486

Quelet, R.; Method for the Synthetic Preparation of *alpha*-Chloroethyl Derivatives of Phenolic Ethers; Application to Synthesis of Vinylanisoles; *Compt. rend.* (1934) 199: 150-152; *Chemical Abstracts* (1934) 28: 6125

Quelet, R.; Chloroalkylation of Anisole. Synthesis of Vinylanisoles.; *Compt. rend.* (1936) 202: 956-958; *Chemical Abstracts* 4158

Quelet, R.; Chloroalkylation of Phenolic ethers; 1. Synthesis of Methoxystyrenes; *Bull. soc. chim.* (1940) 7: 196-205; II. Synthesis of Vinylanisoles and Derivatives of Methoxy(*alpha*-hydroxyethyl)benzenes; *Bull. soc. chim.* (1940) 7: 205-215; *Chemcial Abstracts* (1940) 5425

Rahrs, Emii J.; Method for Producing Chlorinated Ketones (1941) *US 2,235,562*

Rahrs, Emii J.; Stablization of Chloroacetone (1941) *US 2,263,010*

Rangaswami, S.; Rao, V.S.; Preparation of Amyl Nitrite; *Indian Journal of Pharm.* (1952) 14: 64-66; *Chemical Abstracts* (1953) 3225; *US Dispensatory*, 22nd ed. p 135

Rao, K.V.; Seshadri, Thiruvengadam, T.R.; Synthesis of Myristicin and Elemicin; *Proc. Indian Acad. Sci.* (1949) 107-113

Rao, M.G.S.; Srikantia, C.; Iyengar, M.S.; *J.of the Chem. Society* (1929) pg. 1578

Rao, B.S.; Subramaniam, K.; ß-Asarone; *J. of the Chem. Soc.* (1937) 1338-1340

Raschig, F,; Preparation of the Alkali Salts of Hydroxylaminedisulphonic Acid and of Hydroxylamine: *Journal of the Chemical Society* (1888) 54: 913-914.

Reidel, J.C.; Propane to Nitroparaffins. Vapor-phase Nitration Used by Commercial Solvents Corp.; *The Oil and Gas Journal* (1956) 110-114

Reitsema, R.H.; Allphin, N.L.; Chromate Oxidation of Alkylaromatic Compounds; *Journal of Organic Chemistry* (1962) 27: 27-28

Renz, J.; The Preparation and Antibacterial Activity of Nuclear-substituted Derivatives of Gentisyl Alcohol; *Helv. Chim. Acta.*; (1947) 30: 124-139; *Chemical Abstracts* (1947) 41: 4128-4129

Ricaurte et al.; *Brain Research* (1982) 235: 93-103

Ricaurte, G.A.; Studies of MDMA Neurotoxicity in Nonhuman Primates: A Basis for Evaluating Long-Term Effects in Humans; In *Pharmacology and Toxicology of Amphetamine and Related Designer Drugs*, (1989)

Ridley, D.D.; Ritchie, E.; Taylor, W.C.; Chemical Studies of the Proteaceae; *Australian Journal of Chemistry* (1968) 21: 2979-2988

Riegel, B.; Wittcoff, H.; Pyridinium Analogs of the Pressor Amines. I. The Benzene Series; *Journal of the American Chemical Society* (1946) 68: 1805-1806

Ritter, J.J.; Kalish, P.P.; A New Reaction of Nitriles. 1. Amines from Alkenes and Mononitriles; *Journal of the American Chemical Society* (1948) 70: 4045-4048

Ritter, J.J.; Kalish, P.P.; A New Reaction of Nitriles. 2. Synthesis of t-Carbinamines; *Journal of the American Chemical Society* (1948) 70: 4048-4050

Ritter, J.J.; Murphy F.P.; N-acyl-ß-phenethylamines, and a New Isoquinoline Synthesis; *Journal of the American Chemical Association* (1952) 74: 763-765.

Rorig, K; Johnson, J.D.; Hamilton, R.W.; Telinski, T.J.; *p*-Methoxy-phenylacetonitrile; *Organic Syntheses Col. Vol* 4: 576-579.

Rothrock, J.W.; Converting Veratraldehyde to L-(-)3,4-Dimethooxyphenylacetyl Carbinol; (1967) *US 3,338,796*

Rubenstein, l.; Substitution in Derivatives of Quinol Ethers; *Journal of the Chemical Society* (1925) 127: 1998-2004

Rubin, M.; A Carbonyl Reduction by Potassium Hydroxide in Ethanol; *Journal of the American Chemical Society* (1944) 66: 2075-2076

Saito, N.; 1998; Process for production of ketone: *US 5,750,795* (1998)

Sander, A.; Thoenen, H.; Model Experiments on the Molecular Mechanism of Action of 6-Hydroxydopamine; *Molecular Pharmacology* (1970) 7: 147-154

Sanders-Bush, E.; Neurochemical Evidence that Hallucingenic Drugs are 5-HT1c Receptor Agonists: What Next?; In *Hallucinogens: An Update*; (1994)

Sanders-Bush, E.; Steranka, L.A.; Immediate and Long Term Effects of *p*-Chloroamphetamine on Brain Amines; *Annals of the New York Academy of Sciences* (1978) 305: 208-221

Sannerud, C.A.; Brady, J.V.; Griffiths, R.R.; Self-Injection in Baboons of Amphetamines and Related Designer Drugs; In *Pharmacology and Toxicology of Amphetamine and Related Designer Drugs* 1989.

Sauer, W.; Fliege, W.; Dudeck, C.; Petri, N.; Preparation of aromatic and araliphatic aldehydes (1980) *US 4,224,254*

Scheel-Krüger, J.; Behavioral and Biochemical Comparison of Amphetamine Derivatives, Cocaine, Benztropine and Tricyclic Antidepressant Drugs; *European Journal of Pharmacology* (1972) 18: 63-73

Schiitte, Jandirk; Anorexigenic Propiophenones (1961) *US 3,001,910*

Schmidt, C.J.; Taylor, V.L.; Acute Effects of Methylenedioxymethamphetamine (MDMA) on 5-HT Synthesis in the Rat Brain; *Pharmacologist* (1987) 29, Abs. #224

Schwenk, Erwin; Bloch, Edith; A New Modification of Willgerodt's Reaction; *Journal of the American Chemical Society*; (1942) 64: 3051-3052

Schwenk, Erwin; Papa, Domenick; Preparation of Aryl Aliphatic Acids by The Modified Willgerodt Reaction; *Journal of Organic Chemistry* (1946) 11: 798-802

Seaton, M.Y.; Activated Magnesia and Method of Making; (1940) *US 2,219,726*

Seiden et al.; *Biochem. Behav.* (1984) 21: 29-31

Semon, W.L; Hydoxylamine Hydrochloride and Acetoxime; *Organic Syntheses* (1923) 3: 61-66

Sepulveda, S.; Valenzuela, R.; Cassels, B.K.; Potential Psychotomimetics. New Bromoalkoxyamphetamines; *Journal of Medicinal Chemistry* (1972) 15 (4): 413-415

Shaw, K.N.F.; Armstrong M.D.; McMillan, A; Preparation of *m*-Hydroxyphenyl-L-and D-Lactic Acids and Other Compounds Related to *m*-Tyrosine; *Journal of Organic Chemistry* (1956) 21: 1149-1151.

Shields, J.R.; Barnebey, H.L.; Process and Apparatus for Recovering in the Form of Alkali Metal Salts the Oxides of Nitrogen From Gases Containing the Same: *US 2,467,274* (1949)

Shih, J.C.; Chen, K.; Gallaher, T.K.; Structure and Function of Serotonin 5-HT2 Receptors; In *Hallucinogens: An Update*; (1994)

Shishido, K.; Kuyama, H.; Synthesis of Antioxidants for Fats and Oils. I; *Bull. Inst. Chem. Research, Kyoto Univ.* 25: 73-74 (English); *CA* 47: 120 f-i

Shiu, H. S.; Rogers, P. L.; *Biotechnol. Bioeng.*, (1996) 49:52-62

Shulgin, A.T.; The Separation and Identification of the Components of the Aromatic Ether Fraction of Essential Oils by Gas-Liquid Chromatography; *Journal of Chromatography* (1967) 30: 54-61

Shulgin, A.T.; Mescaline: The Chemistry and Pharmacology of its Analogs; *Lloydia* (1973) 36 (1): 46-58

Shulgin, A.T; A Protocol for the Evaluation of New Psychoactive Drugs in Man; *Methods and Findings in Experimental and Clinical Pharmacology* (1986) 8(5): 313-320

Shulgin, A.T.; History of MDMA; In *Ecstasy: The Clinical Pharmacological & Neurotoxicological Effects of the Drug MDMA*; (1990)

Shulgin A.T.; Synthesis of the Trimethoxyphenylpropenes; *Canadian Journal of Chemistry* (1965) 43: 3437-3440

Shulgin, A.T.; *Chemical & Engineering News* (8/29/83) pgs. 22-33

Shulgin, A.T.; Designer Drugs - Where We are, and Where We Are Going; *JFSS* 1991; 31(2): 231-232

Shulgin, A.T.; Sargent,T.; Psychotropic Phenylisopropylamines Derived from Apiole and Dillapiole; *Nature* (1967) 215: 1494-1495

Shulgin,A.T., Sargent, T.; Naranjo, C.; Structure-Activity Relationships of One-Ring Psychotomimetics; *Nature (London)* (1969) 221: 537-541

Sloane, P.D.; Mathew, L.J.; Scarborough, M.; Desai, J.; Koch, G.G.; Tangen, C.; Physical and Pharmacologic Restraint of Nursing Home Patients with Dementia; *JAMA* (1991) 265 (10): 1278-1282

Slotta, K.H.; Muller, J.; Ueber den Abbau des Mescalins und Mescaline-ahnlicher Stoffe in Organismus; *Hoppe-Seyler's Z. Physiol Chem.* 238: 14-22 (1936)

Slotta, K.H.; Szyszka, K.; Über ß-Phenyl-äthylamine; *J. prakt. Chem.*, (1933) 137, 339; *The Alkaloids* (3) 326-327

Small, G.H.; Minnella, A.E.; Hall, S.S.; Lithium-Ammmoia Reduction of Benzyl Alcohols to Aromatic Hydrocarbons: An Improved Procedure; *Journal of Organic Chemistry* (1975) 40(21): 3151-3152.

Smallridge, A; Yeast-based process for production of l-pac; (2001) *US 6,271,008*

Smith; C.A.; Theiling, L.F. Jr.; Production of Propiophenone; (1979) *US 4,172,097*

Smith, D.E.; Wesson, D.R.; Buffum, J.; MDMA: "Ecstacy" as An Adjunct to Psychotherapy and a Street Drug of Abuse; *California Society for the Treatment of Alcoholism and Other Drug Dependencies News* (1985) 12: 1-3

Smith, R.L.; Dring, L.G.; Patterns of Metabolism of ß-Phenylisopropylamines in Man and Other Species; In *Amphetamines and Related Compounds* (1970)

Smythies; *Neurosci. Res. Program Bull.* (1970) 8: 79

Smythies, J.R.; Johnson, U.S.; Bradley, R.J.; Bennington, F., Morin, R.D.; Clark, jun., L.C.; *Nature* (1967) 216: 128

Snyder, S.H.; Yamamura, H.I.; Antidepressants and the Muscarinc Acetylcholine Receptor; *Archives of General Psychiatry* (1977) 34: 236-239

Soine, W.H.; Contamination of Clandestinely Prepared Drugs with Synthetic By-Products; In *Problems of Drug Dependence* 1989

Soloveichik, S.: Nitrous Ester: *US Patent 2,714,606; CA* (1956) 7122

Standridge, R.T.; Howell, H.G.; Gylys, J.A.; Partyka, R.A.; Phenylalkyamines with Potential Psycho-therapeutic Utility. 1. 2-Amino-1-(2,5-dimethoxy-4-methylphenyl)butane; *Journal of Medicinal Chemistry* (1976) 19 (12): 1400-1404

Steranka, L.R.; Rhind, A.W.; Effect of Cysteine on the Persistent Depletion of Brain Monoamines by Amphetamines, *p*-Chloro-amphetamine and MPTP; *European J. of Pharm.* (1987) 133: 191-197

Steranka, L.R.; Sanders-Bush, E.; Long Term Effects of Continuous Exposure to *p*-Chloroamphetamine on Central Serotonergic Mechanisms in Mice; *Biochemical Pharmacology* (1978) 27: 2033-2037

Sternbach, H.; The Serotonin Syndrome; *Amer. J. of Psychiatry* (1991) 148 (6): 705-713

Stinson, S.C.; Psychoactive Drugs; *Chemical & Engineering News*; 10/15/90; pgs. 33-68

Stone, D.M.; Hanson, G.R.; Gibb, J.W.; GABA-transaminase Inhibitor Protects Against Methylenedioxymethamphetamine; Hambourger; *JAMA* (1939) 112: 1340

Stone, D.M.; Johnson, M.; Hanson, G.R.; Gibb, J.W.; A Comparison of the Neurotoxic Potential of Methylenedioxyamphetamine (MDA) and Its N-methylated and N-ethylated Derivatives; *European Journal of Pharmacology* (1987) 134: 245-248

Sugasawa; *Journal of the Chemical Society* (1934) pg. 1483

Sugasawa, S.; Hino, T.; Synthesis of 1-(3,4-Methylenedioxyphenyl)-3,5-dimethyl-7,8-methylenedioxyisoquinoline; *Pharm. Bull. (Japan)* (1954) 2: 242-246 *Chemical Abstracts* (1956) 50: 1016-1017

Sugasawa, S.; Kakemi, K.; VI. Synthesis of 3-Methylisoquinoline Derivatives; *Journal of the Pharmaceutical Society (Japan)* (1937) 57:172-180 (in English 24-27) *Chemical Abstracts* 33: 9307

Sugasawa, S.; Okuda, K.; Preparation of Phenylacetone; *Journal of the Pharmaceutical Society (Japan)* (1952) 72: 117-118 *Chemical Abstracts* (1952) 46: 11145-11146

Sugasawa, S.; Sakurai, K; Synthesis of Compounds Related to Papaverine. V. Syntheis of 1-(3,4-Methylenedioxybenzyl)-3-methyl-6,7-methylene-dioxyisoquinoline and Similar Compounds; *Journal of the Pharmaceutical Society (Japan)* (1936) 56: 563-569 *Chemical Abstracts* 33: 9307

Sugino, K.; Ohdo, K.; Electrolytic Preparation of Ephedrine; *Japan Patent 3308* (51') June 26; *Chemical Abstracts* (1953) 1510 e-f

Sullivan, A.C.; Guthrie, R.W.; Triscari, J.; (-)-*threo*-Chlorocitric Acid-A Novel Anorectic Agent with a Peripheral Site of Action; in *Anorectic Agents; Mechanisms of Aciton and Tolerance* (1981)

Surry, A.R.; Pyrogallol 1-Monomethyl Ether; *Org. Syn. Col.* 3:759-760

Sussman, N.; Neurochemistry of Serotonin and Depression; *Primary Psychiatry* (1995) 28-33.

Suter, Chester M.; Preparation of Phenylalkylamines with Excess Condensing Agent; (1948) *US 2,443.206.*

Suter, C.M.; Weston, A.W.; Some Fluorinated Amines of the Pressor Type; *Journal of the American Chemical Society* (1941) 63: 602-604

Sy, W.; By, A.; Nitration of Substituted Styrenes with Nitryl Iodide; *Tetrahedron Letters* (1985) 26 (9): 1193-1196

Tanka I.; Seki, T.; A New Synthetic Method for N-alpha-Dimethyl-2-methoxy-phenylethylamine; *Yakugaku Zasshi* (1957) 77: 310-311; *C A* (1957) 51: 11278-11279

Taylor, D.; Ho. B.T.; Neurochemical Effects of Cocaine Following Acute and Repeated Injection; *J. Neurosci. Res.* (1977) 3: 95-101

Tiffeneau, M.; Syntheses of Estragol and of aromatic derivatives containing an unsaturated side chain.; *Comp. rend.* (1904) 139: 481-482; *J. Chem. Soc.* (1904) I, 872.

Tindall, J.B.; 1958; Process for the Production of Secondary Amines: *US 2,828,343*

Tohzuka, Ohsaka, Y.; Method for Isomerization of Fluorinated Epoxy Compounds; (1980) *US 4,238, 416.*

Tomita, M.; Fujitani, K.; Aoyagi, Y.; Kajita Y.; Studies on the Alkaloids of Menispermaceous Plants CCXLIV. Synthesis of *dl*-Cepharanthine; *Chem. Pharm. Bull* (1968) 16(2) 217-226

Trikojus, V.M.; White, D.E.; The Synthesis of Myristicin; *J. Chem. Soc.* (1949) 436-439

Turek, I.S.; Soskin, R.A.; Kurland, A.A.; Methylenedioxyamphetamine (MDA) Subjective Effects; *Journal of Psychedelic Drugs* (1974) 6: 7

Turner, J.; Manufacture of Nitrite of Soda; *Journal of the Society of Chemical Industry* (1915) XXXIV (11): 585-586

US vs. Forbes, DC Colo. No. 92-CR-105. 11/20/92; Drugs - Controlled Substance Analogue - Statutory Vagueness

Van Atta, R.E.; Zook, H.D.; Elving, P.J.; Synthesis of Monochloroacetone; *Journal American Chem. Soc.* (1954) 1185-1186

Vanderbilt, B.M.; Hass, H.B.; Aldehyde-Nitroparaffin Condensation; *Industrial and Engineering Chemistry* (1940) 32 (1): 34-38

Vanion, L. (1925).- *Präparative Chemie, 3rd Ed.*, Vol. 1., 325.

Velenyi, L.J.; Krupa, A.S.; Isomerization of Aldehydes to Ketones; (1982) *US 4,329,506.*

Wachter, A., and Smith, S.S. (1943).-*Ind. Eng. Chem.*, 35:366.

Wagner *et al.*; *Brain Research* (1980) 181: 151-160

Wassink, B.H.G.; A Synthesis of Amphetamine; *Journal of Chemical Education* (1971) 51: 671.

Wasserman, D.; Dawson, C.R.; Cashew Nut Shell Liquid. III. The Cardol Component of Indian Cashew Nut Shell Liquid with Reference to the Liquid's Vesicant Activity; *Journal of the American Chemical Society* (1948) 70: 3675-3679

Weinstein, H.; Zhang, D.; Ballesteros, J.A.; Hallucinogens Acting on 5-HT Receptors: Toward a Mechanistic Understanding at Atomic Resolution: In *Hallucinogens: An Update* (1994)

Wellocme Foundation Ltd.; Improvements Relating to the Bromination of Phenones; (1948) *GB 607,538.*

Werner, E.A.; Methylation by Means of Formaldehyde. Part I. The Mechanism of the Interaction of Formaldehyde and Ammonium Chloride; The Preparation of Methyl-amine and of Dimethylamine: *Journal of the Chemical Society* (1917) 111: 844-853.

Wilbert, G.; Sosis, P.; (Nepera Cehmcial Co.); Method of Producing 2-Amino-1-phenyl-1-propanol hydrochloride; *US 3,028,429*

Willis, J.; On Making it through The Night; HHS Pub. No. (FDA) 80-3095

Windholz et al.; Merck & Co. Inc.; Phenylalanine Deriviatives; *Chemical Abstracts* (1963) 59:175

Winter, J.C.; A Comparison of the Stimulus Properties of Mescaline and 2,3,4-Trimethoxyphenylethylamine; *J. of Pharmacol. Expt. Therapeutics* 185 (1): 101-107 (1973)

Winter, J.C.; *Psychopharmacology* (Berlin) (1980) 68: 159

Witkop, B.; Foltz, C.M.; Studies on the Stereochemistry of Ephedrine and pseudo-Ephedrine; *Journal of the American Chemical Society* (1957) 79: 197-201

Wyeth Labs. Inc.; *Science* (1971) 171: 1032-1036

Yensen, R.; DiLeo, F.B.; Rhead, J.C.; Richards, W.A.; Soskin, R.A.; Turek, B.; Kurland, A.A.; MDA-Assisted Psychotherapy with Neurotic Outpatients: A Pilot Study; *J. of Ner. Ment. Dis.* (1976) 163: 233-245

Yakovlev, V.G.; Syntheses of *dl*-2,5-Dihydroxyphenylalanine From Phenols and Aromatic Hydroxy Aldehydes; *CA* (1950) 44: 6831 a-f *Zhur. Obshchei Khim (J. Gen. Chem.)* (1950) 20: 361-357;

Young, H.S.; Renolds, J.W.; Catalytic Syntheses of Ketones from a Mixture of an Aldehyde and an Acid; (1969) *Pat. 3,466,334.*

Young, R.; Glennon, R.A.; Cocaine-Stimulus Generalization to Two New Designer Drugs: Methcathinone and 4-Methylaminorex; *Pharmacology Biochemistry and Behavior* (1993) 45(1):229-231

Yunker, M.H.; Higuchi, T.; Stabilization of Alkyl Nitrites; *US Patent 2,927,939*; *Chemical Abstracts* 54: 11992

Zaputryaev, B.A.; Velitskays, O.Ya.; Glikina, L.S.; Khaletskii, A.M.; Modifcation of methyl benzyl ketone synthesis; *Med. Prom. S.S.S.R.* (1960) 14 (1): 48-51. *Chemical Abstracts* 54: 22464 c-e.

Zenitz, B.L.; Macks, E.B.; Moore, M.L.; Preparaton of *alpha, alpha*-Dimethyl- and N, *alpha, alpha*-Trimethyl-*beta*-cyclohexylethylamine; *Journal of the American Chemical Society* (1948) 70: 955-957.

Zettlemoyer, A.C.; Walker, W.C.; Stump, W. L.; Preparation of Ketones by Hydrocarboxylation of Carboxylic Acids; (1952) *US 2,612,524.*

Zhingel, K.Y.; Dovensky, W.; Crossman, A.; Allen, A.; Ephedrone: 2-Methylamino-1-phenylpropane-1-one (Jeff); *Journal of Forensic Sciences* (1991) 36 (3): 915-920

INDEX

A

N

T

U

V

W

Y

Z

OXY

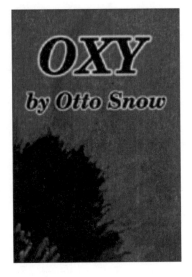

by Otto Snow

OXY stands for OxyCodone (narcotic agonist) easily created from Garden Poppies and varieties of Oriental Poppies. United States consumes 90% of the world's supply of oxycodone, placing a strain on the essential precursor (thebaine) of oxycodone & naltrexone; narcotic antagonist. Many countries have considered increasing the cultivation of Oriental Poppies in the event of terrorist attack, meteor strike, plague, drought or other natural disaster. Hundreds of *Papaver* species/alkaloids described & referenced. DEA and global drug intelligence.

Preparation of Oxycodone and Etorphine from Thebaine.
Thebaine Extraction and Purification from Oriental Poppies.
Extraction of Crude Thebaine from Dried Oriental Poppy Pods.
Extraction of Morphine Alkaloids from Poppy Straw and/or Capsules.
Morphine from Codeine. Also includes:

The Opium Poppy and Other Poppies by Charles C. Fulton
        The Opium Poppy. Distinction of the opium poppy from other commonly cultivated poppies. The closest relatives of *Papaver somniferum*. Principal species of poppies in American horticulture. Opium alkaloids. and characteristic opium products which occur in other plants.

Opium Poppy Cultivation and Heroin Processing in Southeast Asia by the DEA.   Reproduction from actual intelligence report.
        Cultivation Methods. Opium Harvesting. Extraction of Morphine from Opium. Morphine to Heroin. Production using metal barrels.

OXY is packed with references and pharmacology, photos, extractions and chemistry in both English and German. An asset to the survivalist student or anyone interested in the facts. A book for the hope chest. Future generations may find this book a life saver.   6" x 9" 256 pages
LC: 2001118636 ISBN: 0-9663128-2-1 Limited Edition. List $31.95

Distributed by: Homestead Book Co.   Phone: 1-800-426-6777
                        homesteadbook.com   davet@homestead.com
Also distributed by Baker & Taylor Books   btol.com
Available from FS Book Co. Phone:1-800-635-8883   fsbookco.com